The Tyranny of the Normal

Literature and Medicine

MARTIN KOHN, CAROL DONLEY, AND DELESE WEAR, EDITORS

The Tyranny of the Normal
An Anthology

EDITED BY CAROL DONLEY
& SHERYL BUCKLEY

THE KENT STATE UNIVERSITY PRESS
Kent, Ohio, and London, England

© 1996 by The Kent State University Press, Kent, Ohio 44242
All rights reserved
Library of Congress Catalog Card Number 95-36898
ISBN 0-87338-535-7
Manufactured in the United States of America

03 02 01   5 4 3 2

Due to the length of the permissions acknowledgments, a continuation of the
copyright page appears on pages 373–76.

Library of Congress Cataloging-in-Publication Data

The tyranny of the normal : an anthology / edited by Carol Donley and Sheryl
    Buckley.
        p.   cm. — (Literature and medicine ; v. 2)
    Includes bibliographical references and index.
    ISBN 0-87338-535-7 (pbk. : alk. paper) ⊚
    1. Body, Human—Social aspects. 2. Body, Human—Literary
collections. 3. Abnormalities, Human—Social aspects. 4. Abnormalities, Human—Literary collections. 5. Obesity—Social aspects. 6. Obesity—Literary collections. I. Donley, Carol C. II. Buckley, Sheryl, 1946–. III. Series:
Literature and medicine (Kent, Ohio) ; v. 2.
HM110. T9 1996
573.8—dc20
                                                                95-36898
                                                                     CIP

British Library Cataloging-in-Publication data are available.

Contents

❧

Preface

❧

THE IDEA FOR a course on normality, what it is and how we define it, arose from a conversation we had about genetic engineering. Those working in this exciting field are now saying that in as little as twenty years it will be possible for a couple wishing to have a child to select not only traits like hair color, eye color, and adult height and weight, but also more complex traits like intelligence, athletic ability, and musical talent. This led us to imagine what choices those future parents would make. One thing seemed certain: no one would deliberately choose to have an "abnormal" child. But abnormality covers an enormous range. There are the grossly deformed and disfigured, and no one could be blamed for wanting to spare a child the pain of being deformed. But what about those who dislike the shape of their nose or wish to be three or four inches taller? Do they qualify as "abnormal"? We [*their own self perception*] considered the role of variety in nature. Not only humans but animals and plants come in an amazing variety of sizes, shapes, and colors. It is too easy to envision a future where all humans have blond hair, blue eyes, a similar height, and a trim, athletic build. But would this bland homogeneity be an improvement on the human race as naturally constituted? Are we wise enough to make choices that would improve humankind? Whose values would those choices be based upon and for what morally significant reasons?

The project of deliberately refashioning humankind should make us pause to consider what makes us human now and what potential changes in the future would render an individual other than human. Direct genetic manipulation allows us for the first time in history the opportunity to mix human genes with those of other species, something that nature does not permit [*against natural order*] but modern laboratories do. Already transgenic mice with some human genes exist. How many human genes would render a mouse as something other than a mouse? What would that something be? How many human genes make something human?

These are momentous questions, but since the technology of genetic engineering already exists, society as a whole must decide, and in short order, too, what limits will be imposed on the uses of this technology. The genie is already out of the bottle, and genetic engineering offers the opportunity to correct genetic defects associated with terrible suffering, such as the defect that causes cystic fibrosis. But we are called upon to decide how this technology will be used. Nothing less than the definition of what it means to be human is at stake.

This anthology has developed from our experiences over several years of team-teaching an interdisciplinary literature and medicine course called "What's Normal?" As we gathered readings for the course and tried them out in the crucible of the classroom, certain works stood out as especially thought-provoking and stimulating for class discussion and written arguments in student papers. Those are the works we have assembled here. The introduction to this text describes the theories that have guided our thinking as we teach.

Our intention has been to collect different perspectives on the lives of people whose physical appearance places them outside cultural norms. Some of the perspectives are those of health care professionals and medical ethicists. Some perspectives are fictional—imaginative creations of the experience of those "others" whose body size or appearance triggers fear, pity, antagonism, or shock in so-called normal people. Insofar as these "others" suffer rejection, silencing, and subjugation, their experiences may be analogous to those of other groups who do not match the cultural norms for race, religion, gender, or sexual preference. In this anthology, we have concentrated on physiological abnormalities and have not sought to be comprehensive in representing all marginalized people.

We would like to thank the many people who have contributed to the making of this anthology. First, we are grateful for our students, who have taught us as much as we have taught them. Most of our students are adults in Hiram's Weekend College; they bring to the class years of experience, including for some of them the responsibility of caring for members of their own families who are deformed or disabled. Their thoughtful responses to the readings and discussions have helped shape the class and this text.

We also want to thank several people who helped enter the text in the computer and spent considerable time and effort assisting us with editing, seeking permissions, and proofreading. They include Seth Green, Maryann

Maczac, Ruth Wegener, and most especially Joe Ruffner and Jeanne Weis, without whose patient and consistent help we would never have completed this project.

Special gratitude goes to the late Nancy Moeller, dean of Hiram's Weekend College, who always encouraged and supported us in our teaching, and whose infectious, "can do" attitude carried us through some slumps.

And we want to thank our families, especially Marge Buckley and Al Donley, for keeping their sense of humor and bearing with us as we completed this project.

Introduction

In the Greek legend, Procrustes placed all people who fell into his hands on an iron bed. If they were longer than the bed, he chopped off the overhanging parts; if they were shorter, he stretched them until they fit. The legend has become a metaphor for a tyrannical force-fitting of people to one standard. While the myth presents an absurd extreme, in everyday life we usually exert pressures to normalize those who are outside our culture's standards. We half believe fairy tales, where beasts can become charming princes; the ugly ducklings, swans. In fact, we think they should make those changes. If we cannot somehow repair or transform abnormal people, we tend to cast them out because they disturb us deeply. Leslie Fiedler, whose article "The Tyranny of the Normal" provides the title for this anthology, writes that our reaction to freaks reveals a recognition in our secret selves of how grotesque we ourselves sometimes feel. So we want our Rumplestilkskins to disappear, our Quasimodos to stay out of sight. Leviticus 21 orders that none of Aaron's descendants "who has a deformity shall draw near . . . the veil or approach the altar . . . that he may not profane my sanctuaries." In our religious and cultural traditions, we tend to equate beauty with goodness and deformity with evil, justifying our rejection of those who aren't like us.

Our reaction to extremely abnormal people is to pity them and fear them. Fiedler points out that what begins with a "fear of difference eventuates in a tyranny of the Normal. . . . The grosser abnormalities [are] prevented, repaired, aborted, or permitted to die at birth so that those of us allowed to survive by the official enforcers of the Norm will be free to become even more homogeneously beautiful." Sometimes the dominant culture enforces normality and exterminates those who don't fit—as we have seen happen in Nazi Germany and many other places. Sometimes the cultural pressures are psychologically enforced through advertising and other media. In the United States, for instance, a norm of slimness and youth drives many people to desperate diets, exercise programs, cosmetics, and plastic surgery.

Now that new medical technologies and the human genome project bring us the ability to make abnormal people more like us, we are faced with decisions for which we have no precedents. For instance, now that we can tell that a fetus is abnormal, we are faced with the threat of insurance companies refusing to pay for its care if it is born with its pre-existing condition, adding more complications to the question of abortion. Soon we will be able to "fix" abnormal genes and abnormal people through genetic engineering, growth hormones, and surgery. We will be able to "design" our own children, selecting not only healthy genes but also genes for gender, skin color, height, and endless other qualities. Our ability to normalize people is already far ahead of our thinking about who decides what is normal and abnormal, who decides whether normalizing someone is the best thing to do, who has the authority or the right to make any of the possible changes, and, last but not least, who is going to pay for it.

This anthology is a collection of fiction and nonfiction about people whose physical abnormalities make them disturbingly deviant from cultural norms. Part 1 includes essays and articles that explore the problems faced by these "others" as they try to find a place in society. Perhaps their biggest difficulty is the recognition that most normal people find them too deformed to accept, too ugly to love—and they suffer what Jonathan Sinclair Carey calls the "Quasimodo Complex." Barbara McFarland and Tyeis Baker-Baumann, in the excerpt from *Shame and Body Image: Culture and the Compulsive Eater,* discuss how women especially feel shame when they fall short of an ideal image or an idealized version of themselves. Sometimes compulsive overeating or undereating (anorexia) is a numbing response to anger, hurt, or fear. Mary Briody Mahowald suggests that anorexics are trying both to conform "to a socially induced unhealthy stereotype, and [to refuse] to accept the sexist connotations of being female." Fiedler's initial essay describes well the tyranny of the social norms, not only over the psyche of the deformed person but also over the behavior of the normal population toward those who are different. He asks us to consider what is lost when we modify, shun, or eradicate differences.

Part 2 of the anthology collects stories, poems, and plays about three groups of abnormalities: weight, including obesity and eating disorders; height, with particular focus on dwarfism; and deformity or disfigurement, whether a birthmark or a whole body deformity, such as that suffered by the Elephant Man. In all three of these sections, major writers from Kafka and Poe to

Welty and Morrison explore the conflicts and concerns of their abnormal characters as they struggle with their self-image and their otherness.

The theories that have guided our selection of readings are expressed in the articles and essays of Part 1. The authors are literary critics, theologians, philosophers, psychologists, sociologists, physicians, and educators who write in the context of theories within their discipline. Leslie Fiedler writes that freaks "who at first appear to represent what is most absolutely 'Other' (thus reassuring us who come to gape that we are 'normal') are really a revelation of what in our deepest psyches we suspect we recognize as the Secret Self." In the excerpt from his *Freaks: Myths and Images of the Secret Self*, he points out that in our childhood we are often confused about limits of scale, of our sexuality and sexual roles, and of what distinguishes us from animals. We seem dwarfed by adults, but we're giants compared to a new baby. We often seem more like our pets than our parents. And our stories are full of giants, tiny folk, people changing size, and all kinds of beasts, both threatening and friendly, who speak our language.

These childhood confusions and fears are reinforced by the changes puberty brings on adolescents. Most of us as teenagers feel ourselves freakish, with bodies that swell and change out of our control; we may feel "monstrously deficient or excessive—too tall, too short, too fat, too thin." Genital changes and growth of body hair make us feel different from our childhood selves, yet very uncertain of who or what we are becoming.

The people, Fiedler points out, whom we place outside the physiological norms, to whom we react with pity, fear, and shock, tend to address our "primordial fears . . . about scale, sexuality, our status as more than beasts, and our tenuous individuality." All the selections in Part 2 of this anthology, whether they be about eating disorders, dwarfism, or deformity, reflect aspects of these "primordial fears."

It is sobering to consider how instinctive our reactions seem to be. As Carey writes in his description of the "Quasimodo Complex," deformed people read the extent of their abnormality not in mirrors but in interactions with other people. He defines the Quasimodo Complex as the "self-perception and identity formation of concealed and unconcealed deformities engendered from the implicit and explicit reactions of others." In our interactions with deformed individuals, we provide "the means for [their] ultimate self-judgment and self-perception." Needless to say, all of us who meet and work with deformed people ought to control the reactions that would hurt those reading our verbal and nonverbal messages about them. As Arlette Lefebvre comments in her response to "The Quasimodo Complex," "There is a great deal of social finesse and human interaction skill that [the beholder and] the beheld can learn and master. . . . That is the main therapeutic lesson that this paper and clinical experience bring forth: one can learn to get beyond the immediate reaction and to focus on the social interaction."

In an anthology like this, we immediately confront problems with language. So many terms used to describe people outside physiological norms are negative and stigmatizing—freaks, mutants, monsters, and mistakes of nature, among others. And the clinical terminology, such as "terata," seems euphemistic. Even the terms *abnormal, disabled, malformed, deviant* begin with a negative prefix that puts the person being described in opposition to the normal, the able, the formed, those on the right path. The term "others," of course, is also exclusive, though in the present decade it includes the majority of the population that feels, for one reason or another, denied effective power or voice.

In Carol Tavris's *The Mismeasure of Woman,* she shows how women have been measured against male standards, even when women claim equality or superiority. In a similar way, those with abnormal body appearance are always measured against the normal and are always, by definition, outside the bell curve. That we have not found a neutral term, let alone a positive one, indicates how powerful the "tyranny of the normal" is in our culture. Our language shapes our thinking, and if we do not have words to include people, we are likely to leave them out.

We also need to be sensitive to language in other ways. As Joanne Trautmann Banks points out in her commentary on "The Quasimodo Complex," we use literary eponyms to collect a group of concepts under one term. Borrowing the name of a literary character to name an entity has a long history, including such well-known examples as narcissism and the Oedipus Complex. For some, the term *Quasimodo Complex* might explain "the complicated psychosocial accompaniments of deformity," but it could also "freeze the imagination" and put focus on the label rather than the individual. Any label, as we all know, tends to serve as a shortcut and reduces our thinking and awareness. We are likely to believe that once we have named something or someone, we understand it.

While the articles in Part 1 challenge us to examine our own assumptions and behavior, the creative literature in Part 2 engages our imagination and takes us out of ourselves for awhile. The stories and poems about eating disorders are some of the most moving in the anthology. Sharon Olds's poem about her eighty-two-pound mother forcing herself to eat "small spoonful by / small spoonful, so you would not die and / leave us without a mother" is narrated by a family member helplessly watching a loved one suffer. And Pamela White Hadas's powerful "Diary of an Anorexic" puts the reader within the experience of the teenage girl in the grips of the disease. Stories and poems about compulsive overeating and the reactions of society to obesity range from assumptions of the fat person's "moral failure" to control eating, as in Raymond Carver's "Fat," to a recognition of his beauty, as in Jack Coulehan's "The Six Hundred Pound Man."

In the section devoted to abnormal height, particularly dwarfism, several of the stories and poems are narrated by the dwarf, giving the reader insight to his or her anger and bitterness for being treated like a child or a clown or some freakish amusement rather than a real person. Edgar Allan Poe, Rainer Maria Rilke, and Pär Lagerkvist give us extraordinary portraits from the dwarf's perspective. Ray Bradbury's story is narrated by a sensitive woman who realizes that the dwarf goes into a hall of distorted mirrors to see himself transformed into a normal-looking man—a remarkably ironic variation of the narcissus myth and the opposite of what normal people do in a fun house.

In the third section, the stories, poems, and selections from drama portray those who are disfigured and deformed. For example, the excerpt from *The Elephant Man* lets the reader vicariously share John Merrick's experience in the London hospital where he is on show for the aristocrats much as he had been as a freak in a sideshow. He's better fed and cared for, certainly, but people still approach him as an object of horror or pity or wonder or charity rather than as a real person. Even Dr. Treves, who says his aim is "to lead him to as normal a life as possible," treats him like a child and forbids him to have an adult male relationship with Mrs. Kendal.

While their abnormalities differ markedly from each other, the characters in all three sections share similar experiences of the tyranny of the normal. Most suffer the pain and loneliness of rejection. In some stories, people get beyond the surfaces to love the real people inside; but in most of the works, the abnormal surfaces prevent a welcome into the community.

All the stories help us as readers experience through imagination what these abnormalities mean to those who have them. While we do not claim that we become more humane and understanding simply by reading, we do agree with Joanne Trautmann Banks's position that "when a group of people interpret a piece of literature together—when they work out their responses in trial-and-error, in debate with their peers, and sometimes in concert with them—then the chance of literature changing their behavior towards patients is greatly enhanced." For these reasons, we believe this anthology is most useful in a classroom or in a setting where group discussion occurs.

PART ONE

Nonfiction Articles, Essays, and Excerpts from Books

The Tyranny of the Normal

LESLIE A. FIEDLER

I EMBARK UPON this essay with a sense that I am an amateur writing for professionals, a dilettante addressing the committed. I am not a doctor or a nurse or a social worker, confronted in my daily rounds with the problem we discuss here; not even a lawyer, philosopher, or theologian trained to deal with its moral and legal implications. I am only a poet, novelist, critic—more at home in the world of words and metaphor than fact, which is to say, an expert, if at all, in reality once removed. I feel therefore like a Daniel in the Lions' Den, or perhaps I mean rather a Lion in the Daniels' Den—more victim than witness. Yet you have called upon me to testify and, with whatever fear and trembling, I have accepted.

Indeed, I have been asked several times recently to write on these topics because, I presume, not so very long ago I published a book called *Freaks: Myths and Images of the Secret Self*. I was primarily interested in exploring (as the subtitle declares) the fascination of "normals" with the sort of congenital malformations traditionally displayed at Fairs and Sideshows: and especially the way in which such freaks are simultaneously understood as symbols of the absolute Other and the essential Self. But in the long and difficult process of putting that study together (it took almost six years of my life and led me into dark places in my own psyche I was reluctant to enter), I stumbled on the topic treated here, "the care of imperiled newborns."

How dangerous a topic this was I did not realize, however, until just before my book was due to appear. I was at a party, in fact, celebrating the imminent blessed event when I mentioned offhand to one of my fellow-celebrants, a young man who turned out to be an MD, one of the discoveries I had made in the course of my research. It seemed to me, I innocently observed, that in all probability more "abnormal" babies were being allowed to die (in effect, being killed) in modern hospitals than had been in the Bad Old Days when they were exposed and left to perish by their fathers. And I went on to declare that in my opinion at least this was not good; at which point, my interlocutor screamed at me (rather contradictorily, I thought) that what I asserted was simply not true—and that, in any case, it was perfectly all right to do so. Then he hurled his Martini glass at the wall behind my head, barely missing me, and stalked out of the room.

He did not stay long enough for me to explain that our disagreement was more than merely personal, more than the traditional mutual misunderstanding and distrust of the scientist and the humanist. Both of our attitudes, I wanted to tell him, had deep primordial roots: sources far below the level of our fully conscious attitudes and the facile rationalizations by which we customarily defend them. It is, therefore (I would have explained to him as I am now explaining here), to certain ancient myths and legends that we must turn—and here my literary expertise stands me in good stead—to understand the deep ambivalence toward fellow creatures who are perceived at any given moment as disturbingly deviant, outside currently acceptable physiological norms. That ambivalence has traditionally impelled us toward two quite different responses to the "monsters" we beget. On the one hand, we have throughout the course of history killed them—in the beginning ritually at least, as befits divinely sent omens of disaster, portents of doom. On the other hand, we have sometimes worshipped them as if they were themselves divine, though never without overtones of fear and repulsion. In either case, there was a sense of wonder or awe attached to anomalous humans: a feeling that such deviant products of the process by which we continue the species are mysterious, uncanny, and hence "taboo."

Though it may not be immediately evident, the most cursory analysis reveals that not merely have the primitive wonder and awe persisted into our "scientific," secular age; but so also have the two most archaic ways of expressing it. We still, that is to say, continue to kill, or at least allow to die, monstrously malformed neonates. We euphemize the procedure, however, disguise the superstitious horror at its roots, by calling what we do "the removal of life-supports from nonviable *terata*" (*terata* being Greek for "monsters"). Moreover, thanks to advanced medical techniques, we can do better these days than merely fail to give malformed preemies a fair chance to prove whether or not they are really "viable."

We can detect and destroy them before birth; even abort them wholesale when the occasion arises, as in the infamous case of the Thalidomide babies of the '6os. That was a particularly unsavory episode (which we in this country were spared), since the phocomelic infants carried by mothers dosed with an antidote prescribed for morning sickness were in the full sense of the word "iatrogenic freaks." And the doctors who urged their wholesale abortion (aware that less than half of the babies lost would be deformed, but why take chances?) were in many cases the very ones who had prescribed the medication in the first place.

To be sure, those responsible for such pre-infanticide did not confess, were, indeed, not even aware—though any poet could have told them—that they were motivated by a vestigial primitive fear of the abnormal, exacerbated by guilt. They sought only, they assured themselves and the rest of the world, to spare years of suffering to the doomed children and their parents; as well as to alleviate the financial burden to those parents and the larger community, which would have to support them through what promised to be a nonproductive lifetime. We do, however, have at this point records of the subsequent lives of some of the Thalidomide babies whose parents insisted on sparing them (a wide-ranging study was made some years later in Canada), which turned out to have been, from their own point of view at least, neither notably nonproductive, nor especially miserable. Not one of them, at any rate, was willing to confess that he would have wished himself dead.

But such disconcerting facts do not faze apologists for such drastic procedures. Nor does the even more dismaying fact that the most whole-hearted, full-scale attempt at teratacide occurred in Hitler's Germany, with the collaboration, by the way, of not a few quite respectable doctors and teratologists, most notably a certain Etienne Wolff of the University of Strasbourg. Not only were dwarfs and other "useless people" sent to Nazi extermination camps and, by logical extension, parents adjudged (on grounds since totally discredited) likely to beget anomalous children sterilized. But other unfortunate human beings regarded—at that time and in that society—as undesirable deviations from the norm were also destroyed: Jews and Gypsies, first of all, with blacks, Slavs, and Mediterraneans presumably next in line. It is a development that should make us aware of just how dangerous enforced physiological normality is when the definition of its parameters falls into the hands of politicians and bureaucrats. And into what other hands can we reasonably expect it to fall in any society we know or can imagine in the foreseeable future?

Similarly, as the ritual slaughter of Freaks passed from the family to the State, the terrified worship of Freaks passed from the congregation to the audience, from the realm of Religion to that of entertainment and art. From the beginning, the adoration of Freaks was in the Western world a semirespectable, even an underground, Cult. Think, for instance, of the scene in Fellini's *Satyricon,* in which a Hermaphrodite is ritually displayed to a group of awe-stricken onlookers, who regard him not just as a curiosity though not quite as a god either. After all, the two reigning myth-systems of our culture, the Hellenic and the Judeo-Christian, both disavowed the portrayal of the divine in disguise; regarding as barbarous or pagan the presentation of theriomorphic, two-headed, or multilimbed divinities. By the Hebrews the portrayal of the divine was totally forbidden, while the Greeks portrayed their gods in idealized human form, i.e., the "Normal" raised to its highest power.

Yet there would seem to be a hunger in all of us, a need (without fulfilling which we would somehow feel ourselves less than human) to behold in wonder our mysteriously anomalous brothers and sisters. For a long time, this quasireligious need was satisfied in Courts for the privileged few, at fairs and sideshows for the general populace, by collecting and exhibiting Giants, Dwarfs, Intersexes, Joined Twins, Fat Ladies, and Living Skeletons. Consequently, even in a world that grew ever more secular and rational, we could still continue to be baffled, horrified, and moved by Freaks, as we were able to be by fewer and fewer other things once considered most sacred and terrifying. Finally though, the Sideshow began to die, even as the rulers of the world learned to be ashamed of their taste for human "curiosities"; but fortunately not before their images had been preserved in works of art, in which their implicit meanings are made manifest.

Walk through the picture galleries of any museum in the western world and you will find side by side with the portraits of Kings and Courtesans equally immortal depictions of the Freaks they kept once to amuse them (by painters as distinguished as Goya and Velasquez). Nor has the practice died out in more recent times, carried on by artists as different as Currier and Ives (who immortalized such stars of P. T. Barnum's sideshow as General Tom Thumb) and Pablo Picasso (who once spent more than a year painting over and over in ever shifting perspectives the dwarfs who first appeared in Velasquez' *Las Meninas*). Nor did other popular forms of representation abandon that intriguing subject. Not only have photographers captured on film the freaks of their time, but after a while they were portrayed in fiction as well. No sooner, in fact, had the novel been invented, than it too began to portray the monstrous and malformed as objects of pity and fear—and, of course, wonder, always wonder. Some authors of the nineteenth century, indeed, seem so freak-haunted that we can scarcely think of Victor Hugo, for instance, without recalling the grotesque Hunchback of Notre Dame, any more than we can recall Charles Dickens without thinking of his monstrous dwarf, Quilp, or our own Mark Twain without remembering "Those Incredible Twins." And the tradition is continued by modernists like John Barth and Donald Barthelme and Vladimir Nabokov, who, turning their backs on almost all the other trappings of the conventional novel, reflect still its obsession with Freaks.

In the twentieth century, however, the images of congenital malformations are, as we might expect, chiefly preserved in the art form invented during that century, the cinema: on the one hand, in Art Films intended for a select audience of connoisseurs, like the surreal fantasies of Fellini and Ingmar Bergman; and on the other, in a series of popular movies from Tod Browning's thirties' masterpiece, *Freaks,* to the more recent *Elephant Man,* in its various versions for large screen and small. Browning's extraordinary film was by no means an immediate success, horrifying, in fact, its earliest audience and its first critics, who drove it from the screen and its director into early retirement. But it was revived in the sixties and has ever since continued to be replayed all over the world, particularly in colleges and universities. And this seems especially appropriate since in the course of filming his fable of the Freaks' revenge on their "normal" exploiters, Browning gathered together the largest collection of show-freaks ever assembled in a single place: an immortal Super-Sideshow, memorializing a popular art form now on the verge of disappearing along with certain congenital malformations it once "starred" (now routinely "repaired"), like Siamese Twins.

Precisely for this reason, perhaps, we are these days particularly freak-obsessed, as is attested also by the extraordinary success of *The Elephant Man* on stage and TV and at the neighborhood movie theatre. The central fable of that parabolic tale, in which a Doctor, a Showman, the Press, and the Public contend for the soul of a freak, though it happened in Victorian times, seems especially apposite to our present ambivalent response to the fact of human abnormality. It serves indeed to remind us of what we now otherwise find it difficult to confess except in troubled sleep, though the arts have long tried to remind us of it: that those wretched caricatures of our idealized body image, which at first appear to represent what is most absolutely "Other" (thus reassuring us who come to gape that we are "normal") are really a revelation of what in our deepest psyches we suspect we recognize as the Secret

Self. After all, not only do we know that each of us is a freak to someone else; but in the depths of our unconscious (where the insecurities of childhood and adolescence never die) we seem forever freaks to ourselves.

Perhaps it is especially important for us to realize that finally *there are no normals,* at a moment when we are striving desperately to eliminate freaks, to normalize the world. But this impulse represents a third, an utterly new response to the mystery of human anomalies—made possible only by the emergence of modern technology and sophisticated laboratory techniques. Oddly enough, however (and to me terrifyingly), it proved possible for experimental science to produce monsters long before it had learned to prevent or cure them. And to my mind, therefore, the whole therapeutic enterprise is haunted by the ghosts of those two-headed, three-legged, one-eyed chicks and piglets that the first scientific teratologists of the eighteenth century created and destroyed in their laboratories.

Nonetheless, I do not consider my enemies those first experimenters with genetic mutation, for all their deliberate profanation of a mystery dear to the hearts of the artists with whom I identify. Nor would I be presumptuous, heartless enough to argue—on esthetic or even moral grounds—that congenital malformations under no circumstances be "repaired," or if need be, denied birth, to spare suffering to themselves or others. I am, however, deeply ambivalent on this score for reasons, some of which I have already made clear, and others of which I will try to make clear in the conclusion of these remarks. I simply do not assume (indeed, the burden of evidence indicates the contrary) that being born a freak is *per se* an unendurable fate. As I learned reading scores of biographies of such creatures in the course of writing my book, the most grotesque among them have managed to live lives neither worse nor better than that of most humans. They have managed to support themselves at work that they enjoyed (including displaying themselves to the public); they have loved and been loved, married and begot children—sometimes in their own image, sometimes not.

More often than not, they have survived and coped; sometimes, indeed, with special pride and satisfaction because of their presumed "handicaps," which not a few of them have resisted attempts to "cure." Dwarfs, in especial, have joined together to fight for their "rights," one of which they consider to be *not* having their size brought up by chemotherapy and endocrine injections to a height we others call "normal," but they refer to, less honorifically, as "average." And I must say I sympathize with their stand, insofar as the war against "abnormality" implies a dangerous kind of politics, which beginning with a fear of difference, eventuated in a tyranny of the Normal. That tyranny, moreover, is sustained by creating in those outside the Norm shame and self-hatred—particularly if they happen to suffer from those "deformities" (the vast majority still) we cannot prevent or cure.

Reflecting on these matters, I cannot help remembering not merely the plight of the Jews and Blacks under Hitler, but the situation of the same ethnic groups—more pathetic-comic than tragic, but deplorable all the same—here in theoretically nontotalitarian America only a generation or two ago. At that point, many Blacks went scurrying off to their corner pharmacy in quest of skin bleaches and hair straighteners; and Jewish women with proud semitic beaks (how it has all changed since Barbra Streisand) sought plastic surgeons for nose-jobs. To be sure, as the case of Streisand makes clear, we have begun to deliver ourselves from the tyranny of such ethnocentric Norms in the last decades of the twentieth century; so that looking Niggerish or Kike-ish no longer seems as freakish as it once did, and the children of "lesser breeds" no longer eat their hearts out because they do not look like Dick and Jane in their Primers.

But the Cult of Slimness, that aberration of Anglo-Saxon taste (no African or Slav or Mediterranean ever believed in his homeland that "no one can be too rich or too thin"), still prevails. And joined with the Cult of Eternal Youth, it has driven a population growing ever older and fatter to absurd excesses of jogging, dieting, and popping amphetamines—or removing with the aid of plastic surgery those stigmata of time and experience once considered worthy of reverence. Nor do things stop there; since the skills of the surgeon are now capable of re-creating our bodies in whatever shape whim and fashion may decree as esthetically or sexually desirable: large breasts and buttocks, at one moment, meagre ones at another. But why *not*, after all? If in the not so distant future, the grosser physiological abnormalities that have for so long haunted us disappear forever—prevented, repaired, aborted, or permitted to die at birth, those of us allowed to survive by the official enforcers of the Norm will be free to become even more homogeneously, monotonously beautiful; which is to say, supernormal, however that ideal may be defined. And who except some nostalgic poet, in love with difference for its own sake, would yearn for a world where ugliness is still possible? Is it not better to envision and work for one where all humans are at least *really* equal—physiologically as well as socially and politically?

But, alas (and this is what finally gives me pause), it is impossible for all of us to achieve this dubious democratic goal; certainly, not in the context of our society as it is now and promises to remain in the foreseeable future: a place in which supernormality is to be had not for the asking, but only for the buying (cosmetic surgery, after all, is not included in Medicare). What seems probable, therefore, as a score of science fiction novels have already prophesied, is that we are approaching with alarming rapidity a future in which the rich and privileged will have as one more, ultimate privilege the hope of surgically, chemically, hormonally induced and preserved normality—with the promise of immortality by organ transplant just over the horizon. And the poor (whom, we are assured on good authority, we have always with us) will be our sole remaining Freaks.

From Freaks:
Myths and Images of the Secret Self

LESLIE A. FIEDLER

WE LIVE AT a moment when the name "Freaks" is being rejected by the kinds of physiologically deviant humans to whom it has traditionally been applied: Giants, Dwarfs, Siamese Twins, Hermaphrodites, Fat Ladies, and Living Skeletons. To them it seems a badge of shame, a reminder of their long exclusion and exploitation by other humans, who defining them thus have by the same token defined themselves as "normal." Like all demands on the part of the stigmatized for a change of name, this development expresses itself as a kind of politics. But it remains a politics without a program, unlike the analogous efforts of those once called "niggers" and "colored" to rebaptize themselves first "Negroes," then "blacks"; or of former "ladies" and "girls" to become "women"; or of ex-"faggots" and "dykes" to transform themselves into "gays."

There is, that is to say, no agreement among those traditionally called Freaks about what they would like for programmatic reasons to be called now; only a resolve that it be *something else.* Those who still earn their living by exhibiting themselves in side shows apparently prefer to be known as "entertainers" and "performers," like tightrope walkers and clowns. But larger numbers of "strange people" do not want to be considered performers or indeed anything special or unique. They strive, therefore, to "pass," i.e., to become assimilated into the world of "normals," either by means of chemotherapy, like certain Dwarfs and Giants, or difficult and dangerous operations, like some Hermaphrodites or joined twins.

Meanwhile, the name Freak which they have abandoned is being claimed as an honorific title by the kind of physiologically normal but dissident young people who use hallucinogenic drugs and are otherwise known as "hippies," "longhairs," and "heads." Such young people—in an attempt perhaps to make clear that they have *chosen* rather than merely endured their status as Freaks— speak of "freaking out" and, indeed, urge others to emulate them by means of drugs, music, diet, or the excitement of gathering in crowds. "Join the United Mutations," reads the legend on the sleeve of the first album of the Mothers of Invention. And such slogans suggest—as the discontent of circus performers does not—that something has been happening recently in the relations between Freaks and non-Freaks, implying just such a radical alteration of consciousness as underlies the politics of black power or neo-feminism or gay liberation.

Some Freaks have been trying to shuffle off their invidious name for a long time—ever since January 6, 1898, at least, when, according to a publicity release used as advance ballyhoo throughout Europe, the members of a traveling troupe from the Barnum and Bailey Circus held a protest meeting in London. Called by Miss Annie Jones, the Bearded Lady, it was chaired by Sol Stone, the Human Adding Machine, and its minutes recorded with his feet by the Armless Wonder. But like most of their successors, they, too, were at a loss for an appropriate substitute for the "opprobrious" name under which they had long suffered, and appealed to the public for possible alternatives. Some three hundred names were suggested, but none pleased the protesters, until the Bishop of Winchester urged that they be billed as "prodigies," and with near unanimity they concurred. In America, however, that name never caught on; and in any case, the whole affair may have been dreamed up by the Barnum and Bailey public relations staff. Yet this, too, would have been appropriate, since what Barnum called "humbug" is as intrinsic to "Freak shows" as pathos and wonder.

In his *Autobiography,* Barnum refers to human anomalies not as Freaks but as "curiosities," lumping them with other attractions which may seem to us of a quite different kind: the "Woolly Horse," for instance, a "genuine Mermaid," "Jumbo the Elephant," and Joice Heth, a black woman who claimed to be 161 years old and to have been the slave of George Washington's father. "Curiosity" is a typically Victorian word, memorialized in the title of Charles Dickens' most Freak-obsessed work, *The Old Curiosity Shop,* and reminding us that in that era the interest in Freaks had reached a high point. Indeed, Queen Victoria was quite as curious about Barnum's curious charges as was her favorite novelist. And in America the situation was much the same, with such eminent transatlantic Victorians as Abraham Lincoln and Mark Twain proving equally ready to take time off from a war or a book to receive and swap jokes with a Dwarf.

By the twentieth century, however, the reigning figures in politics had begun to break off the dialogue with Freaks which had lasted for millennia, surviving the fall of ancient empires, the emergence of modern nation-states, the invention of gunpowder and printing, and the extension of literacy and suffrage. Indeed, Victorian sentimentality and morality had already begun to undercut the possibility of continuing such a dialogue, even as Victorian curiosity was bringing it to a climax. And that surviving by-product of the era, Socialism, was eventually to spell its doom. The exhibition of Freaks was, for instance, forbidden by law in Hitler's "National Socialist" Germany, and is still prohibited in the Soviet Union.

Indeed, a sense of the Freak show as an unworthy survival of an unjust past spread everywhere in the early twentieth century, so that for a while it seemed as if those of us now living might well represent the last generations whose imaginations would be shaped by a live confrontation with nightmare distortions of the human body. But there has been a revival of the side show at carnivals and fairs which threatens to reverse the trend; though in the end it may prove merely a nostalgic and foredoomed effort, human curiosities having, for most Americans, passed inevitably from the platform and the pit to the screen, flesh becoming shadow. But the loss of the old confrontation in the flesh implies a trauma as irreparable as the one caused by the passage of the dialogue between King and Fool from the court to the stage: a trauma which is, in fact, a chief occasion for this book.

Perhaps, then, the very word "Freak" is as obsolescent as the Freak show itself, and I should be searching for some other term, less tarnished and offensive. God knows, there are plenty: oddities, malformations, abnormalities, anomalies, mutants, mistakes of nature, monsters, monstrosities, sports, "strange people," "very special people," and *phenomènes*. "Monsters" and "monstrosities" were until very recently the standard terms used in medical treatises on the subject, and "monster" is the oldest word in our tongue for human anomalies. But a quite recent book by Frederick Drimmer, who finds even "strange people" too reminiscent of outmoded prejudice, notes piously that "people may be different from everyone else but they don't enjoy being called monsters"; and goes on to observe that though "in circus sideshows they may jokingly refer to each other as 'freaks' . . . they don't relish it when anyone else applies that epithet to them." "Very special people" is his preferred alternative—a term so unfamiliar that he feels obliged to gloss it in his subtitle as "Human Oddities." R. Toole Scott, on the other hand, though similarly motivated, uses as a heading in his splendid bibliography *Circus and Allied Arts* the French term *phenomènes,* presumably because no English word seems to him neutral or inoffensive enough.

For me, however, such euphemisms lack the resonance necessary to represent the sense of quasi-religious awe which we experience first and most strongly as children: face to face with fellow humans more marginal than the poorest sharecroppers or black convicts on a Mississippi chain gang. No wonder that novelists and poets have sought to evoke that aboriginal shudder—Carson McCullers, for instance, describing the feelings of Frankie, girl heroine of *The Member of the Wedding,* before the Half Man/Half Woman, "a morphodite and a miracle of science"; or Carl Sandburg, his own child-self confronting "a sad little shrimp of a Dwarf" and "Jo-Jo, the dogfaced boy, born 40 miles from land and 40 miles from sea."

"She was afraid of all the freaks," Mrs. McCullers says of Frankie, "for it seemed to her that they had looked at her in a secret way and tried to connect their eyes with hers, as though to say: *we know you. We are you!*" But Sandburg's key word is "bashful" rather than "afraid." "When you're bashful," he writes, "you have that feeling of eyes following you and boring through you. And there were at the sideshow these people, the freaks—and the business, the work of each one of them was to be looked at . . ." To him, Freaks represent an absolute other, "mistakes God made," forced to exhibit themselves until death delivers them; whereas Carson McCullers finds them revelations of the secret self.

Yet both render the experience as a visual one, though of a very special kind—a kind which Marshall McLuhan defines in the course of attempting to define the mask. "The mask," he writes, "like the sideshow freak is not so much pictorial as participatory in its sensory appeal." But "participatory" suggests a link with the peep show and the blue movie as well: the sense of watching, unwilling but enthralled, the exposed obscenity of the self or the other. And only "Freaks," therefore, seems a dirty enough word to render the child's sense before the morphodite or Dog-faced Boy of seeing the final forbidden mystery: an experience repeated in adolescence when the cooch dancer removes her G-string and he glimpses for the first time what (as the talkers say) "you'll never see at home." And the sense of the pornographic implicit in all Freak shows is doubled in what has been called more grandly "The Show of Life," though carnival people refer to it as "pickled punks": a display of preserved fetuses in jars. This ultimate invasion of privacy, revealing what travesties of the human form even the normal among us are at two, three, or four months after conception, has sometimes outdrawn, though in the long run it has, of course, failed to replace, shows at which full-grown oddities have looked down out of living eyes to meet the living eyes of the audience.

That a much newer form of popular drama, the cinema, would attempt to capture and preserve the horror of such encounters was inevitable enough, though it was not until 1933 that Todd Browning (who a year before had brought *Dracula* to the screen) attempted to do so in a movie called quite simply *Freaks*. In the midst of the Great Depression, Browning gathered from circuses and side shows, carnivals and dime museums, scores of human anomalies to act out for an already terrified audience a terrifying fable of their condition and ours. And his movie has played and replayed itself in my troubled head so often that merely recalling it, I call up again not only its images, but the response of my then fifteen-year-old self.

That, despite its effect on me, it failed at the box office is hardly surprising, for it was bound to turn off an audience which thought of itself as already having troubles enough; and which, in any case, had no taste for either the kinky erotic thrills it boasted of giving or the quasi-religious awe it did not confess it evoked. We all firmly believed in those days that "science," which had failed to deliver us from poverty but was already providing us with weapons for the next Great War, had desacralized human monsters forever. Three decades later, however, Browning's *Freaks* was to be revived for a new audience capable of recognizing in the Bearded Lady, the Human Caterpillar, and the Dancing Pinhead, Slitzie, the last creatures capable of providing the thrill our forebears felt in the presence of an equivocal and sacred unity we have since learned to secularize and divide.

Moreover, within the last two or three years, it has been used as the prototype for an updated version called *Mutations*, in which a cast of natural monstrosities is supplemented by others produced in the laboratory—as if to make clear our current sense that science creates new terrors rather than neutralizes old ones. In the end, however, the manufactured Freaks of *Mutations*, in part because they are palpable and not very convincing illusions, move the audience to snicker in embarrassment and condescension instead of crying out in terror. Yet beneath the laughter some dim sense of the sacred survives, since the ridiculous and the monstrous are not really incompatible. Indeed, the very word "Freak" is an abbreviation for "freak of nature," a translation of the Latin *lusus naturae*, a term implying that a two-headed child or a Hermaphrodite is ludicrous as well as anomalous.

Even now, many normals laugh not just in the presence of unconvincing Freaks but of any Freaks at all, making traditional jokes at their expense. Some, like the weary quip "How's the air up there?" shouted at Giants by backwoods wits, can never have been very funny; while others, like the observation that marrying female Siamese Twins is at least a way of getting two wives and only a single mother-in-law, can still extract a sexist grin.

Not only the words of anonymous jokesters, however, testify to the amusement men have always found in Freaks. As early as the second century A.D., Pliny wrote smugly that "formerly hermaphrodites were regarded as ominous signs, but today they seem merely entertainments." And in the court records of seventeenth-century Spain, Dwarfs are referred to, along with Negroes and Fools, as *gente de placer,* amusements for the bored aristocracy. We know that in the midst of the Civil War, Abraham Lincoln suggested his cabinet members take time out to swap jests with a Midget called Commodore Nutt, an episode dwelt on in a recent TV show about his life. And only a little earlier, Queen Victoria and her entire retinue had bellowed at the comical encounter of her pet poodle and Nutt's fellow Dwarf and friend, General Tom Thumb. But the laughter of "normals" must always have been ambiguous and defensive, like the titters of a contemporary undergraduate audience at a horror show. If Freaks are, indeed, a joke played by a "Nature" as bored and as heartless as any small boy or feudal lordling, the joke is on *us!*

Indeed, the more archaic levels of our own minds suggest that perhaps such creatures not only are not bad jokes, much less products of random chemical changes in our genes, as we have more recently been persuaded to believe, but omens and portents—as the oldest word used to name them in our tongue indicates. "Monster" is as old as English itself, and remained the preferred name for Freaks from the time of Chaucer to that of Shakespeare and beyond. The etymology of the word is obscure; but whether it derives from *moneo,* meaning to warn, or *monstro,* meaning to show forth, the implication is the same: human abnormalities are the products not of a whim of nature but of the design of Providence.

In the ancient world, such signs were deciphered by experts in fetomancy (prophecy by means of fetuses) or teratoscopy (divination based on examination of abnormal births), as subtle in interpreting their meaning as those who read omens in the flight of birds or the entrails of sacrificed beasts. Indeed, the oldest surviving "document" dealing with monsters is a Babylonian lexicon of monsterology, inscribed on clay tablets which date from about 2800 B.C. All three traditional subclasses of monsters are represented in the tablets, *monstres par excès, monstres par défaut,* and *monstres doubles.* The first always seem to portend ill ("When a woman gives birth to an infant who has six toes on each foot, the people of the world will be injured"). The second are more ambiguous—a child without a penis and nose, for instance, signifying that "the army of the king will be strong," but one without a penis and belly button indicating that there will be "ill will in the house." Similarly with the third—the birth of androgynes, for instance, bodes ill, while a janicepts baby is a good omen ("When a woman gives birth to an infant that has a head on the head . . . the good augury shall enter into the house"). The Romans, on the other hand, thought of all three classes as ill-omened.

And there were among them priestly executioners who dispatched monstrous children at birth by exposure or ritual sacrifice. Indeed, among all ancient peoples there have been such destroyers of malformed children. This history tells us, and the response we feel in the presence of Freaks confirms. But that was elsewhere or at least elsewhen, we assure ourselves. The most celebrated of joined twins, Chang and Eng, may have barely escaped such a fate not much over a century ago in Siam, but in America they became rich and famous. And though the mummy of a Dwarf, dug up out of the sands of Egypt quite recently, may have originally been killed with due rites and ceremonies as was fitting in his culture, we merely display his remains in a museum as is fitting in ours.

Even the ritualized murder of Freaks, however, seemed in ancient times to verge on sacrilege, and its incidence, therefore, was much lower than we might suppose. Sometimes, indeed, they were preserved and worshipped, as was clearly the case of a hideously distorted *shamanka* (female medicine woman) found in an underground cave in Czechoslovakia in the midst of ritual splendor 25,000 years after her interment. And even the Emperor Augustus, convinced that all Freaks, especially Midgets, possessed the Evil Eye, nonetheless had created for his court a gold statue with diamond eyes representing his pet Dwarf, Lucius.

So there never was in earlier times any total genocidal onslaught against Freaks like that launched by Hitler against Dwarfs in the name of modern "eugenics." And it is even likely that fewer monsters were denied a chance to live in older "priest-ridden" societies than in an AMA-controlled age like our own, in which "therapeutic abortions" are available to mothers expecting monstrous births, and infanticide is practiced under the name of "removal of life supports from non-viable major terata."

At any rate, the word "monster" retains much of the awe once felt in the presence of newborn malformations, and the word, therefore, along with its variant form, "monstrosity," has never disappeared from the working

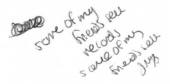

vocabulary of carnivals and side shows. Indeed, I can still replay in my head the spiel of a Freak show "talker," familiar to me since childhood. *Jo-Jo, the Dog-faced boy,* that ghost of a voice keeps saying, *the greatest an-thro-po-log-i-cal mon-ster-os-i-ty in captivity. Brought back at great expense from the jungles of Bary-zil. Walks like a boy. Barks like a dog. Crawls on his belly like a snake.* And at the drawled five syllables of *mon-ster-os-i-ty,* I feel my spine tingle and my heart leap as I relive the wonder of seeing for the first time my own most private nightmares on public display out there.

Why have I not used the word "monster," then, to describe those "unnatural" creatures whose natural history I am trying to write? In 1930, C. J. S. Thompson called a similar study *The Mystery and Lore of Monsters.* But over the more than four decades since its appearance, the term "monster" has been preempted to describe creations of artistic fantasy like Dracula, Mr. Hyde, the Wolf Man, King Kong, and the nameless metahuman of Mary Shelley's *Frankenstein.*

Around these imaginary creatures there has been created a cult, which, beginning as a parodic protest against the stuffy established churches, has assumed the status of a genuine religion, albeit one celebrated in the catacombs of contemporary pop culture, which is to say, in movie houses and underground comic books. It was there that characters created chiefly by Victorian writers of popular fiction were metamorphosed into demons and demigods by a congregation high on grass and sporting buttons which read DRACULA LIVES.

The classic films which they continue to watch and from which the iconography of the comics is derived were made, however, not in the late 1960s when certain physiological normals who called themselves Freaks took to the streets, but during the Great Depression; so that even now it is difficult to imagine Dr. Frankenstein's Monster except as he was played by Boris Karloff, his face stiff under pounds of makeup and the ends of bolts protruding from his shaven skull. Moreover, no matter how many times we have seen the gaunt and beclawed Dracula of Franz Murnau's earlier *Nosferatu* or Christopher Lee's later, more svelte version of the same character, the Vampire Voivode remains for most of us the pallid and black-cloaked villain acted by Bela Lugosi in Todd Browning's 1931 movie with which the Revival of Monsters began. But though Browning also redeemed Freaks for the movies, we must not confuse the two.

Certainly the freaky young do not. Even stoned out of their minds at the latest horror show of some campus film series, or alone in their rooms watching the Fright Night feature on TV, they are aware that monsters are not "real" as Freaks are; i.e., their existence is not granted by a consensus which includes "straights" as well as "heads," the waking consciousness as well as the dreaming one. Whatever margin of ambivalence a particular viewer may feel toward such monsters, they are experienced in the main as other, alien, even hostile. If they project any experience of the self, it is of that self dissolving in the depths of a nightmare or a particularly bad "trip." They evoke in us chiefly fear and loathing, which we may, indeed, need as therapy or *askesis,* but from which we gladly awake.

To be sure, monsters have a mythological dimension like Freaks, and in this respect they are unlike the category of unfortunates whom early French teratologists called *mutilés:* the blind, deaf, dumb, lame, crippled, perhaps even hunchbacks and harelips, though these are marginal; along with amputees, paraplegics, and other victims of natural or man-made disasters. Children who are born legless or armless, their limbs amputated by a tangled umbilical cord, are sometimes hard to tell from true phocomelics, or sealchildren, with vestigial hands and feet attached directly to the torso. But once identified, they are primarily felt as objects not of awe but of pity.

The true Freak, however, stirs both supernatural terror and natural sympathy, since, unlike the fabulous monsters, he is one of us, the human child of human parents, however altered by forces we do not quite understand into something mythic and mysterious, as no mere cripple ever is. Passing either on the street, we may be simultaneously tempted to avert our eyes and to stare; but in the latter case we feel no threat to those desperately maintained boundaries on which any definition of sanity ultimately depends. Only the true Freak challenges the conventional boundaries between male and female, sexed and sexless, animal and human, large and small, self and other, and consequently between reality and illusion, experience and fantasy, fact and myth.

To be sure, no actual Freak threatens all of these limits at once. Dwarfs and Giants, for instance, challenge primarily our sense of scale, Hermaphrodites our conviction that the world neatly divides into two sexes, and so on. In the sixteenth century, however, a kind of total monster called the "Monster of Ravenna" was conceived, in which men continued to believe for three centuries, just as they believed in six-legged calves or joined twins. Its picture, fixed and unchanging, appeared in all the major teratological works of the time, side by side with conventionalized engravings of actual monsters.

Of it, Ambroise Paré writes at the end of a chapter called "Examples of the Wrath of God": "Another proof. Just a little while after Pope Julius II sustained so many misfortunes in Italy and undertook the war against King

Louis XII (1512), which was followed by a bloody battle fought near Ravenna, there was born in the same city a monster with a horn on its head, two wings and one foot like that of a bird of prey, an eye at the knee cap, and participating in the nature of male and female. . . ." The accompanying illustration clarifies the last detail, showing the monster with budding female breasts and, just above the beginning of its single scaly leg, a rather infantile penis canted to the right to reveal the hairless vulva beside it. And Pierre Boaistuau (as translated by Edward Fenton in 1519) not only specifies that "it was double in kind, participating both of the man and woman," but adds that it had "in the stomach the figure of a *Greke* Y, and the form of a crosse."

Not content to leave this creature "so brutall and farre differing from humaine kinde" as a general symbol for the wrath of God, Boaistuau explains the horn as signifying pride and ambition, the wings lightness and inconstancy, the lack of arms want of good works, the eye in the knee too much love of worldly things, the "ramping foot" usury and covetousness, and the double sex "the sinnes of the *Sodomites.*" The added epsilon and the cross, he makes clear, are signs of salvation, indications of a way out of the calamity portended by so monstrous a birth.

To a modern eye, however, the composite creature seems not so much an allegory specially created by a vengeful but ultimately merciful God exasperated by Italian moneychangers and pederasts, as a quite human attempt to sum up in a single iconic form the essential nature of all Freaks. It is not only a *monstre par défaut,* lacking one leg and foot, but also a *monstre par excès,* possessing an oddly displaced third eye, as well as a supernumerary horn on its otherwise human head. And it is especially a *monstre double,* a multiple hybrid of bird and beast, beast and man, man and woman: a pictorial myth of the super-monster.

There has long been a debate in learned circles about which came first: such grotesque fantasies, which were in due course identified with malformed humans who resembled them; or anomalous births, miscarriages and abortions, which bred nightmares, later transmogrified into deities or demons. Men have hewn out of rock and painted on the walls of caves freaklike figures ever since art began, and these have usually been considered idols or icons based on the human form but distorted for symbolic purposes. One of the most ancient and celebrated is the so-called Willendorf Venus, a barely iconic mass of petrified female flesh, traditionally interpreted as a fertility symbol.

A scholarly article which appeared in 1973, however, contends that it portrays with almost clinical accuracy a typical Freak: the victim of "diencephalendocrine obesity with parasymptomatic hypertonia, infertility and libido-reduction." Moreover, the author of the article goes on to argue, other monsters, long believed purely fantastic, may represent analogous attempts to represent anomalies found only in aborted fetuses. He cites as one example the Skiapodes, creatures with a single foot large enough to use as a parasol, believed by Herodotus to be inhabitants of India, where—needless to say—they have never been found. And certainly the drawing of a mermaid-like fetus, or "Sirenoform symmelic miscarriage *(sympus monopus),*" which he reproduces strongly resembles the Renaissance engraving of the "imaginary" Indian monster which he prints alongside it.

Such evidence lends credence to the theory that the observation of human malformations preceded the creation of mythic monsters. We are given pause, however, by the fact that there exist certain long-lived fantasy creatures with *no* prototypes among actual Freaks, fetal or full-grown. Among them are those ostrich- or crane- or goose-necked men, sometimes bird-beaked as well, and occasionally bearded, whom medieval and Renaissance illustrations never tired of portraying. Most notable among them, perhaps, are the celebrated "men whose heads do grow between their shoulders," of whom Othello speaks to Desdemona. We have, indeed, testimony to the existence of such Blemmyae far more reliable than the words of a fictional character, since St. Augustine assures us that in his youth he had seen a "monstrum acephalon," which is to say, a headless monster, with his own eyes. And there are in the libraries of the Western world hundreds of illustrated texts in which we can still see them with ours.

What monsters men have needed to believe in they have created for themselves in words and pictures when they could not discover them in nature. And it is with that psychic need, then, that we should begin; seeking prototypes neither in history or anthropology, nor in embryology or teratology, but in depth psychology, which deals with our basic uncertainty about the limits of our bodies and our egos. More precisely, it is with the psychology of childhood that we must start, for in childhood such uncertainty is strongest and the distinction between the dreams it begets and the reality to which we wake hardest to maintain.

Not psychology textbooks, however, but children's literature, books written for boys and girls or usurped by them, provide the essential clues. Reading any of L. Frank Baum's Oz books, for instance, or James Barrie's *Peter Pan,* or *Alice in Wonderland,* or *Gulliver's Travels,* we cross in our imaginations a borderline which in childhood we could never be sure was there, entering a realm where precisely what qualifies us as normal on the one side identifies us as Freaks on the other. And after returning, we may experience for a little while the child's constant confusion about what really is freakish, what normal, on either side. For children the primary source of such confusion is scale, as Jonathan Swift and Lewis Carroll both make quite clear. And the living metaphors for the nightmare of relative size are Giants and Dwarfs, Fat Men, Fat Ladies, and Living Skeletons—by all odds the best-remembered, and sometimes even best-loved, of all Freaks.

Even before he has seen such side show Freaks or read about them, the child may have come to feel that compared to an adult, he is himself a Midget, while compared to a baby or his last year's self, he is a Giant. In his deep consciousness, he is forever growing bigger and smaller, depending on the contest and the eye in which he sees himself reflected. "But am I really and truly big or small, or just right?" he continues to ask himself, even after he has ceased to grow—and begins, he may suspect, to shrink.

Scale is, however, not the only major identity problem with which children must contend. Born unhousebroken and half wild, dabbling in their own feces and popping into their mouths whatever unlikely object they can grab, they remain for a long time unsure—as the Alice books everywhere imply and Book IV of *Gulliver* explicitly states—whether they are beasts or men: little animals more like their pets than their parents. And the embodiments of the Freaks they feel themselves to be in this regard are the Wild Man of Borneo, Jo-Jo the Dog-faced Boy, or that quasi- or half-imaginary Freak, the "Geek," gobbling down live chickens and rats.

There is, in addition, the problem of child sexuality created by the bisexual, polymorphous, perverse nature of pre-pubescent children, and aggravated by the adult workers changing views of their sexual viability. Obviously, a child's notion of himself is derived from such views. How different, then, a young boy's attitude toward his own body in the heyday of Hellenistic pederasty, when his sexual ambiguity was considered erotically attractive, and that of a male child in, say, Victorian times, when he was deemed "innocent" until puberty and pointed from birth toward the achievement of exclusive male genitality. And how equally different a young girl's attitude toward herself since Vladimir Nabokov's *Lolita* glorified the sexually aggressive "nymphet," and that of a twelve-year-old in the days when Lewis Carroll might, without suspicion of lubricity, ask her parents for permission to photograph her in the nude.

Yet whatever the sexual codes of his culture, pre-Freudian or post-Freudian, repressive or permissive, the child is bound to feel some monstrous discrepancy between his erotic nature and the role expectations of his era. And the incarnate symbols of his distress in this area are the sex Freaks: the Monorchid, the Eunuch, the girl without a vulva, the Hottentot Venus with labia halfway down her thighs, and especially the Hermaphrodite: Joseph-Josephine, Half Man/Half Woman.

Typically, however, children's books, being rooted not in the nightmares of sleep but in half-waking reveries, do not stop with this distress and confusion, but move on to a Happy Ending represented by waking up or growing up, or both. In Baum's *The Land of Oz*, for instance, the protagonist enters the scene as a boy but exits as a girl: a princess, in fact, restored to her throne once her true sex has been released from a witch's spell, i.e., once she has passed over the threshold of puberty. The Alice books, too, are about "growing up," though that process is not rendered in such explicit sexual terms. For Lewis Carroll the process of female maturation implies learning to make oneself, rather than chance or circumstance, the arbiter of scale: learning to be just the right size for every occasion. Only then can a girl be "queened," and thus entering into full womanhood, distinguish the real from the make-believe, the human from the pseudo-human. What children's books tell us, finally, is that maturity involves the ability to believe the self normal, only the other a monster or Freak. Failing to attain such security, we are likely to end by not growing up at all, like Lemuel Gulliver, whom we leave at his story's end in a stall with beasts—his sole refuge from full adulthood, home, and the family.

But this was never the conscious point of the classic Freak show. A Victorian institution it is, like Victorian nonsense, intended to be finally therapeutic, cathartic, no matter what initial terror and insecurity it evokes. "*We are the Freaks*," the human oddities are supposed to reassure us, from their lofty perches. "Not you. Not *you!*" It is primarily to the actual children before them, along with what remains of the child in the hearts of their adult audience, that they speak. To this day circus people call such exhibitions "kid shows." Asked why, they say sometimes that the word "kid" means not child but put-on or send-up or hoax; or they may insist that it refers to those on display rather than those who have paid to see them, Freaks being notoriously—at least according to their exploiters— "just like children." But it is clearly actual boys and girls that the word intends, since no exhibitor can be unaware that the core of his audience is made up of children.

But the myth of monsters is twice-born in the psyche. Originating in the deep fears of childhood, it is reinforced in earliest adolescence by the young adult's awareness of his own sex and that of others. The young male finds that even after his whole body has ceased to grow and his scale vis-à-vis the

rest of the world seems fixed once and for all, his penis disconcertingly continues to rise and fall, swell and shrink—at times an imperious giant, at
others a timid dwarf. For girls at puberty, the growth of breasts is similarly
traumatic. It is a rare young woman who in the crisis of adolescent shame-
facedness does not feel herself either too flat-chested or too generously en-
dowed, and in either case a Freak. So, too, burgeoning boys, in the locker
room or at the urinal (and in an age of X-rated films, at the picture show as
well), are moved to compare the size of their penises with those of others.
And, of course, the whole body as well, at a point in life when one feels himself primarily a sex machine, is felt by both male and female as monstrously
deficient or excessive, too tall, too short, too fat, too thin—still fixed in its
freakishness though childhood has at long last been left behind.

Moreover, passing the line of puberty means for boys and girls alike the
growth of hair around the genitals, more like animal fur than that on their
heads; and for the boys, on face, chest, and belly as well. Both may have longed
for the appearance of such signs of full maturity, but for both it stirs doubts
about their place on the evolutionary scale. And when young women find
what they are taught to regard as "excess hair" growing between their breasts,
on the upper lips, in their armpits, or on their legs, they may doubt their full
femininity as well as their full humanity. A whole industry, indeed, has grown
up by exploiting this fear: advertising painless electrolysis, sure-fire depila-
tories, and dainty mini-razors for women eager to de-freakify themselves
before a night of partying or a day on the beach.

Especially, however, it is at the sight, real or imagined, of each other's
genitals that newly mature men and women endure traumas which reinforce
the myths of monstrosity. It is the child's glimpse of his parents' huge and
hairy genitals which perhaps lies at the origin of it all. Freud has argued that
our basic sense of the "uncanny," which is to say, the monstrous, the freakish, arises from seeing for the first time the female genitals. But Freud's view
is partial, since clearly the primordial model for our notions of the monstrous is each sex's early perception of the other's genitalia in adult form. A
very young man looking at a vulva is likely to feel its possessor a *monstre par
défaut*, while a very young woman looking at his penis may find him a *monstre
par excès*. Or reflexively, he may feel himself a *monstre par excès*, she herself a
monstre par défaut.

Finally, therefore, each sex tends to feel itself forever defined as freakish in
relation to the other. And from our uneasiness at this, I suppose, arises the
dream of androgyny. Through most of the course of Western history, how-

ever, that dream has been undercut by a profound fear of being unmanned or unwomaned, and by guilt for desiring such an event; so that actual Hermaphrodites seem to both sexes the most grotesque of all side show Freaks, a *monstre double* more terrifying than the fears it should presumably allay. Only very recently has our ambivalence in this regard begun to tilt toward the positive side, making the notion of "unisex" not just a useful come-on for barbers and clothes designers but the source of political slogans with wide appeal to the disaffected young, particularly the women among them. Still, as late as Fellini's *Satyricon* and Russ Meyer's *Beyond the Valley of the Dolls,* the image of a Hermaphrodite, naked or half-naked on the screen, continues to stir in the general audience a shudder of revulsion and fear, and a therapeutic titter.

It is, at any rate, the mythic monsters—those who, before they were exhibited at fairs and the courts of kings, already existed in fable and legend because they projected infantile or adolescent traumas—who most deeply move spectators to this very day. I myself, for instance, have recently made a pilgrimage to the Circus World Museum in Baraboo, Wisconsin, ". . . where circus history comes to life . . . 33 acres of displays, shows, demonstrations. . . ." And there, in the midst of old circus wagons, a mechanical gorilla in a cage, a real, live tightrope walker, and a herd of performing elephants, I found the side show tent, where, fixed on a platform forever, stood the plaster images of representative Freaks. The sign before the entrance read "Congress of Strange People," a term which belongs to the twentieth century, and the statues inside were dressed, appropriately enough, in Victorian garb. But I was not surprised to discover that the choice of figures to occupy that limited space responded to our basic insecurities, the sort of primordial fears which I have been examining, about scale, sexuality, our status as more than beasts, and our tenuous individuality.

To represent the first—the child's oldest and deepest fear—were a Fat Lady, a Human Skeleton, a Giantess supporting on one hand a Dwarf, and the "Cardiff Giant," which was, of course, a notorious fraud. There was no Hermaphrodite to stand for the second fear, perhaps out of a sense that the Circus Museum was a family show; but a Bearded Lady did well enough. The third was doubly figured forth, in the form of Lionel the Lion-faced Man and Jo-Jo the Dog-faced Boy; while the fourth was embodied by Chang and Eng, the original "Siamese Twins," looking in formal nineteenth-century dress very respectable, and a little bored by the ligature to which they owed their fame and fortune.

Confronting them, I could feel the final horror evoked by Freaks stir to life: a land of vertigo like that experienced by Narcissus when he beheld his image in the reflecting waters and plunged to his death. In joined twins the confusion of self and other, substance and shadow, ego and other, is more terrifyingly confounded than it is when the child first perceives face to face in the mirror an image moving as he moves, though clearly in another world. In that case, at least, there are only two participants, the perceiver and the perceived; but standing before Siamese Twins, the beholder sees them looking not only at each other, but—both at once—at him. And for an instant it may seem to him that he is a third brother, bound to the pair before him by an invisible bond; so that the distinction between audience and exhibit, we and them, normal and Freak, is revealed as an illusion, desperately, perhaps even necessarily, defended, but untenable in the end.

The Quasimodo Complex:
Deformity Reconsidered

JONATHAN SINCLAIR CAREY

The body
Eternal shadow of the finite Soul,
The soul's self-symbol, its image of itself.
Its own yet not itself.

S. T. Coleridge

I am uneasy to think I approve of one object,
and disapprove of another; call one thing
beautiful, and another deform'd; decide
concerning truth and falshood, reason and
folly, without knowing upon what principles
I proceed.

David Hume, *A Treatise of Human Nature*

INTRODUCTION

SAINT PAUL AND the hunchback Quasimodo shared more in common than perhaps meets the eye. For both suffered from deformities of the human body, albeit of different clinical manifestations.[1] Biblical scholars and physicians, in numerous books and articles, assume that the apostle suffered from temporal lobe epilepsy[2] or from some other recurring internal problem, based on their medical exegesis of "there was given to me a thorn in the flesh" (2 Cor. 12:7) and other related verses.[3] Anyone familiar with Victor Hugo's classic *Hunchback of Notre Dame*, through reading the original (1831) novel or through viewing any of the silent or sound cinematic renditions, even a ballet, recognizes the nightmarish extent of his hideous external congenital afflictions.

What may not be so easily recognized, be it in theory or in practice, are the multifarious ramifications—psychological, philosophical, theological, moral, cultural, and legal, to name but a few—of what I identify as the Quasimodo Complex. This complex, which I shall conceptually define and develop through the course of this essay, refers to the self-perception of concealed and unconcealed deformities engendered from the implicit and explicit reactions of others. The deformed body, and its accompanying soul, to allude to Coleridge's verse, have stood relatively neglected too long in the shadows of what is commonly called narcissism or the narcissistic complex in psychoanalytical literature. It is time that deformity itself—its theoretical and practical meaning and significance in affected human lives and its relation to the art and science of healing—is reconsidered more fully in its own stark light.

FLESHLY PERFECTION AND IMPERFECTION

Both Saint Paul and Quasimodo undoubtedly suffered in the flesh; and both might well have had their own theological interpretations of, or psychological responses to, Jesus' exhortation that "it is better to enter into life crippled or lame than to have two hands or two feet and be thrown into the eternal fire" (Matt. 18:8).[4] In this increasingly secular and technologically capable society, however, where both the present moment and physical appearance are considered primary factors for personal acceptance and even worldly success (or what has also been called an individual's "efficacy"),[5] before any explicit eschatological beliefs or psychological coping devices were developed, such a declaration may not altogether suffice. In fact, judging from empirical evidence and statistical studies pertaining to deformity and to the deformed in society, it may represent a crueller fiction than that written by Victor Hugo.

Whether in employment or in daily social exchanges, discrimination or prejudice on earth based on the stigma of deformity may be a far more intolerable hell and reality than any other imaginable. Had Saint Paul's affliction been apparent, as a thought-provoking example of what could have had far-reaching historical, if not theological, repercussions on the course of world events, he would have been denied his priestly employment, based on Leviticus 21:1–24:

> And the Lord said to Moses, "Say to Aaron that none of your descendants throughout their generations who has a deformity shall draw near, a man blind or lame, or one who has a mutilated face or a limb too long or a man who has an injured foot or an injured hand, or a hunchback or dwarf, or a man with a

defect in his sight or an itching disease . . . he shall not come near the veil or approach the altar because he has a deformity, that he may not profane my sanctuaries; for I am the Lord who sanctify them."[6]

Holiness was equated with the beautiful and perfect; God was not to be defiled by those with corporeal imperfections, irregularities, or impediments of any sort, no matter how pure their confessions of faith. This argument based on physical appearance, or physicalism as it has been called, pertains not only to employment but also to what constitutes being considered a human being, a person, in certain traditions. Some societies in recorded history, from the Spartans in 600 B.C. to the Nazis of this century, put their deformed infants to death, rather than allowing them to overtax the resources of a country.[7]

Roman Catholic manuals of moral theology in the past three or more centuries frequently contained sections labeled *De baptizandis monstris*, in which certain complex and troublesome questions pertaining to physical deformities were considered by casuists; they considered whether such deformed neonates, many of whom were stillborn or died soon after delivery, should be baptized (that is, considered to be human and entitled to the sacraments). Such manuals also exist in this century and contain the Levitical prohibitions against those who are considered to be "irregular from defect" and who cannot "becomingly" minister at the altar. As one pre-Vatican II manual, originally published in 1929 and reprinted in 1959, states about those candidates for the priesthood with "irregularities and impediments":

Accordingly, those are irregular who have no thumb or index finger; who tremble in such wise that there is danger of their spilling the Precious Blood; whoever has an artificial leg, in as far as this defect cannot be concealed; the blind or mute, the deaf who cannot hear the answers of the server; those who stammer so as to excite laughter or derogatory remarks; those who are seriously deformed by mutilation, or otherwise, e.g., if the last three fingers are missing; those so hunchbacked that they excite laughter, or who cannot stand upright.—The absence of the left eye does not constitute an irregularity if the deformity can be rendered unnoticeable by an artificial eye.[8]

Concealed afflictions might also cause serious problems. Those candidates for the priesthood with epilepsy, according to the same manual, might have to apply for a special dispensation from their bishop.[9]

In some countries, modern campaigns for advocating equal opportunity for all, be it in the religious vocation (for example, for eliminating spiritual discrimination) or in any form of employment, may be more of a political myth than people realize.[10] Given this contemporary world and its demands, the sensitive British writer, Richard Jeffries, declared "Let me be fleshly perfect"[11] in his autobiography, *The Story of My Heart* (1883). His statement expresses a fairly universal hope, yearning, even prayer, shared by a majority of people—religious or otherwise—throughout the world, whatever their particular cultural aesthetics of fleshly perfections.

Western civilization has certainly developed its own understanding of fleshly perfection and its importance in the arts and sciences, with far-reaching consequences. The first-century Roman architect Vitruvius, for example, argued that the symmetry necessary for designing temples and other buildings "must have an exact proportion worked out after the fashion of the members of a finely-shaped human body."[12] Fra Luca Pacioli (1445–1517) in *De Divina Proportione* (1509) also wrote about the symbolic importance of the proportionally perfect human body,[13] as did Leonardo da Vinci (1452–1519).[14] Frequently the (male) Apollo or (female) Venus served as paradigms for the beautiful and virtuous, as portrayed by many artists, philosophers, and theologians in their respective disciplines through the following centuries. As Kenneth Clark states in *The Nude*, about this western anthropocentricity, the major concern was with the "design" of the body, not with its being "a living organism."[15] For all of the contemporary interest in the person and his rights, however, fleshly perfection may be more important than imagined.

CALOCAGATHIA

As one facet of this "aesthetic" tradition, some Greek and Roman philosophers considered the design of the body also to be an essential indicator of a person's virtue—or latent immorality. Physical attractiveness in the male or female was equated with moral goodness *(calocagathia)*, and its absence was a potential sign of innate depravity or moral ugliness.[16] In other words, the human soul was thought to assume the shape of the human being. The physical condition of the body was therefore critically important. Plato and his followers argued that a mediocre physical condition or congenital defect could inhibit the ascension of the soul.[17] As Cicero also wrote several centuries later in his *Tusculan Disputations,*

> It matters greatly to the soul by what sort of body it is placed; for there are many conditions of the body that sharpen the mind, and many that blunt it.[18]

A deformed body, whether from congenital or accidental defect, or from a failure to nourish it or exercise properly, could not help but to prejudice the soul and human flourishing. It is for this reason that Juvenal (first century A.D.), reflecting the Western classical tradition, stated his familiar maxim of *mens sana in corpore sano*: a healthy mind in a healthy body. Muscular development was one thing: the flourishing of the soul, another matter.

Later church fathers, concerned with how the flesh related to salvation, or indeed if the flesh represented the "hinge" of salvation as believed by Saint Tertullian, even debated whether deformed individuals possessed "reasonable souls" and if they were capable of resurrection.[19] Saint Augustine, for example, discussed the meaning of monstrous births in *The City of God* as an exercise in theodicy, concluding that such births must be the will of God and that "God forbid that any one should be so besotted as to think the Maker erred in the creation of this, though we know not why He made it thus."[20] Such births, though, still troubled him, and his concern was with the divine meaning of the event and not with the import of the deformity upon the life itself. Saint Jerome, as another example, was said to be "grieved in his time to see the deformed and lame offering up spiritual sacrifices to GOD in religious houses."[21] Saint Gregory the Great, in his influential *Pastoral Care* shows how his cure of souls *(cura animarum)* had its own revealing theological interpretation of the deformed, as in the particular case of the individual born with a hunchback:

> The crookbacked is one who is weighed down by the burden of earthly cares, so that he never looks up to the things that are above, but is wholly intent on what is underfoot in the lowest sphere. If at any time he hears something good about the heavenly fatherland, he is so weighed down by the burden of evil habit, that he does not raise up the face of his heart; he just cannot lift up the cast of his thought, being kept bowed down by his habitual earthly solicitude.[22]

According to Saint Gregory, such deformities must be understood as "sins" when no cure of bodies is possible because they are *contra naturam;* against nature. Such deformed individuals are "forbidden to offer loaves of bread to the Lord. The reason is obvious: a man who is still ravaged by his own sins, cannot expatiate the sins of others."[23] From the distorted appearance results the symbolic conclusion that the deformed body, and hence the soul, must be spiritually incapable of experiencing the beatific vision or transcendental thoughts, physically trapped, as Saint Gregory says, "underfoot in the lowest spheres."

PHYSIOGNOMY

Such arguments with their implicit and explicit assumptions about the body and soul relied more on physiognomy than on theological principles. To be sure, the Bible mentions that "a man may be known by his look" (Eccles. 19:29), and the Judeo-Christian heritage has long been concerned with debating the meaning of the *imago Dei et hominis* (image of God and man). But how accurate are such claims to know others by their appearances? Physiognomy, promoted as an exact science by many philosophers and scientists from Aristotle[24] to Karl Jaspers and Carl G. Jung, developed centuries ago as one popular means of assessing human personality on the basis of appearance.[25] Physiognomists thought that by reading the face, the hands, the eyes, and the posture much could be determined about the "inner man," in both his design and as a living organism, and about a person's past and future. Johann Kaspar Lavater's *Essays on Physiognomy* (first appearing in French in four volumes between 1775–1778; in English between 1789–1798) has been considered to be the most important example of this approach.[26] As Lavater (1741–1801), a Swiss Reformed pastor, conceived of physiognomy, instead of analyzing the components of the soul and all its facets and "execrescences," he proposed to concentrate on outward appearances to deduce the qualities of a man's soul from the shape of his head and the features of his face.

In the course of his massive study, so admired by Goethe especially for its combination of anatomy and the classical elements of physiognomics, Lavater considered the effects of deformity on the inner man, producing what he called his "theorem" on deformity:

> The beauty and deformity of the countenance is in a just and determinate proportion to the moral beauty and deformity of the man. The morally best, the most beautiful. The morally worst, the most deformed.[27]

His underlying indebtedness to Greek (especially neoplatonism) and Roman philosophy should be apparent, even if his idiosyncratic work is hardly academically rigorous and systematic. Barbara Maria Stafford has explored Lavater's underlying theological premise behind physiognomics.[28] According to her research, Lavater's man is created in the image and likeness of "a simple, luminous, and homologous God," but through his sin produces blemished offspring that reflect their "heterogeneous birthmark" and individualism. Stafford concludes:

This creative error, identical to the monstrous, is, Lavater tells us, an imperfection resulting from a mother imprinting her unborn child through the force of an impure and covert longing. It represents a grotesque deviation from the norm—the continuous and gradual procession of being—into the formless, the disproportionate, the indeterminate.[29]

In other words, physical deformity basically "turns a person inside out," in Lavater's words, and challenges the goodness of creation itself.

What troubled Lavater, incidentally, as it had Montaigne and other earlier writers, was that the philosopher Socrates was an obvious exception to the scientific validity of Lavater's statements. Tradition ascribed great physical ugliness to him, however attractive his metaphysics. As Montaigne, for example, wrote:

> It grieves me that Socrates, who was a perfect pattern of all great qualities, should, as reports say, have had so ugly a face and body, so out of keeping with the beauty of his soul, seeing how deeply he was enamoured of beauty, how infatuated by it! Nature did him an injustice.[30]

But evidently, according to one credible account, his appearance enriched his philosophy. Diogenes Laertius (third century A.D.) recorded that Socrates used to recommend that young men should be constantly looking into mirrors in order to determine their appearance. If they were handsome, then they should act virtuously so as to be worthy of their beauty; and if they were ugly, they should conceal their unsightly appearance by their moral accomplishments.[31] Lavater, in some of his more convoluted prose and logic, is at pains to reconcile his science of physiognomy with this Socratic anomaly:

> The sharp, compressed, and heavy parts shocked, or bedimmed, the eye of the Greek, accustomed to consider beauteous forms, so that the spirit of the countenance escaped his penetration.[32]

Although the word "physiognomy" is infrequently used these days, and many of Lavater's findings have been discredited as conjecture or historical "oddity,"[33] physiognomy itself survives, in various forms. Many, if not all, cultures still believe that by one's face and body one shall be known. In other ways, too, that "knowing" may be influenced consciously or unconsciously by a modern form of the ancient Greek concept of *calocagathia*, or *dysmorphophobia*.[34]

UNCONCEALED ANOMALIES

The grossly misshapen Quasimodo could do little to hide his many unconcealed deformities—including his contorted hands and legs, his almost crippling kyphosis, and his extensive maxillofacial and *fons cranii* malformations (one can only speculate on the various other concealed abnormalities of skeleton, muscles, vessels, nerves, and viscera)[35]—from himself or from others. He would have presented a physiognomist's dream—or nightmare—to the practitioner attempting to ascertain the inner man of the hunchback of Notre Dame.

By all medical odds, Quasimodo should have been stillborn, or died shortly after birth, baptized or unbaptized by his Roman Catholic Church, and buried simply and anonymously as another *terata* or *monstrum*.[36] As recompense for his unlikely survival, he might at least have been spared his mental anguish by being born autistic or severely retarded, to keep him from awareness of his own lack of fleshly perfection. The cumulative morphological portrait of his assorted physical abnormalities is that perhaps there would have been more poignancy, or even dramatic irony, if Quasimodo, instead of Saint Paul (who was plagued by a largely concealed "thorn in the flesh," that inflicted physical and psychological suffering even though few people were aware of the condition), had stated about his lifelong awareness of who or what he was: "For now we see in a mirror dimly, but then face to face. Now I know in part; then I shall fully understand, even as I have been fully understood" (1 Cor. 13:12). He defied the very meaning of being human, as most people would consider it, based on the expected average design of the human body and its function as a living organism. Yet Quasimodo, it could be argued, was very much a person.[37]

It was one thing for Saint Paul to confront himself (and his theology) in a mirror, literally and figuratively speaking, and quite another matter for the hunchback to face himself. The mirror reflected no mythological Narcissus in his psychological confrontation with Self, who—in the poetic words of Ovid—"did chance to spy the image of his face, / the which he did with fervent love embrace."[38] Rather, Quasimodo recognized overwhelmingly that he was grotesquely deformed, and indeed had lived daily since birth with this reality as mirrored in the horrified faces of others. He was repulsively ugly—to the point of suffering maternal rejection at birth, perhaps the cruelest fate of them all.

Narcissism

Despite Quasimodo's monstrous appearance, he remained a rational, sentient human being, complete with a reasonable soul. He yearned for love (of God and La Esmeralda alike) and for acceptance of his mind and of his physical appearance. But in vain. All in all, consider him tragedy incarnate—a *homo sapiens* who truly and painfully came to know himself and who came to understand only too clearly the seemingly inescapable bounds of his contorted flesh and self-loathing. His was quite a different situation from that confronting the handsome Narcissus, despite the fact, and the irony, that his self-love of his attractiveness ultimately and directly led to his self-destruction.

Despite the deep-rooted origins of the myth of Narcissus and frequent allusions to it, it is worth recalling how surprisingly modern the concept really is, and also how its meaning in psychoanalysis is still debated. Ellis[39] and Nacke,[40] in separate publications (1898 and 1899), first introduced the term and concept of narcissism in psychoanalysis to describe the attitude of a person who treats his or her own body in the same way in which the body of a sexual object is ordinarily treated. In Freud's important 1914 essay on the topic, written to advance his own psychology of the ego (ego-interest), he identifies narcissism, or what he calls "the egoism of the instinct of self-preservation," as when the libido that has been withdrawn from the external world has been devoted to the ego.[41]

Psychoanalytical psychology, especially influenced by Freud, Ferenczi, Kohut, and Kernberg,[42] has attempted, albeit to a variety of conclusions, to identify what constitutes healthy and unhealthy narcissism. Much of the research has centered on trying to describe the origins of narcissism in the earliest stages of infant and child development. As Louis A. Gottschalk of the University of California states:

> So long as there are no abrupt or disruptive external stimuli by surrounding human caretakers, the infant's evolving sense of consciousness and reality proceeds smoothly. Under these circumstances, the environment of the infant is perceived as nearly unconditionally supporting, nurturing, and accepting.[43]

Yet, where a disruption occurs, of whatever sort and by whatever means, the development of the child is affected, sometimes quite profoundly. Quasimodo the hunchback becomes a reminder of this fact in ways that no symbolic psychoanalysis of Apollo, Venus, or Narcissus can adequately treat. Yet Quasimodo's psychological development was never abruptly disturbed; rather, his entire life (that is, his ego) was at continuous physical odds with the world due to his congenital deformities. Notre Dame, for the sake of the argument, might have offered him conditional support, nurturing, and acceptance as his home and symbolic mother (literally his *alma mater,* his nourishing mother); still however, Quasimodo had to interact with other people. It was precisely at this point that Quasimodo's burden became the most recognizable.

No doubt Quasimodo, after such societal encounters, might have strongly echoed William Blake's poetic lamentation:

> O why was I born with a different face?
> Why was I not born like the rest of my race?[44]

For how well Quasimodo recognized, objectively and subjectively, in his own eyes and in the eyes of those around him, that he was indeed different. He was physically different in his face and in his entire body, not approximating any western expectations of fleshly perfection or even the plainness to be lost in a crowd (*pace* Blake). And how difficult it is for others, poets and psychiatrists alike, to comprehend conceptually what such an overwhelming and omnipresent awareness of being different means in the life and in the daily survival of a deformed person.

Certainly deformed people differ in their own awareness and responses to their deformities, however deformity itself may be defined and in whatever relative form. One physical deformity may psychologically cripple one person, and have a negligible influence on another person. Psychological defense mechanisms such as denial, displacement, or projection may serve to assist a deformed individual unconsciously to shield himself from himself. But still the confrontation with judgmental society itself is inevitable. For all the defense mechanisms, the public realm still exerts its influence on the individual's private realm. The plastic surgeon Robert M. Goldwyn rightly identifies the importance of appearance in most societies:

> The concern with appearance is not a peripheral matter for most human beings. Every society has a standard of beauty, a hierarchy of values pertaining to what is pleasing or ugly to the eye. Admittedly there is great variation among societies but within each culture, standards of attractiveness are not ambiguous.[45]

Compiling such a hierarchy of values for a society is probably far easier than predicting the reactions of those people who would appear to fall short of such values of beauty or even of acceptability. Negative reactions, as a matter of fact, have had, until fairly recently, enforceable legal protection. Many major American cities had what were called "ugly laws," usually part of their vagrancy laws.[46] For example, until its repeal in 1974 as a violation of the Constitution's Fourteenth Amendment guaranteeing equal protection of citizens, Chicago (like other cities) could impose fines on anyone appearing in public who was "diseased, maimed, mutilated, or in any way deformed so as to be an unsightly or disgusting object."[47] With such laws, Quasimodo should at least have been grateful for his medieval French origins. Even without such explicit laws, whatever the era, "facial justice" is hardly guaranteed.[48] The Fourteenth Amendment still produces few *de facto* guarantees of acceptance of those people with physical differences.

Whatever the outward prejudice or discrimination, it is also true that no hierarchy of deformities can be developed in which to predict with scientific accuracy the impact of a deformity on a life. For example, it would be unfair to suggest that epilepsy should be seen as lower on a scale than a kyphosis, the external deformity gaining more prominence than an internal abnormality. Deformity, whether congenital or acquired, may have tremendous implicit and explicit consequences, both to the individual concerned and to society.

QUASIMODO COMPLEX

The Quasimodo Complex, by my definition, refers to the self-perception and identity formation of concealed and unconcealed deformities engendered from the implicit and explicit reactions of others. It stands in contradistinction to narcissism. Society, in the form of one or more directly and/or indirectly interacting persons, provides the means for the ultimate self-judgment and self-perception by the deformed. Narcissus, by contrast, adjudged himself fleshly perfect while alone, admiring his own reflection in a mirror. That "mirror," however, must be carefully understood. Carol Gilligan notes that

> From George Herbert Mead's description of the self as known through others' reflection and Cooley's conception of the "looking-glass self," to Erikson's emphasis on the discovery of the self in others' recognition, and the current psychoanalytic fascination with the process of "mirroring," the relational con-

text of identity formation has repeatedly been conveyed. But the recurrent image of the mirror calls attention to the lifelessness in this portrayal of relationships.[49]

Gilligan argues that a far more effective means than such mirroring is the use of the "experience of connection" and "interaction, the responsiveness of human engagement." In social intercourse, and especially through dialogue, the true nature and consequences of deformity are realized. Quasimodo became acutely aware of the extent of his deformities when removed from the inner sanctum company of the silent, inanimate gargoyles and his beloved bells, and when forced to interact with other human beings. Inevitably, he was then verbally and physically tormented, alienated, taunted and tortured, and treated as less than human, with unending verbal and nonverbal reminders of his difference when close to the maddening crowd.

Motivations for such culturally conditioned and unconditioned responses, which range from humor to violent actions against the deformed, would certainly present a study in itself and are outside the scope of this essay. Yet it is interesting to see that in Henri Bergson's philosophical essay *Laughter* (1899), he considers a hunchback in his philosophical analysis of a "comic physiognomy."[50] He says that certain deformities occasion the "sorry privilege of causing some persons to laugh; some hunchbacks, for instance." According to Bergson, deformities can be divided into two groups: (1) those that nature has directed towards the ridiculous; and (2) those that absolutely diverge from it. In his analysis he suggests that a hunchback is considered comical because he "suggests the appearance of a person who holds himself badly." What is considered "physical obstinacy" leads to the comic precisely because the hunchback becomes a caricature of a normal human being, and society feels at liberty to laugh. Bergson therefore states what he calls his law that "a deformity that may become comic is a deformity that a normally built person could successfully imitate."[51] His law, however, says nothing about how the hunchback feels about the privilege of being imitated in such means. The hunchback Rigoletto in Verdi's 1851 opera of that name gives one poignant response: "Oh, fury, what a dreadful thing / to be deformed, to be a jester! Tears, the right of all men, are denied me!"[52]

The fact that a hunchback, as one example of a deformed person, can be the object of ridicule, indicates cultural acceptance of this treatment. For whatever reason, the deformed person is considered by some people to be a freak, and judged by physical criteria to be humorous. In a different age and culture such an attitude would have been generally impermissible. In Thomas Fuller's 1642 essay on deformity he remarks:

> Mock not at those who are misshapen by Nature. There is the same reason of the poore and of the deformed; he that despiseth them despiseth God that made them. A poore man is a picture of Gods own making, but set in a plain frame, not guilded: a deformed man is also his workmanship, but not drawn with even lines and lively colours.[53]

Another Puritan divine, Thomas Bedford, revealing his Pauline-Augustinian theology, spoke of deformity as "the special handiwork of God."[54] Still another Puritan opined in his *Certaine Secrete Wonders of Nature* (1569) that deformed neonates

> proceede of the judgement, justice, chastisement and curse of God, which suffreth that the fathers and mothers bring forth these abominations as a horrour of their sinne.[55]

Francis Bacon also devoted a 1625 essay to the topic and encouraged his readers to recognize that the deformed will "seek to free themselves from scorn; which must be either by virtue or malice."[56] That theme was frequently portrayed in seventeenth- and eighteenth-century literature and theater.

John Dryden and Nathaniel Lee, in their 1679 theatrical *Oedipus: A Tragedy,* present an excellent example of this attempt to obviate scorn.[57] The character Creon, in love with Eurydice, is quite deformed. When he expresses his love for her, she rejects him in no uncertain and quite cruel terms, saying that

> Nature her self start back when thou wert born;
> And cry'd, the Work's not mine—
> The midwife stood aghast; and when she saw
> Thy Mountain back, and thy distorted Legs,
> Thy Face itself.[58]

Creon retorts with what amounts to a rhetorical question: "Am I to blame, if Nature threw my Body in so perverse a Mould?" pleading his physiological case that

> The God strook fire, and lighted up the Lamps
> That beautify the Sky, so he inform'd
> This ill-shap'd Body with a daring Soul:
> And making less than Man, he made me more.[59]

Such over-compensation falls on deaf ears as Eurydice responds bluntly: "No; thou art all one Error; Soul and Body," and that deformed people like him "would tempt the Gods / To cut off humane Kind."[60]

By the time Hugo wrote his novel, however, the Romantic era had begun and his story explored the concept of *homo duplex: ange* and *bete*.[61] Teratology, the study of malformations, had established itself as far more of a science in his day,[62] and deformities were not simply seen as divine retribution against the parents because of original sin or as punishment for what was considered to be "filthy and corrupt affections,"[63] as stated in the most common sex manual for some four centuries. The deformed Quasimodo presented a haunting nineteenth-century story of a character caught somewhere between angel and beast; but in twentieth-century terms, Quasimodo represents more than a psychoanalytical study of narcissistic vulnerability, or what is also frequently referred to as a "failure of mirroring."[64] To see the character in these terms alone is to limit its importance as an insight into deformity itself and societal understandings of, and reactions to, the condition.

The sheer presence of the beautiful La Esmeralda provides the ultimate catalyst for Quasimodo's self-realization. After rescuing her from execution, delivering the unconscious gypsy unto sanctuary within the cathedral, and carrying her high up into the safety of the cathedral's tower—all acts we identify as heroic—this teratoid consciously remains sequestered among the shadows or hidden behind granite pillars for fear of frightening the woman he loves (and also for fear of experiencing what he assumes will be rejection). Finally he articulates, as best he can with his speech impediment, his innermost feelings in what constitutes his most succinct self-revelation: "Never have I seen my ugliness as I do now. When I compare myself to you, I feel very sorry for myself, poor unhappy monster that I am! To you I must seem like an animal."[65] No matter how good his acts and his soul, his physical body remains repulsive; and he must resign himself to this truth brought home in La Esmeralda's facial reactions. Expressed succinctly, *Deformitas vincit omnia* (deformity conquers all).

Standing face-to-face before La Esmeralda, where she is forced repeatedly to avert her glance in revulsion, he now fully understands what he had only previously known in part: that he is incapable of experiencing true love (of self or the requited love of another), and that nothing—no religious beliefs or psychological coping devices—can alter or protect him from this reality because of his fleshly imperfections.

DEFORMITY IN LITERATURE

Literature records other memorable scenes of self-perception about deformity and modes of identity and response. Shakespeare's interpretation of the congenitally deformed Richard III has him lamenting that he is "rudely stamp'd . . . Cheated of feature by dissembling nature, Deform'd, unfinish'd, sent before my time into this breathing world, scarce half made up."[66] Dr. Frankenstein's creation recalls in a vivid soliloquy "How was I terrified when I viewed myself in a transparent pool . . . and when I became convinced that I was in reality the monster that I am, I was filled with the bitterest sensations of despondence and mortification."[67] Cyrano de Bergerac confides to a friend that "I have my bitter days, knowing myself so ugly, so alone."[68] No doubt all of these fictitious characters would have produced interesting and revealing results on the recently conceived Narcissistic Personal Inventory (NPI) in such categories as vanity, self-sufficiency, and exhibitionism.[69]

Quasimodo, though, still provides a different and, to my mind, a far more significant perspective on what contributory factors conditioned his own personality and behavior. He gives voice to how he perceives his appearance in relation to others, such as to La Esmeralda, the very incarnation of fleshly perfection to him, and not just while staring alone into a transparent pool or mirror with his own intimations and psychological symptoms of depression, anxiety, despair, and paranoia. He does avoid the bitterness, intentional cruelty, and revenge sought upon the world by such deformed people as Richard III and the notorious Phantom of the Opera, who experiences morbid satisfaction in revealing himself in vengeful acts of murder and in his eventual dramatic unmasking: "See! Look, cast your eyes upon my face, glut yourself upon my soul!"[70] There is little doubt about how deformed the phantom's soul has become due to his acquired bodily deformity. Just what pathos is involved is another matter.

There is also the example of the cruel dwarf in Pär Lagerkvist's masterful *The Dwarf* (1944), who frankly acknowledges that

I have noticed that sometimes I frighten people; what they really fear is themselves. They think it is I who scare them, but it is the dwarf within them, the ape-faced man-like being who sticks up its head from the depths of their souls. They are afraid because they do not know that they have another being inside.[71]

As he concludes his own self-analysis in a powerful use of projection (with other psychological undertones): "And they are deformed though it does not show on the outside." It is also sublime irony: the dwarf who early in the novel brutally murders another dwarf in order to eliminate his only deformed competition at court, inverts the obvious. Rather than defining himself as deformed, it is the others around him who are perceived as errors of nature, not the dwarf himself. Yet his moral ugliness runs rampant throughout the story; his hierarchy of values is at odds with his society.

For all of the examples cited, Quasimodo still presents a unique and important character in literature. This hunchback, this angel and beast, this person provides an excellent paradigm in both his recognition of his deformed appearance, as directly and indirectly influenced by society, and in his attempt to articulate through self-analysis his tragic condition. The Quasimodo Complex itself is meant to provide a theoretical means for assessing the deformed person, the inner man and the outer man, without using the modern concept of narcissism as a basis upon which to comprehend deformity and its self-evident and not-so-self-evident impact upon his life.

APPLICATIONS

Spranger and his colleagues have developed a practical and widely accepted system for classifying dysmorphogenetic events that have a pathogenetic basis.[72] As scientifically and clinically useful as their four classifications are for identifying malformations, disruptions, deformations, and dysplasia, they do not address the obvious and subtle ramifications of such physical conditions affecting the inner man. For no simple equation exists for calculating the impact of the outer man on the inner; or the impact of deformed body upon soul, however such concepts might be used in modern medicine.[73] That is precisely why more work needs to be done in this field.

It could be argued that the Quasimodo Complex applies to people with such congenital conditions as cerebral palsy,[74] microtia,[75] spina bifida,[76] port wine stain,[77] cleft palate,[78] hypospadia,[79] epilepsy,[80] a missing limb,[81] or any of the other conditions identified in such books as Smith's *Recognizable Patterns of Human Deformation* (1981)[82] or its companion volume, Smith's *Recognizable Patterns of Human Malformation* (1970).[83] Whatever the clinical diagnosis, there is still the need to respond to the person involved, whatever the age and stage of development. Recognizing the Quasimodo Complex is not merely an exercise in trying to be sympathetic or sensitive to feelings. More accurately, and this is the challenge, it is meant to enable the health-care practitioner to recognize—theoretically and practically—how both the public and private realms of the individual, the inner and the outer man, are affected. Studies indicate, for example, that the deformed may well have poorly developed psychosocial skills. They may avoid intimacy for fear of discovery of their deformity and rejection.

Deformed people tend to marry five years later on average than their peer group—if, in fact, they do marry. Many do not. The deformed tend to marry in a lower social class than their own. They may also hold an expressed or unexpressed fear of procreation, despite medical reassurance that their deformity is congenital and will not be passed on. Some religious traditions even refuse to allow marriage if certain deformities of the reproductive organs are involved, based on a physicalist argument. Suicide rates run higher where deformity is present. Deformed orphans have a noticeably greater difficulty in finding adoptive parents. Educational achievements may be affected; this may be because of the limiting nature of the deformity itself, or for psychological reasons such as withdrawal. Studies also show that their employment opportunities are limited. Discrimination may be subtle but it is apparent.[84]

As the flesh is injured, so may be the individual's view of the world and his place and function therein. Richard III, for example, vowed that he would seek political and moral revenge upon the world as a direct consequence of his deformity. Psychoanalysts might identify this attitude as entitlement: a restitution sought stemming from suffering and anger. Studies showing a proportionately greater number of deformities among prison inmates than among the general population provide more empirical substantiation of this professed entitlement.[85]

STAGES OF DEVELOPMENT

For all of the great advances in genetic testing and progress in identifying the etiologies of birth defects and attempting to eliminate them, one baby in every forty will be born with some abnormality or defect.[86] And for all of the concern with preventing birth defects, supportive literature for assisting the deformed and for assisting healthcare practitioners remains fairly limited for many deformities and nonexistent for too many others. In fact, the first international conference on congenital malformations was only held in 1960, resulting from the thalidomide tragedy; a classification list of known deformities appeared in 1964. More scientific strides have probably been made in teratology and in establishing the probable etiology of certain congenital abnormalities than in theoretical and practical ways to assist the deformed through the various stages of psychological development as they relate to the Quasimodo Complex. Obviously much more needs to be done in multidisciplinary fashion.

The self-realization of deformity does not simply occur once, before life becomes one of resignation or eventual acceptance. In terms of psychological development, clinical studies indicate that a child becomes conscious very early of various parts of his own body, and conscious of the anatomical parts of others about the age of four. At about this point the deformed child begins to sense being "different," from noticing his anomalous body or anatomical part. Health-care practitioners need to be acutely aware of the important role they can play in assisting both parents and the child in comprehending the deformity in itself, its short-term and long-term implications, and how it might be symbolically understood.

Practitioners must be especially cognizant of their own treatment of the deformed person. For example, one book written for medical personnel on the subject of the malformed infant and child states that "the longer you refrain from touching the child, the more you will learn."[87] Yet, unless the need for this overt medical detachment is comprehended by the child and by the parents, the psychological reaction could be one of experiencing rejection and puzzlement about why the deformity or the deformed person is being treated as an object. It may well be the case that the sooner the child is touched, the sooner the symbolic confirmation of personhood is bestowed upon the deformed. As another example, if the practitioner is not prudent in the choice of words used when speaking of deformity—difference, ugliness, a "bad" body part—he may only reinforce the patient's sense of being different. The choice of adjectives and their use, combined with touch, may be just as important for the child as for the adult, such as the woman having undergone disfiguring surgery.

COSMETIC SURGERY

Times and attitudes would seem to have changed from when John Dryden wrote that "God did not make his Works for man to mend."[88] Surgically speaking, little could be done in the seventeenth century to correct deformities.[89]

Orthopedic surgery in the nineteenth century attempted to correct some conditions, generating interest in the correction of deformity.[90] Twentieth-century cosmetic surgery has attempted with increasing success to help some deformed people to improve their appearances and hence their quality of life. The results, in some cases dramatic, have enabled some of them to live almost normal lives, both in their own eyes and in the eyes of the everjudging society. The wartime surgical work of Sir Archibald MacIndoe and his staff on the badly disfigured members of the Guinea Pig Club provides a familiar example. In more recent days, the French plastic surgeon, Paul Tessier, has pioneered radical surgery to treat patients with terrible congenital mal-formations as well as victims of extensive facial injuries. Tessier's technique has been used to treat hypertelorism and Crouzon disease. For all of the pos-sibilities, cosmetic surgery still raises many ethical questions, especially about motivations for operating. Given the fact that the results may be intended more for societal acceptance than for the sake of the patient who may be unaware of the changes, can such surgery be morally justifiable?

The societal pressure to conform in appearance is so pervasive that, in-creasingly, operations on children with Down syndrome to reduce their fa-cial anomalies are being performed, with proxy consent given by parents. This practice is controversial, because the limited mental functions cannot be corrected, even if the children are made to look more "normal."[91] Some plastic surgeons will argue that such surgery is justifiable because the emo-tional and behavioral reaction to such facially deformed patients is far more positive after such radical craniofacial surgery.[92] What this suggests is that physicalism and physiognomy are still important criteria, as is *calocagathia*, in defining what it means to be human, at least in the public realm. What it also suggests, in all seriousness, is that with all of the technological develop-ments in plastic surgery, there must be concerted ethical care in charting our course in this brave new world to ensure that we never reach the island of Dr. Moreau.

CONCLUSIONS

Classical Greek mythology records that Vulcan fathered a very deformed child named Ericthonius. Athena ordered that he be confined in a box and she also commanded the daughters of Cecrops not to open it at any cost. Curiosity, however, gave way to commandment and they opened the lid. Aghast at the extent of his malformation, they jumped off the Acropolis to their deaths.

Few health-care practitioners will go to such extremes when they confront deformities. Yet, medical history records how previous ages have leapt to various conclusions as to how the deformed should be treated.[93] And what of twentieth-century treatment? Many people have little experience dealing with the deformed, not really knowing what to do or what to say, or even what to think about deformity and its multifarious ramifications. As this essay has shown, there are many such ramifications. The Quasimodo Complex is suggested as a means for identifying and responding to the meaning and significance of deformity in the ongoing development of a deformed life. At stake is not the narcissism of an individual—a self-image—as developed by Freud and by others, but an other-image as defined through societal response. At stake, too, is a means of contributing to the theoretical discussion about what deformity may mean in a life and whether, as Helga Kuhse and Peter Singer argue, "some infants with severe disabilities should be killed."[94]

The hunchback of Notre Dame, who might arguably have been killed at birth, might have experienced some rare unspoken empathy from an eighteenth-century hunchbacked Englishman, William Hay (1695–1755), who wrote of his own "contemptible Carcass" that

> Bodily Deformity is visible to every Eye; but the effects of it are known to very few; intimately known to none but those who feel them; and they are generally not inclined to reveal them.[95]

It is for this reason that fiction and fictitious characters tell us more about the sufferings of the deformed, with varying degrees of sympathy, than the deformed themselves do in direct discourse.[96] For many deformed people, however, the Quasimodo Complex is only too real; and little sanctuary from it can ever exist in the body, let alone in the human soul—despite their prayers or consultations with a cosmetic surgeon to be made fleshly perfect.

ACKNOWLEDGMENT

This article is dedicated to Mr. David Manners, actor emeritus, active sage, and friend, on the happy occasion of his ninetieth birthday. Mr. Manners starred in the 1931 Gothic horror film *Dracula* and, years later, convinced me anew that there was more in heaven and earth than ever imagined by philosophers.

NOTES

1. To spare undue pedantry, this essay will not attempt to define "deformity" in precise detail or as it differs from, say, malformation, abnormality, and disruption.

2. D. Landsborough, "St. Paul and Temporal Lobe Epilepsy," *Journal of Neurology, Neurosurgery and Psychiatry* 50 (1987): 659–64.

3. S. Levin, "St. Paul's Sickness," *Medical Proceedings* 9 (1963): 26–65; and P. T. Manchester and O. T. Manchester, "The Blindness of St. Paul," *Opthamology* 85 (1978): 1044–53.

4. See also John 9 for the story of Jesus curing the blind man, a classic Christian account of a miracle performed in order to magnify the glory of God. Yet notice, for example, Augustine's sobering commentary (in *Contra Julianum* 3, 6) on this biblical text: "These words cannot be applied to the innumerable infants born with such a wide variety of physical and mental handicaps. For many, indeed, are never healed, but die, disabled by their disabilities . . . even in infancy. Some infants retain the disabilities with which they were born, while others are afflicted with even more." Quoted in Elaine Pagels, *Adam, Eve, and the Serpent* (New York: Vintage Books, 1989), 135. Augustine is not so much concerned with theodicy or miracles, but with divine justice itself and the consequences of original sin. Physical handicaps reveal human suffering, which, according to the Bishop of Hippo, proves that sin is passed on from parents to their offspring, contrary to Julian's arguments under discussion here, about the meaning of sin and human suffering.

5. F. Broucek, "Efficacy in Infancy: A Review of Some Experimental Studies and the Implications for Clinical Theory," *International Journal of Psycho-Analysis* 60 (1979): 311–16.

6. Translation based on Revised Standard Edition of the Bible, with slight variations.

7. J. S. Carey, "Of Deformity," *Journal of the Florida Medical Association* 76 (1989): 261–62.

8. H. J. Jone, *Moral Theology* (Cork, Ireland: Mercier Press, 1951), 457; see also P. Palazzini and F. Galen, *Dictionarium Morale et Canonicum* (Rome: Catholic Book Agency, 1966), s.v. "Monstra et Ostenta," 304–5.

9. Jone, *Moral Theology,* 458.

10. See L. P. Hartley, *Facial Justice* (Oxford, 1987; first published in 1960), for a provocative futuristic account of the perfect facial society.

11. R. Jeffries, *The Story of My Heart* (London: Longmans, 1891), 152.

12. Vitruvius, *On Architecture* (London: William Heinemann, 1931), 159–65.

13. Pacioli's work, it might be noted, was highly dependent on Euclidean principles.

14. [L. da Vinci], "On the Proportions and On the Movements of the Human Figure," in *The Literary Works of Leonardo da Vinci* (Oxford: Phaidon Press, 1970), 243–70.

15. K. Clark, *The Nude: A Study of Ideal Art* (London: John Murray, 1957), 11.

16. M. A. Deschamps, *Ce Corps Hai et Adore* (Paris: Tachou, 1988), 37. See also his *L'Invention du Corps* (Paris: Presses Universitaire de France, 1986).

17. Plato, *Symposium,* 201; also, Plato, *Crito,* 48.

18. Cicero, *Tusculan Disputations* 1.xxxii, Loeb Classical Library, no. 14 (Cambridge, Mass.: Harvard University Press, 1927).

19. Pseudo-Aristotle, *The Works of Aristotle* (London, [n.d.]), 28–29.

20. Augustine, *City of God,* 16.viii (translation mine).

21. Cicero, *Tusculan Disputations* 1.24.

22. [St. Gregory the Great], *Pastoral Care* (Baltimore: The Newman Press, 1958), 41–42.

23. Ibid.; see also Aquinas, *Summa Theologiae*, 3a, 14, 4, for his account of *humanos defectus*. Rather than grounding them as a cause of original sin, he states that "there are other disabilities which, not being the cause of original sin, are not common to all humanity, but occur in particular people as a result of special causes—things like leprosy, epilepsy and so on. These disabilities are sometimes caused by men's own fault, as when they do not keep a balanced diet; or at other times by a genetic defect."

24. Scholars debate, it must be said, whether Aristotle did in fact write this essay.

25. G. Tytler, *Physiognomy in the European Novel* (Princeton, N.J.: Princeton University Press, 1958), 41-42.

26. J. C. Lavater, *Essays on Physiognomy; Designs to Promote the Knowledge and Love of Mankind*, 3rd ed. (London: B. Blake, 1840). Yet it is important to realize that physiognomy was not the only "science" of face and features. As Dorothy Johnson demonstrates, the eighteenth century developed the "gestural sublime," especially in French painting, to respond to the tradition of Le Brun's celebrated *Conférence sur l'expression générale et particulierè* (1698), indicating a different understanding of corporeality and morality. See D. Johnson, "Corporeality and Communication: The Gestural Revolution of Diderot, David, and *The Oath of the Horatii*," *The Art Bulletin* 71 (March 1989): 91–113.

27. Ibid., 99.

28. B. M. Stafford, "'Peculiar Marks': Lavater and the Countenance of Blemished Thought," *Art Journal* 27 (Fall 1987): 185–92. See also B. M. Stafford, J. La Puma, and D. L. Schiedermayer, "One Face of Beauty, One Picture of Health: The Hidden Aesthetic of Medical Practice," *The Journal of Medicine and Philosophy* 14 (1989): 213–30.

29. Stafford, "Peculiar Marks," 186.

30. M. Montaigne, *Essays* (London: Penguin Books, 1958), 336.

31. D. Laertius, *The Lives and Opinions of Eminant Philosophers* (London: George Bell and Co., 1901), 69–70.

32. Lavater, *Essays on Physiognomy*, 117.

33. J. Brophy, *The Human Face* (London: G. G. Harrop and Company, 1945), 9.

34. *Dysmorphophobia* is defined in the *Diagnostic and Statistical Manual of Mental Disorders (DSM-II-R)* (Washington, D.C.: American Psychiatric Association, 1987) as a "preoccupation with some imagined defect in appearance in a normal-appearing person" (p. 255). The manual states that this "defect" is not of delusional intensity, and that the occurrence is not exclusively during the course of anorexia nervosa or transsexualism (p. 256). *DSM-III-R* notes that an associated feature may be repeated visits to plastic surgeons or dermatologists. The disorder is relatively short-term, and "social and occupational functioning may be impaired, but marked disruption is uncommon" (p. 256).

It seems to me there is a conceptual, and etymological, confusion operating from the beginning here. First of all, the concept is misnamed: dysmorphophobia literally means a fear of deformed or malformed things (or people). It could just as correctly be used by a person confronting and rejecting someone deformed, such as La Esmeralda in her response to Quasimodo, as with a more general societal response to the deformed. In a more serious vein, dysmorphophobia, as identified in *DSM-III-R*, or any of the other disorders in what they refer to as relating to somatoform, really fails to penetrate into the phenomenological or hermeneutical ramifications of deformity in direct terms.

As used in this essay, dysmorphophobia refers to the individual and group response of people to the deformed, notably in the way of fear. Further studies in psychiatric literature are needed into congenitally deformed "body image" to correct both the prevalent definition and conceptual usage. See also C. S. Thomas, "Dysmorphophobia: A Question of Definition," *British Journal of Psychiatry* 144 (May 1984): 513–16.

35. J. Cox, "Quest for Quasimodo," *British Medical Journal* 291 (1985): 1801–3.

36. *Terata* is the plural of the Greek *teras*, a marvel, a monster. Teratology is the study of malformations, monstrosities, or serious deviations from the normal in growing organisms.

37. A. O'Malley and J. J. Walsh, *Essays in Pastoral Medicine* (New York: Longmans, Green, 1911). See chapter six, "Human Terata and the Sacraments." Consider, too, Aristotle's reflection: "Why is the face chosen for representation in portraits? Is it because the face shows best what the character of a person is? Or is it because it is most easy recognized?" *The Works of Aristotle,* vol. 7, trans. W. D. Ross (New York: Oxford University Press, 1927), 965b. Yet what is to be made of the face, and of the person, when deformity is involved?

38. Ovid, *Metamorphoses,* trans. Mary Innes (New York: Penguin Books, 1955), 3, lines 520–21.

39. H. Ellis, *Studies in the Psychology of Sex* (Philadelphia: Davis, 1898).

40. P. Naecke, *Über die sogenannte Moral Insanity s: Grenzfragen des Nerven - u. Seelenlebens 18—dis Unterbringung giesteskranker Verbrecher gr. 8* (Halle, Germany, 1902).

41. S. Freud, "On Narcissism: An Introduction," *Collected Papers,* vol. 4 (London: Hogarth Press, 1948), 31.

42. S. Ferenczi, "Stages in the Development of Reality," *Internationale Zeitschrift fur Artzliche Psychoanalysis* (1913): 124–38; H. Kohut, *The Analysis of Self* (New York: International Universities Press, 1971); and O. Kernberg, *Borderline Conditions and Pathological Narcissism* (New York: Jason Aronson, 1975).

43. L. A. Gottschalk, "Narcissism: Its Normal Evolution and Development and the Treatment of Its Disorders," *American Journal of Psychotherapy* 42 (1988): 5.

44. G. Keynes, ed., *The Letters of William Blake with Related Documents,* 3rd ed. (New York: Oxford University Press, 1980), 312.

45. P. Regnault and R. K. Daniel, *Aesthetic Plastic Surgery: Principles and Techniques* (Boston: Little, Brown, 1984), 31.

46. "Facial Discrimination: Extending Handicap Law to Employment Discrimination on the Basis of Physical Appearance," *Harvard Law Review* 100 (June 1987): 2035–54.

47. Chicago, *Illinois Municipal Code* (1966) Secs. 36-34 [repealed 1974].

48. Burgdorf and Burgdorf, "A History of Unequal Treatment: The Qualifications of Handicapped Persons as a 'Suspect Class' Under the Equal Protection Clause," *Santa Clara Law Review* 15 (1975): 855, 863.

49. C. Gilligan, "Mapping the Moral Domain: New Images of Self in Relationship," *Cross Currents* 39 (Spring 1989): 53. See also C. F. Alford's enlightening and important discussion of "the culture of narcissism" in *Narcissism: Socrates, the Frankfurt School, and Psychoanalytic Theory* (New Haven: Yale University Press, 1988).

50. H. Bergson, *Laughter: An Essay on the Meaning of the Comic* (London: Macmillan and Co., 1911), 22.

51. Ibid., 23.

52. "O rabbia! esser difforme! / O Rabbia! esser buffone! Non dover, non poter altro che ridere! / Il retaggio d'ogni uom m'e tolto, / il pianto!" (*Rigoletto,* act 1, sc. 1). The opera was based on Hugo's 1832 work *Le Roi S'Amuse* and the character of the hunchback Triboletto. Verdi's hunchback jester's name was changed to Rigoletto as a deliberate play on the French *rigoler* (to laugh or guffaw), which fits in well with Bergson's position.

53. T. Fuller, *The Holy State* (Cambridge, 1642), 190. Compare this with an ancient Jewish prayer to be used "On seeing strangely formed persons, such as giants and dwarves": "Blessed art Thou, O Lord our God, King of the Universe, who variest the forms of thy creatures." From J. H. Hertz, *The Authorized Daily Prayer Book,* rev. ed. (New York: Bloch Publishing, 1948), 993.

54. T. Bedford, *A True and Certain Relation of a Strange Birth* (London, 1635). Compare this with the attitude of the American Puritan Cotton Mather (1663–1728) when he commented on the antinomian "heresy" of Anne Hutchinson (*c.* 1600–1643) and its effect on a pregnancy that this "erroneous gentlewoman, convicted of holding about thirty monstrous opinions, growing big with child, and at length coming to her time of travail, was delivered of about thirty monstrous births at once; whereof some were bigger, some were lesser; of several figures; few if any perfect, none of any human shape." In R. Boas and L. Boas, *Cotton Mather: Keeper of the Puritan Conscience* (New York: Harper and Brothers, 1928), 41. When Mather's own son was born in 1693, incidentally, he lacked an anus and died within three days. In this case, Mather suspected witchcraft as the cause of this deformity, writing to his father that several weeks before birth his wife had been frightened by a *"Spectre."* The implication is of course that the deformity was not caused by any sin on the part of the Mathers.

55. E. Penton, *Certaine Secrete Wonders of Nature, Containing a Description of Sundry Strange Things, Seming Monstrous in Our Eyes and Judgement, Because We are not Privie to the Reasons of Them* (London: Henry Bynneman, 1569), 3. For a remarkable historical account of "monsters" and attitudes toward them during this era, see K. Park and L. J. Daston, "Unnatural Conceptions: The Study of Monsters in Sixteenth- and Seventeenth-Century France and England," *Past & Present* 90–93 (1981): 20–54.

56. [F. Bacon], "Of Deformity," in *The Works of Francis Bacon* (London, 1826), 347.

57. [J. Dryden and N. Lee], "Oedipus: A Tragedy," *The Dramatic Works of Mr. Nathaniel Lee* (London, 1734).

58. Ibid., I:i.

59. Ibid.

60. Eurydice's statement about deformed body and accompanying soul is a rare identification of the dual effects of deformity.

61. That is, "two-fold man, angel and beast," from W. D. Howarth, "From Classical Tragedy to Romantic Drama: The Monstrous Demythologized," in *The Monstrous: Durham* [England] French Colloquies 1 (1987): 7–25.

62. T. V. N. Persaud, A. E. Chudley, and R. G. Skalko, *Basic Concepts in Teratology* (New York: Alan R. Liss, Inc., 1985), 1–11. For a classic, if not Romantic, study of teratology, see Isidore Geoffroy Saint-Hilaire, *Histore Generale et Paniculaire des Anomalies de l'Organisation Chez L'Homme et les Animaux* (Paris, 1832). Published a year after *The Hunchback of Notre Dame* appeared, this book was the most important study to appear on the topic since teratology as a science developed in the first half of the eighteenth century. See also the writings of Mery, Duverney, Haller, Morgagni, Hirst, and Piersol.

63. Pseudo-Aristotle, *The Works of Aristotle,* 29.

64. Broucek, "Efficacy in Infancy," 317–24.

65. V. Hugo, *Notre-Dame de Paris* (London: Penguin Books, 1987), 368.

66. Shakespeare, *Richard III,* I:i.

67. M. Shelley, *Frankenstein or, The Modern Prometheus* (London: Penguin Books, 1985), 203.

68. E. Rostand, *Cyrano de Bergerac,* trans. B. Hooker (New York: Bantam Classics, 1987), I:v.

69. R. Raskind and C. S. Hall, "A Narcissistic Personality Inventory," *Psychoanalytical Reports* 45 (1979): 590.

70. G. Leroux, *The Phantom of the Opera* (London: W. H. Allen, 1985), 141.

71. P. Lagerkvist, *The Dwarf* (London: Chatto & Windus, 1953), 20.

72. J. Spranger, K. Benirschke, and J. G. Hall, "Errors of Morphogenesis: Concepts and Terms," *Journal of Pediatrics* 100 (1982): 160–65.

73. See Milton T. Edgerton, "Deformity as A Disease," *Transactions and Studies of the College of Physicians of Philadelphia*, 4th ser., 41 (October 1973): 124–30. Edgerton attempts, albeit not satisfactorily, to explore what impact a deformity has on a patient; and what change may be brought about through surgical intervention. Obviously, classifying some deformities as diseases has pragmatic consequences, such as in convincing insurance companies to pay for what might otherwise be classified as elective—and therefore nonreimbursible—cosmetic surgery.

74. J. Magill and N. Hulbut, "The Self-Esteem of Adolescents with Cerebral Palsy," *American Journal of Occupational Therapy* 40, no. 6 (1986): 402–7.

75. J. S. Carey, "Microtia: A Personal Case Study," *Aesthetic Plastic Surgery* 9 (1985): 197–206.

76. A. Pearson et al., "The Self Concept of Adolescents with Spina Bifida," *Zeitschrift fur Kinderchirurgie* 40, supp. 1 (December 1985): 27–30.

77. H. Collyer, *Facial Disfigurement: Successful Rehabilitation* (London: Macmillan, 1984), 26–60.

78. B. J. McWilliams, "Social and Psychological Problems Associated with Cleft Palate," *Clinics in Plastic Surgery* 9 (July 1982): 317–26.

79. M. Duskova and H. Helclova, "The Problem for Timing Surgical Treatment for Hypospadia from the Surgeon's and Psychologist's Points of View," *Acta Chirurgiae Plasticae* 29, no. 4 (1987): 228–48.

80. P. Valerio, G. D'Amorosio, A. De Rose et al. "Living with Epilepsy: Medical and Social Considerations," *Monographs in Neural Science* 5 (1980): 245–49.

81. M. S. Pinzur, G. Graham, and H. Osterman, "Psychological Testing in Amputation Rehabilitation," *Clinical Orthopedics and Related Research* 229 (1988): 236–40.

82. J. M. Graham, Jr., *Smith's Recognizable Patterns of Human Deformities* (London: W. B. Saunders, 1988).

83. D. W. Smith, *Recognizable Patterns of Human Malformations* (London: W. B. Saunders, 1970).

84. "Facial Discrimination," 2036.

85. See, for example, R. L. Kurtzberg, M. L. Lewin, N. Cavior, et al. "Psychologic Screening of Inmates Requesting Cosmetic Operations: A Preliminary Report," *Plastic and Reconstructive Surgery* 39 (April 1967): 387–96.

86. A. Fern, "When a Baby is Handicapped," *Nursing Times* 84, no. 33 (August 17, 1988): 66.

87. R. M. Goodman and R. J. Gorlin, *The Malformed Infant and Child* (New York: Oxford University Press, 1983), 3.

88. John Dryden, as quoted in William Hay, *Deformity: An Essay* (London, 1754), 7.

89. The deformed English poet Alexander Pope (1688–1744) provides a case in point. Frequently painted or depicted in sculpture, his image certainly did not reflect his deformities, especially his obvious hunchback. As Sir Oliver Piper writes in *The Image of the Poet: British Poets and Their Portraits* (New York: Oxford University Press, 1982), 58: "[V]anity was intensified by the need to rectify the tragic twisted reality of his crippled body with an image of the

lucid, beautifully articulated construction and spirit of his poetry—the need very literally to put the image straight. When the sum of his portraits is surveyed [more than sixty distinct types, matched during Pope's lifetime only by royalty], it reads like a willed highly controlled projection by Pope of his person into posterity—." Pope was not alone, it must be said. History records that such famous persons as Byron, Descartes, Mirabeau, William III, and Henrietta Maria also had evident deformities that were ignored in formal portraits. (Velasquez, however, was a notable exception with his portraits of several deformed people and dwarves. See also the works of the nineteenth-century Chinese painter Lam Qua for even more vivid examples.) For a stimulating modern discussion of how our perception of the monstrous affects aesthetic comprehension of "the human," see "Notes on Monsters" in Rudolph Arnheim, *Toward a Psychology of Art: Collected Essays* (Berkeley: University of California Press, 1966). Arnheim writes: "Monsters have been made in all epochs of art. . . . Today, we have been made to recognize evil as a part of our own behavior, and thus the monster has become a portrait of ourselves and the kind of life we have chosen to lead" (pp. 256–57).

90. W. J. Little, *On the Nature and Treatment of the Deformity of the Human Form* (London, 1853), 5. Little wrote that "the attempt to cure deformity is no longer disdained by medical men of eminence."

91. L. Rozner, "Facial Plastic Surgery for Down's Syndrome," *Lancet* 1 (1983): 1320–23; D. J. Hatch, "Facial Reconstruction in Down Syndrome," *Journal of the Royal Society of Medicine* 81 (January 1981): 1; and H. Hohler, "Changes in Facial Expression as a Result of Plastic Surgery in Mongoloid Children," *Aesthetic Plastic Surgery* 1 (1977): 245.

92. R. C. Barden, M. E. Ford, W. M. Wihelm, et al., "Emotional and Behavioral Reactions of Facially Deformed Patients Before and After Craniofacial Surgery," *Plastic and Reconstructive Surgery* 82, no. 3 (1988): 409–18.

93. G. M. Gould and W. L. Pyle, *Anomalies and Curiosities of Medicine* (London: W. B. Saunders and Co., 1900).

94. H. Kuhse and P. Singer, *Should the Baby Live? The Problem of Handicapped Infants* (New York: Oxford University Press, 1985), v.

95. Hay, *Deformity*, 2.

96. See R. Rorty's *Philosophy and the Mirror of Nature* (Princeton, N.J.: Princeton University Press, 1979), 320–21, for his distinctions between normal and abnormal discourse. It could be argued that such linguistic distinctions have relevant phenomenological bearing on any discussions pertaining to deformity, especially since the understanding of an affliction can never be purely based on an epistemological or psychological foundation.

Self-Help for the Facially Disfigured:
Commentary on "The Quasimodo Complex"

Elisabeth A. Bednar

As an adult disfigured from birth and the director of a self-help network for individuals who are facially disfigured, I read Jonathan Sinclair Carey's article and was overwhelmed by the injustice of centuries of judgment based on appearance. What a burden this has wrought on those of us who, by circumstance of birth, disease, or trauma, assume a countenance that is less than acceptable to some elusive and unquantifiable norm! *ability to overcome*

Indeed we do have, as Quasimodo did, an "overwhelming and omnipresent awareness of being different." We know that in the place where personal adjustment and acceptance come face-to-face with the reality of acceptance in the public realm, there is a chasm of misunderstanding. Whether we are shopping, riding the subway, or eating in a restaurant, all of which are casual day-to-day social encounters, there is the initial stare, then the look away, before a second, furtive glance inevitably puts the beheld immediately in a separate class. For those who experience this discrimination, the question of the moral justification of surgery to increase societal acceptance is merely rhetorical. There can be no greater wish than to melt into the crowd or to walk into a room unnoticed. *we all want to fit in but appearances won't do that*

And discrimination by appearance is reinforced in advertising. We are led to believe that if we look great, happiness, success, and romance are bound to follow. For the individual who cannot achieve that "perfect 10" facial appearance, the outlook can only be bleak. Yet, is it not the whole person who gives off an aura of beauty? And what of our definition of beauty? What if those we see as disfigured misfits of our planet were cast as a different humanoid race? Would they then, by other standards, be beautiful? And would we, the earth humans, find it acceptable to view them as perfect—good without and within?

As an ethical issue, perhaps the greatest challenge is to abandon the "either/or" approach and recognize that the best results can be achieved by working on both society's attitudes *and* the individual's self-perception at the same time. Certainly there is evidence that a two-sided approach is most expedient in other situations. For example, we install a water filter on the tap, but we don't cease trying to clean up the lake while we prevent further contamination with stricter antipollution laws. Fixing the outcome does not preclude working on the source.

Indeed, at About Face this is the structure we have adopted in offering information, support, and programs of public education. Five years old, About Face is dedicated to meeting the needs of individuals who are disfigured as a result of a birth defect, a disease, or an accident. Through linking people with similar concerns, those who have felt alone often find, for the first time, that they are not. Developing printed material relating to psychosocial issues and describing syndromes and anomalies which cause disfigurement serve to inform, empower, and assist decisions. But all of this must be combined with a social-awareness initiative. To feel better about oneself, but to be met with a constant reminder at each and every chance encounter that one is different, to face the myths associated with this form of discrimination—that the soul and brain are also afflicted—is an incalculable attack on the self-esteem. By teaching in schools, educating physicians and other health-care providers about their unspoken communication during treatment, and talking candidly to journalists, our aim is to dispel these misconceptions, to implore others to look past our flawed package, and to cultivate an environment of understanding and acceptance. As playwright Jean Rostand wrote in *Cyrano de Bergerac,* "The best way to fight your enemy is to educate him." Through education we can learn to walk together to the rhythm of circumstance.

For information, contact AboutFace, 99 Crowns Lane, Third Floor, Toronto, ONT M5R 3P4, Canada, Telephone: 416-944-FACE.

[Handwritten marginal notes:]
interesting idea

do it is normal to be abnormal, abnormal is just a feeling

you can overcome your own feelings,

be in reality, everyone has some abnormality, which is why they feel insecure and shun out others

A Brief Response to "The Quasimodo Complex"

HARRY YEIDE, JR.

JONATHAN SINCLAIR CAREY's essay represents exactly the kind of work that scholars in the humanities like to see, the use of sacred texts and high literature to stimulate reflection on the human condition in a way that provides direct entry into practical, and in this case clinical, concerns. While these same scholars will insist that there are additional reasons for dealing with these texts, few would find this kind of venture foreign to their own interests. The essay reminded me of a long-forgotten footnote by Rollo May on the training of psychologists:

> Many of us made the discovery in those college days that we learned a good deal more about psychology—that is, man and his experience—from our literature courses than we did from our psychology itself. The reason, of course, was that literature could not avoid dealing with symbols and myths as the quintessential forms of man's expression and interpretation of himself.[1]

Understandably, May regards the recovery of this insight as one of the gifts psychoanalysis has shared with other forms of psychological study and therapy.

Having affirmed the general thrust of Carey's essay, I wish to discuss several points that seem to me in need of correction or elaboration. Carey could have developed the material in Corinthians regarding St. Paul's "thorn in the flesh" in a way that contributes more substantively to the discussion. The real context for Paul's reference to this "thorn" is not the issue of perfection and deformity, but rather strength and weakness. Indeed many Bible scholars regard the "thorn" as a useful metaphor rather than a clinical description. (The persisting but unresolved search for a clinical diagnosis grew out of an epoch of biblical scholarship driven by theories of psychological reductionism; while some biblical scholars continue to be interested in such possibilities, I believe most regard the materials as recalcitrant to such analysis and find other modes of analysis more illuminating.)

Paul wants to convince the Corinthians that strength, as measured by "the world" (or in less loaded language, the surrounding culture), is less deserving of our allegiance than the weakness of God. The embodiment of this weakness is, in turn, discussed in terms of the crucifixion of Jesus and Paul's own unimposing personal presence. The argument climaxes: "When I am weak, then I am strong."

Whether Paul was deformed or simply ordinary, the theme of weakness is, of course, potentially related to the problem of physical deformity and ugliness. The New Testament writers often make this connection. One of the primary texts used in interpreting the crucifixion of Jesus comes from the prophetic book of Isaiah. There we find a series of statements about a "suffering servant," where the suffering is explained in terms of weakness and ugliness.

> He had no form or comeliness that we should look at him, and no beauty that we should desire him. He was despised and rejected by men . . . and as one from whom men hide their faces he was despised. (Isa. 53:2–3)

But in Isaiah, as in Paul, God is judged to be *especially* present in the ugly and weak servant; here is where the deepest, most real power manifests itself. While the world generally associates power with strength and beauty and the way in which these traits enable humans to at least influence and possibly dominate others, power is here associated with the capacity to suffer with and for others, including the ugly and deformed. Indeed, the suffering servant is empowered to join the company of those that the strong and the beautiful despise and avoid. The agonizing, contorted, deformed Jesus in Grünewald's painting of the crucifixion catches well this stream of tradition.

Carey is certainly correct in pointing out that the Bible gives rise to or supports prejudice against deformity, and that this prejudice is justified by concern for ritual purity and/or the belief that deformities are evidence of divine wrath. But there is another quite different stream of tradition that also flows through the Bible and is visible in the writings of Paul.

Indeed, the conjoining of deformity and the divine does not seem confined to the biblical tradition. If, as the essay suggests, epilepsy belongs to the range of deformities to be considered regarding the Quasimodo Complex, it is often asserted that the holy power of shamans is evidenced in part by their manifestation of symptoms we would likely interpret as epilepsy. It has also been asserted that some of the Egyptian pharaohs had elongated heads, a deformity that was associated with their divine status. (Indeed, a similar deformity in the paintings of El Greco does not always seem to elicit a negative response by viewers in our Western culture.) There is an early Taoist tradition in which the crafting of features on the blank face gives rise to death; a blank face is better. A whole host of physical objects of worship in many cultural histories are simultaneously anthropomorphic and radically distorted. Certain ascetic practices knowingly lead to permanent deformity. Additional reflection on these matters would give greater depth to the concept of the Quasimodo Complex. While this brief response can hardly develop this "suspicion," the traditions noted above minimally suggest a larger variety of possible cultural responses than we see in the hunchback's experience. It does not occur to the hunchback that deformity and ugliness are not so much deviations from the beautiful as their necessary partners in the grand scheme of things.

Furthermore, there is an interesting parallel between the approach of the author and that of Saint Paul. Both wish to do battle with the notion of strength as defined by the relevant culture. As Carey asserts, a beautiful or at least ordinary appearance confers strength in our culture. He presents various data to demonstrate the disadvantaged state of the deformed. But he does not conclude that things are as they should be. Rather, he argues for various therapeutic interventions that will at least modify their destiny for the better; there is something "wrong" with what he takes to be the prevailing social view on these matters. A more direct attack on cultural evaluation of physical perfection and deformity is a conceivable extension of his point of view.

There are many other points about which I would like to know more. I am, for instance, puzzled by use of "Pseudo-Aristotle" as important in the witness of the later Church Fathers. "Pseudo-Aristotle" is the name given to approximately one hundred documents wrongly attributed to Aristotle. They originate in many different languages and centuries; some of the best known were first composed in Arabic and unknown in Christian Europe until the sixteenth century. All of this fits ill with our conventional designations of the Church Fathers.

But there are also less intellectual, more clinical matters about which I would like to know more. Most importantly, is the definition of the Quasimodo Complex sufficiently detailed to apply to clinical practice at this stage?

(It seems more like an ideal type as it stands.) Are the definitions of body and soul sufficiently precise and consistent to clarify particular cases? Despite questions of this sort, I remain completely persuaded that we have much to learn from the hunchback of Notre Dame, and am grateful for the stimulus thereto contained in this essay.

NOTE

1. R. May, *Symbolism in Religion and Literature* (New York: G. Braziller, 1960), 13.

A Response to "The Quasimodo Complex"

FRANCES COOKE MACGREGOR

CONSIDERING THE VAST differences in orientation, training, and objectives between the disciplines of science and theology, it is, in my opinion, a form of arrogance or naïveté to assume the role of commentator about the paper by Jonathan Sinclair Carey. But in view of my years of research as a medical sociologist-anthropologist on the social, psychological, and cultural problems associated with facial deformities, I believe a response is in order.

Since World War II, the effect of both congenital and acquired physical deformities upon human beings has been a subject of increasing interest and research from a variety of clinical and academic perspectives, such as medicine, surgery, psychiatry, anthropology, sociology, and psychology. One is intrigued, therefore, by a paper written from the perspective of theology—a discipline that neither shuns the subjective nor avoids moral precepts and value judgments. Such prerogatives, however, are not included in the armamentarium of science which, in addition to other basic differentials, makes discourse difficult.

In 1967, two physicians, F. W. Masters and D. C. Greaves, defined "The Quasimodo Complex."[1] It is characterized by "anxiety, hostility, social withdrawal and abnormal personality traits—produced by emotional reaction to physical deformity." Jonathan Carey has added another dimension: the "accompanying soul." This dimension, he contends, has been too long neglected, specifically in psychoanalysis with its focus on narcissism (a problem, it should be noted, more intrapsychic than interpersonal).

While the author has made an admirable effort to address the tragedy of "looking different" in a world that, since recorded history, has scorned and stigmatized those who do not conform physically to the accepted standards of their particular culture, the result, unfortunately, is not as cogent as it might be. Instead, his attempt to encompass too many disparate facets in this large and complex area of human suffering results in superficial treatment.

For example, in human relationships there is a vast difference between the kinds of social and psychological problems associated with physical handicaps (such as a paralyzed leg or the loss of an arm) and those stemming from deviations or distortions of the face (a symbol of one's identity and persona)—which evoke adverse reactions and social rejection. This is a special irony with which facially disfigured persons must contend and which those who work in the field of disabilities and rehabilitation have for too long failed to take into account. As a victim of ocular hypertelorism (a congenital craniofacial deformity characterized by defective development of the sphenoid bone and greater breadth of the nose with correspondingly great width between the eyes) said: "What is my crime? I am strong, I have two arms, I can work—but I can't get a job. I can't go out in the world—wherever I go people stare."

Carey's main concern is based on his claim that the impact and meaning of physical malformation on what he calls the "inner" and "outer" man have been neglected by those involved in the art and science of healing. But by recognizing the Quasimodo Complex, he claims, health practitioners will be helped to recognize how both the inner and outer man are affected. This assertion is followed by a list of examples (with no citations given): the deformed *may* [italics mine] well have poorly developed psychological skills; they *may* avoid intimacy and potential discovery of their deformity; they *may* possess an expressed or unexpressed fear of procreating, despite medical reassurance; their suicide rates are higher. Whether these statements are true of those with bodily or facial deformities, or both, is not specified.

The author makes a plea for greater awareness on the part of health practitioners in their approach to the physically deformed and their families lest they unwittingly reenforce the patient's feeling of being different. This important dimension of medical care and doctor-patient relationships is almost totally lacking in the medical school curriculum and centers of physical rehabilitation. This is not to ignore the attention given to the establishment of good relationships with patients to gain their cooperation and provide a high quality of care. Indeed, health practitioners value sensitivity and intuition, but view them, for the most part, as innate qualities. In short, they place more emphasis on the aims rather than the methods of achieving them.

The high cost of this neglect is exemplified in Shoeph's thorough investigation of doctor-patient interaction in a large reconstructive plastic surgery center for the facially disfigured. She graphically demonstrates the way various parameters in the treatment situation contribute to dissonance in doctor-patient relationships with nontherapeutic consequences.[2]

Dissonance in the doctor-patient relationship that is traceable to problems of communication occurs far more often than most people realize. I am referring here not to verbal communication alone, but to "nonlexical" behaviors—the messages conveyed from one person to another on nonverbal levels. These include, for example, the kinesic level (body movements and tonus, gestures, facial expressions, eye movements, and so forth), the paralinguistic level (tone and pitch of voice, yawns, sighs, rate of speech, and so forth), and the proxemic level (spatial arrangements, movements towards or away from one another, and so forth). Called the "silent language,"[3] they are dimensions of communication that, while usually received on a subliminal level, can have significant positive or negative effects on doctor-patient interaction and the therapeutic outcome.

There is little attention given to the high sensitivity of malformed and disfigured persons as to how they are perceived while interacting with others. Anxious about the impression they give, they are especially alert to both verbal and nonverbal symbols by which the nondisfigured wittingly or unwittingly convey information; this feedback, in turn, affects their self-image and feelings of self-worth.[4]

In recent years, we have seen a vast improvement in efforts to make life more livable for the physically handicapped, for example, vocational training, modes of transportation, public accommodation, and so forth (which, it should be noted, have little relevance for those with facial deviations). While extremely important, these are but external aids at best. Nor are they enough to prevent or assuage the pain of looking different or ugly in a society not only obsessed with physical perfection but where first impressions can be crucial to social interchange and to the establishment of human relationships. What is essential for improving the quality of life for those who happen to deviate from the norm is a facet of social intercourse that has received small attention. This is the need for a trained sensitivity and awareness of our own modes of communication that can make the difference between conveying acceptance or rejection. But this need is not limited to health practitioners nor to caring laymen. A trained awareness is equally essential for the disfigured who, despite their understandable hypersensitivity, can by their own demeanor and expectation unconsciously affect—either positively or negatively—the quality of interaction with the nondisfigured.[5]

NOTES

1. F. W. Masters and D. C. Greaves, "The Quasimodo Complex," *British Journal of Plastic Surgery* 20 (1967): 204–10.

2. B. G. Shoeph, "Doctor-Patient Communication in the Medical School Social System: A Plastic Surgery Clinic" (Ph.D. diss., Columbia University, 1969).

3. E. T. Hall, *The Silent Language* (New York: Doubleday, 1959).

4. F. C. Macgregor, "Facial Disfigurement: Problems and Management of Social Interaction and Implications for Mental Health," in *Aesthetic Plastic Surgery* (New York: Springer-Verlag, forthcoming).

5. F. C. Macgregor, *After Plastic Surgery: Adaptation and Adjustment* (New York: Praeger Publishers, 1979), 115–18.

Commentary on "The Quasimodo Complex"

Arlette Lefebvre

I found Jonathan Sinclair Carey's paper to be fascinating and somewhat awe-inspiring. Fascinating because it traces the origins of stigma associated with physical disability from Greco-Roman times, through the medieval period, to present psychoanalytic thinking. In addition, it is so comprehensive and detailed in its references and illustrations that it could only have been distilled from a massive literature search and months of intensive study—standards which very few clinicians with a dilettante's interest in ethics will ever be able to meet. And yet, I found myself thinking: Wouldn't it be wonderful to have available to us this kind of panoramic cultural perspective on other controversial issues, such as abortion, euthanasia, and homosexuality?

With eloquence, yet simplicity, the author deftly puts together the pieces of the Quasimodo puzzle, interweaving poetical verse, philosophical theory, religious dogma, and plain bigotry (the "ugly laws") in an intriguing blend of myth and reality, observation and distortion, which seizes the reader's attention by the throat and holds it prisoner until Quasimodo is finally revealed, as he emerges through the distorted mirrors of societal perceptions.

From a psychiatric perspective, several excellent points are brought forth in the discussion. First of all, compiling a hierarchy of social values on what is considered "pleasing" or "ugly" at a given time is a great deal easier than predicting any one individual's adjustment to disability, in particular, visible deformity. Indeed, we seem much better able to measure the effects of intellectual or emotional deprivation, the impact of divorce or bereavement, or even the aftereffects of catastrophic experiences, such as earthquakes or concentration camps, than we are able to conceive of, let alone quantify or predict, the experience of being seen as different every day of one's life. It has certainly been our experience here in Canada, working with over three thousand affected families over a fifteen-year period, that the severity of the disfigurement is the *least significant predictive factor*. Far more significant are the personality strengths of the individual, both in terms of innate ability or talent and acquired interests and hobbies, and the support and acceptance given by family and friends. The eye of others is where we seek the validation of our existence, and this is the yardstick by which we each judge our self-worth. But universal approval, or even acceptance, is far less important than the consistent love and admiration of a few consistent others.

The second brilliant point is the one made by both Carey and Carol Gilligan (who is cited in Carey's article) about the psychoanalytic literature's excessive emphasis on the "mirroring" aspect of relationships: mirroring that accurately describes the initial, immediate social reaction, but underestimates or totally ignores the dynamic elements of "connectedness" in human relationships. Certainly, we may be initially attracted by a particular face or form, but isn't it the twinkle in the eye, the warmth in the laughter, the spontaneity of the gestures, and, ultimately, the attitude of the other person toward us that makes or breaks a relationship? How else can we account for the incredible charisma and charm of certain individuals whose features, examined one by one, have nothing outstanding or beautiful? And how else can we account for the empty disillusionment that besieges us when what looked like a beautiful person turns out to be an empty shell? The heart of the beholder is much more perceptive than we give it credit for, and there is a great deal of social finesse and human interaction skill that the beheld can learn and master to his or her own advantage. That is the main therapeutic lesson that this paper and clinical experience bring forth: one can learn to get beyond the immediate reaction and to focus on the social interaction.

However, strangely enough, it is the scope of the ethical discussion of this paper that leaves me wanting more. "Is that all there is?" and even "Must we accept the status quo?" are two feelings that come to mind. The evidence is certainly overwhelming in favor of universal, cross-cultural bias for attractiveness, and we will probably never be able to eradicate that initial, almost instinctive, but perhaps ethologically programmed and socially reinforced, reaction of shock, curiosity, fear, or pity in different combinations. But beyond that initial reflex, everything can and should be changeable. Look how far we have come in promoting social acceptance and respect for individuals with Down's syndrome, or for the blind and hearing impaired, largely through the impact, I believe, of the powerful medium of television. Look how social attitudes toward smoking and sexual stereotypes have evolved in the past twenty years.

Further, a female astronaut would probably have been inconceivable in my mother's generation, so why give up when it comes to prejudices about facial deformity? Why not take up the challenge of presenting a news anchor person with a very visible facial deformity, in another ten or twenty years?

After all, the excessive narcissism promoted by the *Cosmopolitan* girl is beginning to take its toll on all women; for example, consider the escalating rates of anorexia nervosa and bulimia. And the idealized, superfit, supermale Stallone male role model is probably, although less visibly, affecting the confidence and sexual potency of many men. Isn't it time to shift the emphasis from the external package to the human interaction? From measured performance—in sports, orgasm, or whatever—to living and learning and growing together? From the obsession with achievement and control to the realization that shared embarrassment, shortcomings, and funny moments do more to cement a relationship than a perfect face or track records?

I do believe that it is the responsibility of publications such as *The Journal of Clinical Ethics* to raise these issues, to examine and question the role models we are promoting in the media or to our children and to challenge clinicians' defeatist acceptance of the status quo. The real failure consists in not trying. The unforgivable ethical lacuna is noting the injustice and accepting it as a permanent reality, without challenge.

For as Beverly Sills points out: "You may be disappointed if you attempt it and do not succeed, but you are doomed to failure if you do not try."

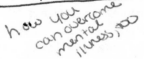

Literature as a Clinical Capacity:
Commentary on "The Quasimodo Complex"

JOANNE TRAUTMANN BANKS

THE EDITOR HAS asked me to comment on Jonathan Sinclair Carey's use of literature and to suggest how literature might generally be valuable to health-care providers. I intend to do so with dispatch—clinical ethicists, I take it, typically do not dawdle over another discipline's theory and trivia—but I request at the outset that my remarks be taken in the light of history. For centuries, after all, literary and medical thinkers have occasionally encountered each other on their mutual mission to understand human suffering and promote well-being. Within the last twenty years, the conjoined force of literature and medicine has been an active, formal presence in American classrooms and clinics, and in journals and books around the world. Therefore, the following remarks include only a few of the literary clinical possibilities that might be drawn from that much larger arena.

I have organized my response into four categories: (1) the use of literary names to describe patients; (2) literature's unique contribution to empathy; (3) how to put literary empathy to work in clinical care; and (4) an alternative literary form for the study of ethics.

LITERARY NAMES FOR PATIENTS

One of the most popular uses of literature in medicine is illustrated by Carey's central figure, Quasimodo. The literary eponym—that is, the borrowing of a character from literature to name an entity—is well known in medicine through such terms as "Oedipus complex," "Munchausen's syndrome," and dozens of other examples. In fact, the authors of a recent book discovered over 350 of them, including other uses of Victor Hugo's Quasimodo.[1] Medical writers reach for literary eponyms for many reasons, and the results are, for the most part, helpful or at least benign. For one thing, a literary eponym is an aid to memory. Second, it offers a creative relief from the sometimes

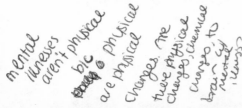

mental illnesses aren't physical b/c are physical are physical these physical changes are changes, chemical changes to brain by mental illness?

stifling neutrality of scientific language. Most important, it reminds us that diseases and disorders and science itself are part of a larger culture from which they take their ultimate meanings.

But a practical clinician, particularly one with interests in philosophy and ethics, needs to ask other questions of the literary eponym. Does it, for instance, truly clarify our understanding of the malady thus named? If when clinicians see a deformed patient, they conjure up the "Quasimodo Complex," do they then move quickly to awareness of the complicated psychosocial accompaniments of deformity, as discussed by Carey, and thereafter appropriate feelings of empathy for the patient? If they do, the literary eponym works well. But an eponym, as opposed to more scientific language, might also freeze the imagination by capturing it and focusing on it too narrowly. For instance, Hugo's Quasimodo was basically a gentle man. Even his violent anger, directed at the evil archdeacon, is seen as heroic. Carey's eponym draws on these qualities. Therefore, thinking Quasimodo Complex, while treating someone whose deformity may have pathologically scarred his mind, could subtly persuade clinicians to stop looking before the patient's real problems have emerged. Likewise, applying the Quasimodo Complex to someone who is really rather ordinary could lead to a misleading overuse of the concept. Clinicians also might even be guided by the terminology to expect too much of the patient. A literary medical eponym (such as "Ondine's Curse," to cite one from outside psychiatry) could induce an unwitting condescension towards the patient based upon our primitive feeling that to name something is to control it. In fact, it is possible that the Quasimodo Complex could prove every bit as deceptive in some instances as Freud's "narcissism"— itself a literary eponym of course—which Carey is at pains to warn us about. In short, those who believe that literary references will help clinicians to avoid scientific reductionism could run into a humanistic reductionism of a similarly worrisome kind.

LITERATURE'S UNIQUE CONTRIBUTION TO EMPATHY

Whatever the benefits or liabilities of the medical literary eponym, it is superficial compared with other claims by literature to clinical turf. Let me now go straight to the largest claim—that literature helps clinicians to develop empathy. To some extent, it too operates in Carey's essay. It begins with the often profound differences between the clinician and the patient. Please imagine two columns headed "we" for clinicians, and "they" for patients.

(The medical score can aptly be kept on something like a bridge tally.) First of all, we are relatively well, and they are sick. We are often young, or younger than they are, more moneyed, more likely to be Caucasian. They are sometimes conventionally unattractive, even deformed Quasimodos, whereas we can walk down the street with, in Erving Goffman's marvelous phrase, the benefit of strangers' "civil inattention."[2] Given these gaps in nature and experience, how are we to understand them? How are we to feel with them? In other words, how are we to develop empathy—that special blend of understanding and feeling that most people find necessary for fully competent medical care?

One of the traditional answers to these questions has been to draw from literature in all its forms—novels, poetry, drama, essays, and film. Different answers have been offered on behalf of the social sciences and the other humanities disciplines. We are told that we can develop empathy by reading psychological, sociological, and economic data about patients. We are urged to read about patients' faith systems and see how attitudes toward illness have changed through time. And these answers are good ones. The humanities and social sciences can provide us with some of the vicarious data we must have to supplement our own lived experience. Literature's unique contribution arises because it is free, within certain conventions, to take data from a wide range of sources and shape them imaginatively according to literary needs. Literature, for instance, can reveal the inner world of a patient's illness, as psychology and religious studies can, while simultaneously portraying society's values about that illness, as sociology or history do. It is true that when compared to other disciplines, literature's methods are indirect. But it is the contention of some people that since indirection demands the involvement of readers, literary methods release readers' own creativity to work on the situation at hand.

There is not a clinical subject, broadly conceived, that has not been investigated by literary writers.[3] Put more practically, no clinician can get through a day without running into several situations that have been "treated" in literature. Carey's references to deformity in literature, for instance, only skim the surface, as I'm sure this well-read man knows. Indeed, Quasimodo—whom some now think a victim of neurofibromatosis—has been resurrected for contemporary audiences in the play, the movie, and several books about John Merrick, the "Elephant Man." Furthermore, for almost every medical subject, there are helpful interpretations by literary critics of the relevant literature. For instance, on the subject of deformity, Leslie Fiedler's brilliant

Freaks comes to mind.[4] Saint Paul's "thorn in the flesh" was possibly epilepsy, as Carey notes. Here, too, literature offers abundant information. Some of the finest examples are from Fyodor Dostoevsky. His temporal lobe epilepsy inspired him to create several characters with seizures. *The Idiot, The Brothers Karamazov,* and other pieces by the man—who is arguably the world's greatest novelist—contain extraordinary instances of Carey's Quasimodo Complex. Do neurologists read Dostoevsky? They should. For that matter, do surgeons read Walt Whitman? Or nurses, Patrick White's *The Eye of the Storm?*[5]

But literature does much more than convey information, and herein lies its vast difference from other sources of knowledge. Literature embodies information in human form. It lures us. It enchants us. It tells a story, and almost everyone loves a good story. Literature has tremendous power to awaken us to the humanity of others. We may even identify with them so that the distance between "them" and "us," as discussed earlier, is suddenly unimportant. Properly produced and optimally read, literature can touch our hearts at the same time that it clears our heads. It can create such a compelling clarity of being that many people seek it as an end in itself.

PUTTING EMPATHY TO WORK

"That's all very well," I hear some busy clinicians saying. "That's all very pretty, but it has never been satisfactorily proven under exacting conditions." This is true. Moreover, so many words have been proclaimed on the ability of literature to make life better that some of us in the literary professions find ourselves wishing that the soapbox would be dismantled. Certainly, most of us can point to some very nasty people whose study of literature appears to have improved their minds while leaving their behavior completely unaltered.

So the working question for the health professions must be this: how can we increase the odds that literary information will lead to more effective patient care?

First, speaking generally, there have been attempts to demonstrate that after studying certain works of literature, readers have been changed for the better. But, to me, these experiments have been inconclusive in that the participants inevitably report their own perceptions or experiences rather than having others observe their behavior. Of course, such observation has its own problems, and perhaps no satisfactory study can be designed at this time. There is, in addition, a large body of reports from individuals about their own literary salvation. John Stuart Mill, for one, gives an account in the *Autobiography* of his transformation through literature from alienated depressive to mature philosopher.[6] And countless numbers of more ordinary people have apparently changed aspects of their behavior as a response to literature and film.

In a sense, the challenge to make literature operative in health care is easier than in the world at large. I can imagine a pediatrician who specializes in infectious diseases sitting down at home one night to read Camus's inspiring novel, *The Plague*. The next day she comes in to treat her AIDS patients. She should have little trouble putting the novel's insights to work. It may be that the physician behaves more selflessly, in the manner of Dr. Rieux. Perhaps she spends the day honing her own ideas about the suffering of innocent children against the ideas of Father Panaloux. It is quite likely that she sees in the reactions of people around her parallels to the ways in which Camus's plague took on metaphorical significance for an entire society.

In medicine we have constantly before us a second text, the suffering patient—whom the psychologist Anton Boisen called a "living human document"—that demands comparison with the literary text. The task for literarily sophisticated clinicians, then, is to go from the clinical text to the literary text and back again to the first, checking the data of one against the other. It is not necessary for the clinicians always to match a particular work of literature with a particular patient. (Realistically, the Camus-AIDS example cannot be reproduced on a regular basis.) It is essential only that they continue to develop an awareness of the human condition through literature while simultaneously seeing counterparts in everyday life. Their consequent behavioral change toward patients is related to their literary thinking in much the same way that, in psychoanalytically influenced therapy, "working through" follows insight. When we medical educators ask students to read Leo Tolstoy's *The Death of Ivan Ilych* and afterwards send them to talk to patients with terminal cancer and their families, we are initiating this dual-text process. We hope that it will form the basis for patterns of learning and behavior throughout the students' future careers.[7]

As effective as this individual learning may be, I believe that it is far less predictable than that which occurs in groups. I do not wish to deny that literary bonding occurs primarily between one author and one reader. Nor am I saying that a teacher's presence is essential for a work of literature to be properly understood. That would be suspiciously self-indulgent. What I am suggesting is that when a group of people interpret a piece of literature together—when they work out their responses in trial-and-error, in debate with their peers, and sometimes in concert with them—then the chance of that literature changing their behavior toward patients is greatly enhanced.

I have observed this process over many years. Medical students who sign up for a course on aging, for instance, or—to return to Carey's concern—handicaps, frequently state at the beginning that they are there for negative reasons. That is, young, able-bodied medical students know that they are ignorant about these patients and slightly afraid of them as well. Observing those same students on the clinical floors later in their training, I have seen a degree of comfort with aging and handicapped patients that I would not have expected earlier. This growth seems to be partly an effect of a group of students advancing to the clinical years together after sharing a common experience with literature. Those of us working in humanistic medical education have a great deal of work to do in regularizing these changes, not only for students but for other health professionals.

We may find some help in Carol Bly's introduction to a recently published anthology of short stories about aging people.[8] She, too, is concerned about how the stories, as splendid as most of them are, can actually affect caregivers in the real world. She is charmingly sassy about what literature can and cannot do in directly contributing to the help of people in trouble. Bly asserts that literature

> points out victims, gives us some clear images of their sufferings, and leaves us with either of two responses: if we are sensitive, we feel shamed and a little blamed. If we are insensitive . . . we pause in our constant attending to our own affairs long enough to feel a little ethical flutter, a little *frisson*—and that's all.[9]

The problem is, Bly continues, shaming and blaming doesn't work. So she suggests that literary people learn about the antistereotyping workshops at Cambridge Hospital under the sponsorship of Harvard Medical School, wherein the goal of the group process is to "halt inaccurate abstraction and subjective inference."[10] I have no idea how this workshop accomplishes its goals, but Bly's passing comments seem linked to my own thoughts about the necessity of adding a group process, or at least an understanding of how people change, to the study of literature and medicine. I can imagine that in the case of aging and handicapped people, formalized practice in avoiding inaccurate abstraction could work very well as a bridge between the insights of literature and the treatment of patients. Perhaps the work of the perceptual psychologists about how people make closures could be brought to our assistance. Whatever we do, thanks to Bly, we now have a memorable image of what literature in medicine should not be. It should not under any circumstances be consigned to morally titillating entertainment that provides "little ethical flutters."[11]

AN ALTERNATIVE LITERARY FORM FOR ETHICISTS

Fortunately, there is yet another method for avoiding these lonely palpitations. But here I must leave Carey's interesting paper behind in order to speak directly to the daily concerns of clinical ethicists. I would like ethicists to consider the benefits of literary form apart from content. I realize that they have already settled on a kind of literary form for their work in that the case study is an adaptation of narrative. I suggest that it is not narrative—but drama—that is the ethicist's natural ally.

This is because the essence of a bioethical decision is conflict. Where there is no true conflict, there is no issue. There is only conversation. Likewise, all traditional drama as derived from the ancient Greeks exists for the purpose of elucidating conflict. Conventionally, a hero, or protagonist, pits himself against another person, an antagonist, or perhaps against a force of nature or society. In Sophocles' *Antigone,* for instance, the heroine's values of duty to family and religion are in mortal conflict with the values of the political ruler, Creon, whose first duty is to maintain the stability of the state. As is true in most first-rate dramas, opposing values are given nearly equal weight. In this case, Creon is heard almost as clearly as Antigone, and the whole is an excellent arena in which to play out the timeless conflict of individual rights versus the community's. Readers of the play are able to judge the persuasiveness of each character's arguments in view of Greek norms as well as today's. Nowhere does Sophocles raise a bioethical issue. Yet ethicists who choose to study this play will be practicing their clinical skills as they trace the arguments of the main characters and of affected family members, set those arguments into various systems of justice, disentangle the emotional from the logical strands, and finally make their own statements about the matter at hand.

Ethicists could make equally good use of George Bernard Shaw's *The Doctor's Dilemma.* Here the conflict is overtly bioethical. The question is whom shall the central character, Dr. Ridgeon, treat with his limited but life-saving clinical resources? Should he choose his kind and aging colleague, whose medical career has been undistinguished, or the deeply talented but morally irresponsible young artist? The interesting aspect of this drama is that in its preface, Shaw, writing as social philosopher, complacently asserts that "the man who costs more than he is worth is doomed by sound hygiene as inexorably as by sound economics."[12] But once Shaw the playwright is underway, his pristine ethical pronouncements become entangled with dramatic, emotional, and altogether human considerations that make the ultimate ethical decision far more complicated.

Sophocles and Shaw are both philosophical writers, but any fine traditional drama would serve the ends of clinical ethicists, even where the play is fueled primarily by emotions rather than ideas. It might be preferable, in fact, for ethicists to sharpen their minds amidst passionate emotions that more nearly approximate the muddle into which they are sometimes thrown by clinical realities. Anton Chekhov's masterpiece, *The Three Sisters*, would serve very well. Most people find Chekhov more difficult than Shaw. In Chekhov's play the conflict lies within human nature. In this case, the sisters' provincial inertia conflicts with the yearning of their idealized selves to escape from their increasingly depressing circumstances. Like the runner who practices with heavy boots and then wins the race in his light shoes, medical ethicists who understand the decisions—and, just as important, the absence of decisions—in Chekhov may have less trouble with the simpler matters presented to them clinically.

In addition to conflict, other components of drama may speak directly to ethicists' needs. I am thinking of such matters as role, dialogue, audience interaction, and point of view. For instance, drama can remind ethicists that they too are playing roles in which they have been cast by society. Clinical ethicists may even be in costumes, usually white ones. Their ethical advice may sound something like a play's "set pieces." Certainly they have lines that they regularly repeat in a given situation. And who, one might ask, is the playwright? That is not a frivolous or figurative question. Who has created the language for the ethicists? Are they their own script writers, or have their roles been written for them by their tradition, medical training, and philosophical studies? Are they playing their roles as method actors do—that is, by becoming fully involved in them? Or are they, like English actors, simply using various practiced techniques while all the time keeping their real selves as invulnerable as possible?

Drama also serves clinical ethicists by demonstrating the intimate relationship between the meaning of a play and the reaction of an audience on any given day. After all, a play is not merely the words written on the page any more than an ethical decision consists solely of the language in which it is expressed. A play changes with each audience. As audience members respond to what they are able to hear that day, the actors in turn change their emphases. Thus, drama is constantly reinventing itself in response to the needs of its collaborators. What it gives up in terms of perfection, it gains in terms of humanity. Ethical arguments are unstable in just this way. The same ethical argument will be interpreted differently in various quarters, and the responses of those whom the decision will affect may, and perhaps should, modify the ultimate resolution of the conflict.

One of a clinical ethicist's most useful skills is the ability to hear fully. Put in dramatic terms, it is necessary for an ethicist to be able to follow a dialogue, delineate roles, and understand from what point of view a person is speaking. Words alone are meaningless in drama, as in life, without their personal context. I have frequently heard people quote Polonius's advice to Laertes, "To thine own self be true," as though the words represented Shakespeare's own values, and his most mature, at that. In the context of *Hamlet,* however, Polonius is something of a blathering, self-serving old fool who fails to see what is going on around him, let alone what is of lasting importance. In short, for an ethicist to give proper weight to someone's expressed judgment, it is essential to analyze it in the light of that person's character and perspective.

In the middle of clinical pressures, such analysis is not always easy. The study of drama allows the clinician to step back from the tactical tensions of practice to hone these strategic skills. So does the case study, whose strengths and limits are well-known to readers of this journal. I am merely making a claim for drama as an interesting alternative and—in this commentary as a whole—for literature as a healing art.

NOTES

1. A. E. Rodin and J. D. Key, *Medicine, Literature and Eponyms* (Malabar, Fla.: Robert E. Krieger Publishing, 1989).

2. E. Goffman, *Behavior in Public Places* (New York: Free Press of Glencoe, 1963), 84.

3. See J. Trautmann and C. Pollard, *Literature and Medicine: An Annotated Bibliography,* rev. ed. (Pittsburgh: University of Pittsburgh Press, 1982), which includes over 1,400 entries on 39 medical topics.

4. L. Fiedler, *Freaks: Myths and Images of the Secret Self* (New York: Simon and Schuster, 1978).

5. P. White, *The Eye of the Storm* (New York: Viking Press, 1974).

6. A. Belli discusses the Mill instance and others in "The Impact of Literature Upon Health: Some Varieties of Cathartic Response," *Literature and Medicine* 5 (1986): 90–108.

7. Nothing about this process will surprise medical ethicists or indeed medical educators generally. Their universal challenge is how to take theoretical material (in ethics and in science) and turn it not only into practical, clinical information, but also into daily behavior that will then be regularly revised on the basis of new insights.

8. C. Bly, "Foreword," in *Full Measure: Modern Short Stories on Aging,* ed. D. Sennett (St. Paul: Graywolf Press, 1988), xix.

9. Ibid.

10. Ibid.

11. Ibid.

12. G. B. Shaw, "Preface on Doctors," in *The Doctor's Dilemma* (1913; reprint, Baltimore: Penguin Books, 1954), 87.

Quasimodo and Medicine:

What Role for the Clinician in Treating Deformity?

RONALD P. STRAUSS

THE SOCIAL EFFECTS OF APPEARANCE

JONATHAN SINCLAIR CAREY's paper reconsiders physical deformity by examining literature and history for examples of how physical differences affect identity. The relationship between appearance, social stereotyping, and expectations has been established as one of the most consistent and robust research findings in social science.[1] Deviant appearance, especially facial appearance, is readily noticeable and central. Research indicates that attractiveness has an important effect on psychological development and social relationships.[2]

The bodily signs of being different, known as stigma, carry a moral evaluation—usually a negative one. Goffman's classic work, *Stigma*,[3] has provided a theory of stigmatization and handicap that is useful in understanding the social responses to human difference and health conditions.[4] Persons may be seen as deviant when judged by cosmetic norms or when judged with prejudices about the cause and impacts of congenital conditions.[5] Further, myths, fiction, and legends reveal a cross-culturally shared distress with difference.[6] The "beauty is good" hypothesis has been confirmed across age, race, and varying situations.[7]

By the age of seven, children are able to differentiate between attractive and unattractive children, and to use consistent judgments about attractiveness.[8] Nurses, parents, schoolteachers, and peers rate the attractive infant, child, and adult more positively—nicer, more cooperative, more likable, and better adjusted[9]—and attractive individuals also receive preferential treatment or more attention from caretakers.[10] Appearance has been known to affect school,[11] legal proceedings,[12] hiring and promotion,[13] and psychotherapeutic prognosis.[14]

CLINICAL OBSERVATIONS ABOUT DEFORMITY

As a social scientist–clinician on a facial birth defects treatment team, I have an opportunity to observe how people may respond to deformities. I have been struck with the finding that people with significant deformities often hold the same beliefs about identity as do those with normal appearance. Like others, they feel as though they deserve a "fair break," but they are aware that they are not accepted and that others do not meet them on an "equal ground." This awareness may generalize into feelings of being inadequate or incomplete, or of having failed. In extreme cases, shame and self-derogation may occur, and the person may perceive himself as contaminated.

Perhaps the most surprising observation is that people with severe deformities may be less psychosocially impaired and more resigned to their lives than those with minor defects. One might speculate that persons with obvious and uncorrectable deformities must learn to live with them and accept their appearance. For some persons the defect may be discussed as a blessing in disguise or as a learning experience. Some indicate that by learning through suffering, they experience a deepened awareness of others and develop skills in finding happiness within themselves. Such comments seem to generally reflect self-reliance and not self-pity.

For some people with deformities there is great uncertainty in social interaction. They can never be sure what a new acquaintance will perceive, and each new encounter causes worry about whether they will be accepted or rejected. People with deformities often seem to worry before the initiation of a new social contact. They may develop strategies to allow others to see them from a distance before a conversation begins, thus permitting some time for adjusting to the deformity. Uncertainty may occur in other contexts, as well. Some people with defects say they can never be sure that others will show or tell them what they are *really* thinking about them. People with speech defects, for example, report that others pretend to understand them. The person with the defect may be fully aware of his limited intelligibility and may actually know that the listener really does not understand. The pretense that all is normal may undermine social interaction and make encounters quite uncertain.

Goffman has described how people with stigmas may "break through," by developing special ways to move past initial tactfulness and distance. Such persons may try to move beyond a superficial interaction in order to get

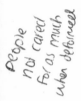

beyond the social reaction to their appearance. Some people with deformities will choose to normalize daily interactions by making what is called "rounds," in which they see the same people and do the same things on a daily basis, so as to elicit predictable reactions.

Uncertainty about social interactions and identity may remain after a defect is corrected by medical means. For persons with invisible or well-repaired defects, there may be the constant worry of discovery. They fear that once their "secret" is discovered, others will relate to them through their deformity as a plight. Where surgical repair of a deformity is possible, what often results is not a fully normal identity, but rather a transformation of the self from someone with a particular blemish into someone with a record of having a corrected blemish.

The stigma and self-perception may not change with a repair. For years the deformity may have been looked upon as a handicap and its importance in social and emotional adjustment may have been global. For some, the deformity is the easiest explanation for all insecurities, inadequacies, dissatisfactions, and unpleasant aspects of social life. The deformity may become a protection from social responsibility and an escape from competition. Surgical repair that is effective may leave the person adrift without the emotional protection or hiding place that the defect once provided. With discomfort and surprise, the person with a corrected defect may discover that life is not easy even for those with ordinary appearance. Sometimes the handicap provides a special status and a shelter from which to cope with life; its removal may cause anxiety and behavioral problems. Clinicians who anticipate the impact of repairing a deformity can help their patients through a possibly difficult, but promising, transition.

APPEARANCE CHANGE AND SOCIAL CHANGES

Discrimination and stigmatization have historically characterized social responses to deformities and physical handicaps. In the extreme, infants who were very unusual were denied nutrition or care, resulting in infanticide. Though the killing of deviant children is illegal in most of the developed world, infanticide or selective neglect is still practiced in a hidden fashion in a number of societies. Often infanticide has been explained by a society's limited ability to feed or care for less than perfect children. In developed modern societies, such resource limitations rarely exist and defective children generally survive and are provided for. The rise of modern medicine and surgery has raised the possibility that deformed or handicapped persons might be offered treatment to improve their situations. The desire to provide treatment and remediation associated with medical activism is characteristic of how Western societies respond to children with birth defects.

Humanists have sometimes criticized society's high value on attractiveness and the degree to which appearance influences opportunity. Advocates of active approaches to remediation of appearance argue that social values are difficult to change and that each person must adapt to the existent cultural context and stereotypes.[15] Health educational interventions in school settings have been shown to alter attitudes on a short-term basis,[16] but pervasive advertising and mass media images continue to bolster the desirability of physical attractiveness.

The surgical improvement of facial appearance has been shown to change social perceptions. One study of photographs, before and after plastic surgery, revealed that observers uniformly found postoperative views to be more attractive, kinder, and more sexually appealing than the preoperative views.[17] Facial surgery has often been used to alter social experience. Reports of the use of rhinoplasty in Jewish patients[18] suggest that people may often strive to accommodate social norms rather than to struggle against discrimination or stigmatization. Naturally, surgery cannot change ethnic origins, nor can it alter the fact of Down's syndrome, but it might enhance social integration and improve self-concept. Surgery and other treatment modalities may create possibilities for growth and change.

Let us take, for example, the case of Down's syndrome and facial plastic surgery. Facial plastic surgery for individuals with Down's syndrome may be recommended along with a number of other possible interventions, in order to enhance the quality of life and to improve opportunities for such persons to be contributing, rather than isolated and marginal, members of society.

The Active Modification approach[19] for the person with Down's syndrome employs a coordinated series of cognitive, behavioral, vocational, speech, medical, and surgical interventions directed toward enhancing the individual's potential. The totality of therapeutic options, including surgery, may be combined into a plan that counters the passive acceptance of the child. The activism directed toward persons with Down's syndrome represents optimism that some deficiencies are changeable or reversible.

One study of social perceptions of the effects of facial surgery for persons with Down's syndrome[20] was designed to examine how public school children (not with Down's syndrome) perceived the faces of nine children with Down's syndrome, eight of whom had facial surgical treatment. This study examined how 277 Israeli school children evaluated these faces and compared ratings of social perceptions of control (without Down's syndrome) faces to the faces of children with Down's syndrome. The basic findings were that children with Down's syndrome were seen as less attractive, intelligent, good-hearted, and socially appealing, than were control children. Though respondents were unaware of the diagnosis or the use of surgery, they did rate children who had facial surgery for Down's syndrome as slightly, but significantly, improved as a group, over their presurgical ratings on all four of the social dimensions. Perhaps most interesting was the finding that in children who appreciated a postoperative improvement in appearance ratings, there was a corresponding linear increase in intelligence ratings offered to them by nonaffected school children. Such findings raise the possibility that surgical alterations in facial appearance may result in improved social and educational opportunity. This study suggests that there are nonapparent social effects of surgery for persons with deformities.

If social effects are demonstrated for surgical approaches to appearance change, why would a clinician not be active in his medical interventions? Why not allow people with deformities, such as those found in Down's syndrome, to have ordinary appearances, if that is possible? If we permit children with minor physical deviances to have orthodontic treatment, why should this be denied to those with more severe defects? The search for aesthetic change is based on the hope that appearance may in part create opportunities for other changes.

Medical Activism and Roles for Clinicians

The control of medical activism and professional power are issues that arise in the treatment of persons with deformities. Being able to medically or surgically treat a condition may alter the social expectations and responses to persons who possess a deviant attribute. Let us look at the treatment of facial deformities. The availability of plastic surgery, facial reconstruction, and orthodontic care have changed American attitudes towards facial appearance. The advent of maxillofacial and craniofacial surgery has made it technically possible to move parts of the face and jaws and to remake faces so that they are more attractive. The possibility of restoring the face has made an unrestored face less acceptable. For example, what was acceptably "bucktoothed" in the 1950s has now become a "dentofacial deformity," and is treated with surgery and orthodontics. Several questions can be asked. Has the advent of new surgery reawakened concerns in persons who had accepted their appearance? Do peers and others interacting with such persons find discomfort in a decision not to correct a deformity that might be altered? What are the legitimate goals of facial surgery? Should surgeons be charged with the social role of remediating frank deformity or should they strive to create acceptable, or even beautiful, faces? What does the desire to "fix" faces say about the acceptance of difference or variance in appearance? Is this society capable of integrating people with deviant characteristics into community life?

American society has chosen to deal with deformity as an illness in a medical context. Indeed, even Carey's paper coins the term "Quasimodo Complex" as though deformity is a psychiatric diagnosis. Medical responses, however, are rarely only directed toward classification; rather, they are directed toward amelioration. Medicine has worked toward covering up or repairing deformity, and plastic surgery has been used as a tool to control human differences. This activism occurs within a health-care marketplace in which the clinician manages or responds to the demand for his or her services. The decision to physically rehabilitate occurs in response to social, economic, and medical forces. Factors that influence the decision are: family and individual demand for services; the desire to prevent people from becoming unproductive or dependent on the social welfare system; financial gain to the provider, hospital, or institution; and a perceived mandate to protect the aesthetic standards of the culture.

Seeing cosmetic surgery as a luxury service, denying it public funds, or ensuring that surgeons are a scarce resource to be carefully allocated, are all steps that would serve to limit public access to such care. Currently, in the realm of treatment for deformity, control over intervention is largely in the hands of the medical and dental professions and their patients. Because medical treatment of this nature is now often covered by health insurance or public welfare programs, the market of potential patients has increased. What once may have been a luxury is now accessible to a wider segment of Americans. As a consequence, the medical profession can control access to cosmetic changes of a surgical nature. The decision whether and on whom to perform surgery is a crucial "gate-keeper" function for the medical profession, especially since physicians have the unusual capacity to develop and manage their own market.

This situation calls upon the profession to regulate itself and to perform surgery only when it is absolutely necessary. Learning when surgical intervention is not necessary becomes very important, for a decision not to operate often implies normalcy. A statement from a surgeon that "this is not serious enough to operate on" may be seen as a guarantee of physical acceptability. In the case of multiple rehabilitative plastic surgical procedures, the surgeon's statement that "there is no more that I can do" permits the patient and family to adapt to limitation and residual disfigurement.

One of the dangers of placing normalization within the medical context is the propensity of well-socialized physicians to intervene whenever requested. Eagerness to perform surgery has caused a great deal of criticism of the medical profession. The basic mode of surgical decision making remains largely the same; the surgeon determines criteria and decides on whom he will operate. Such a physician-based, gate-keeping mechanism is currently undergoing a challenge by insurance carriers and public agencies that fund and scrutinize health care. The use of second opinions and certificates of need point to institutional constraints on who receives elective surgical care. Public welfare and third-party funding agencies may raise the very real questions of "when is a difference a defect?" or "when is it reasonable for a society to bear the burden of providing an operation?" Both questions imply a growing interest in determining surgical need and monitoring surgical endeavors.

The interest in surgical activities from outside the medical profession may signal increasing nonprofessional control over treatment activism. This interest rises from an appreciation that society has limited its ability to set health and social policy, in deference to the medical profession. This change comes at a time when increasing numbers of people are coming to understand the limitations on science's ability to make ethical and value-based judgments for the society. Decisions about medical and scientific activism and about norms (including aesthetic norms) will require input from a variety of sources, including spiritual, economic, and political viewpoints, in order to ensure that moral and equitable choices are made. While fleshly perfection remains unlikely, one wonders how Quasimodo would have fared in the care of contemporary medicine.

The potential for cosmetic and reconstructive surgery to alleviate human suffering is great, yet the endeavor itself has a number of inherent difficulties. Cautious and thoughtful decision making and resource allocation are necessary to avoid the extremes of medical activism or the appeal of normalization. In the process of treating facial disfigurement, one grapples with the basic question of how a society deals with differences. Decisions about whether to integrate, to alter, or to reject differences are political, moral, and ethical choices.

NOTES

1. J. H. Langlois, L. A. Roggman, R. J. Casey, et al., "Infant Preferences for Attractive Faces: Rudiments of a Stereotype?" *Developmental Psychology* 23 (May 1987):363–69.

2. E. Bersheid, "Overview of the Psychological Effects of Physical Attractiveness," in *Psychological Aspects of Facial Form*, ed. G. W. Lucker, K. A. Ribbens, and J. A. McNamara, *Craniofacial Growth Series*, monograph no. 11 (Ann Arbor: Center for Human Growth and Development, 1980), 1–23.

3. E. Goffman, *Stigma: Notes on the Management of Spoiled Identity* (Englewood Cliffs, N.J.: Prentice-Hall, 1963).

4. J. Ablon, "Stigmatized Health Conditions," *Social Science and Medicine* 15B (January 1981): 5–9.

5. F. C. Macgregor, *Transformation and Identity—The Face and Plastic Surgery* (New York: Quadrangle/New York Times, 1974).

6. W. C. Shaw, "Folklore Surrounding Facial Deformity and the Origins of Facial Prejudice," *British Journal of Plastic Surgery* 34 (July 1981): 237–46.

7. M. R. Cunningham, "Measuring the Physical in Physical Attractiveness," *Journal of Personal and Social Psychology* 50, no. 5 (1986): 925–35; and R. P. Strauss, "Culture, Rehabilitation and Facial Birth Defects: International Case Studies," *Cleft Palate Journal* 22 (January 1985): 56–62.

8. J. P. Cross and J. Cross, "Age, Sex, Race and the Perception of Physical Beauty," *Developmental Psychology* 5 (July 1971): 433–39; and C. K. Sigelman, T. E. Miller, and L. A. Whitworth, "The Early Stigmatizing Reactions to Physical Differences," *Journal of Applied Developmental Psychology* 7 (January–March 1986): 17–32.

9. G. R. Adams and P. Crane, "An Assessment of Parents' and Teachers' Expectations of Pre-school Children's Social Preference for Attractive or Unattractive Children and Adults," *Child Development* 51 (March 1980): 224–31; D. Byrne, *The Attraction Paradigm* (New York: Academic Press, 1971); K. Minde, S. Trehub, C. Corter, et al., "Infant Attractiveness and the Infant-Caretaker Relationship," *Pediatrics* 61 (March 1978): 373–79; C. Corter, S. Trehub, C. Boukydis, et al., "Nurses' Judgments of the Attractiveness of Premature Infants," *Infant Behavior and Development* 1 (November 1978): 373–80; and S. A. Nida and J. E. Williams, "Sex Stereotyped Traits, Physical Attractiveness and Interpersonal Attraction," *Psychological Reports* 41 (June 1977): 1311–22.

10. G. R. Adams and J. C. LaVoie, "Teacher Expectations: A Review of the Student Characteristics Used in Expectancy Formation," *Journal of Instructional Psychology Monographs* 4 (January 1977): 1–28.

11. M. Clifford and E. Walster, "Research Note: The Effect of Physical Attractiveness on Teacher Expectations," *Sociology of Education* 46 (Spring 1973): 248–58; and L. C. Richmond, "The Effects of Facial Disfigurement on Teachers' Perception of Ability in Cleft Palate Children," *Cleft Palate Journal* 15 (April 1978): 155–60.

12. H. Sigall and N. Ostrove, "Beautiful But Dangerous: Effects of Offender Attractiveness and Nature of the Crime on Juridic Judgement," *Journal of Personality and Social Psychology* 31 (March 1975): 410–14.

13. R. L. Dipboye, H. L. Fromkin, and K. Wiback, "Relative Importance of Applicant Sex, Attractiveness, and Scholastic Standing in Evaluation of Job Applicant Resumes," *Journal of*

Applied Psychology 60 (February 1975): 39–43; J. Scheuerle, A. M. Guilford, and S. Garcia, "Employee Bias Associated with Cleft Lip/Palate," *Journal of Applied Rehabilitation Counseling* 13 (January 1982): 6–8; and D. Landy and H. Sigall, "Beauty is Talent: Task Evaluation as a Function of the Performer's Physical Attractiveness," *Journal of Personal and Social Psychology* 29 (March 1974): 299–304.

14. R. Barocas and F. L. Vance, "Referral Rate and Physical Attractiveness in Third-Grade Children," *Perceptual and Motor Skills* 10 (September 1974): 731–34.

15. R. P. Strauss, "Ethical and Social Concerns in Facial Surgical Decision Making," *Plastic and Reconstructive Surgery* 72 (November 1983): 727–30.

16. E. M. Arndt, A. M. Lefebvre, P. Klaiman, and J. C. Posnick, "The Impact of Two Educational Programs on Normal High School Students' Impressions of Those with Craniofacial Anomalies," paper presented at the meeting of the American Cleft Palate Association, Williamsburg, Va., April 1988.

17. E. Bersheid and S. Gangestad, "The Social Psychological Implications of Facial Physical Attractiveness," *Clinics in Plastic Surgery* 9 (July 1982): 289–96.

18. F. C. Macgregor, "Social and Cultural Components in the Motivations of Persons Seeking Plastic Surgery of the Nose," *Journal of Health and Social Behavior* 8 (June 1967): 125–35.

19. R. Feuerstein, Y. Rand, M. Hoffman, and R. Miller, "Cognitive Modifiability in Retarded Adolescents: Effects of Instrumental Enrichment," *American Journal of Mental Deficiency* 83 (May 1979): 539–50; and R. Feuerstein, Y. Rand, M. Hoffman, and R. Miller, *Instrumental Enrichment* (Baltimore: University Park Press, 1980).

20. R. P. Strauss, Y. Mintzker, R. Feuerstein, et al., "Social Perceptions of the Effects of Down's Syndrome Facial Surgery: A School-Based Study of Ratings by Normal Adolescents," *Plastic and Reconstructive Surgery* 81 (June 1988): 841–46.

Deformity and the Humane Ideal of Medicine

Robert M. Goldwyn

With erudition and sensitivity, Jonathan Sinclair Carey has described the multiple misfortunes of those who are grossly deformed. Some, literally, are born to suffer, to bear the onus of a major disfigurement, and to experience humiliation, isolation, and alienation. With plastic surgery as well as with the benefits of other medical and surgical specialties, and with the warmth of support groups, many of these unfortunate persons may become active, productive participants in society. Yet very few individuals with visible, severe malformations will ever blend into society. They will always be considered "special"; children may taunt or avoid them, and later peers may reward them less because of their ability than because of the guilt and pity they have aroused in others.

Deformity, if uncorrected and not hidden, is relentless and ubiquitous. Its bearer can neither shed it nor flee it. A few patients have revealed that some of their happiest moments are in dreams when they and others see themselves as normal, free of fate's injustice.

The Quasimodos of the world certainly do not want to be stoned or scorned; they would like more than to be merely tolerated, however. They want acceptance as total human beings. They hope that if others reject them, it will not be on the basis of their physical afflictions, over which they have no control. For some, a trip to the supermarket demands as much courage as did Stanley's expedition to Africa. While most people, except children, will refrain from pointing at them or making hurtful remarks, the individual with the Quasimodo deformity will note people's instinctive facial and body reactions, which betray their surprise and often their revulsion. Indeed, no society can ignore the spectacularly malformed.

Throughout the recorded life of man, various cultures have dealt with these people differently: murder (infanticide), ostracism, deification (a form of isolation that also prevented their reproducing), and grudging acceptance.

The last is most commonly practiced in technically advanced societies, such as ours. To my knowledge, no cultures have accepted a Quasimodo as a "normal" person. Reconstructive surgery has the objective not only of helping an abnormal individual achieve a kind of normalcy, but of ridding, if possible, society of a visible, uncomfortable exception.

Health-care professionals should realize that the first objective in treatment is to accept a patient—to make him or her feel comfortable, to establish a relationship based on understanding and empathy first, and competence later. With a patient who has a significant deformity, it is untruthful and unwise to minimize it. If a physician or nurse, for example, makes light of the patient's problem, he receives the opposite message—the true one—that his disfigurement is so massive that even those supposedly trained to accept it cannot.

Thus far, I, like Carey, have emphasized the overwhelming psychological problems that accompany gross deformity. The fact is, however, that many whom one would expect to be psychological cripples are not. Experts have observed that craniofacially deformed children are usually well-integrated into their families, and often fail to realize the extent of their problem. With age, however, comes the comprehension of their aberration, as they venture outside the home. That is why it is advisable to correct the deformity as much as possible, as soon as possible—before self-esteem is injured or shattered forever. The final anatomic result will also be better.

In studying children with clefts, Lansdown, a clinical psychologist, recently wrote:

> There is really no evidence of overt maladjustment among such children . . . [but] it is a mistake to think that children who do not display overt disturbance or are not maladjusted in a rating scale are perfectly happy. . . . Any kind of facial deformity is likely to lead to an increased psychological strain . . . life is just that little bit harder. . . . But we are not going to find ourselves surrounded by children who are neurotic, aggressive bullies or delinquent.[1]

Lansdown was writing of children with cleft lip and palate. One might imagine that those with grosser deformities, obvious even after multiple reconstructive procedures, might fare less well. While that is generally true, one is regularly surprised by the relative outward emotional stability of these individuals who may inwardly feel far from joyous.

At some point, the person with a congenital deformity, or the parents, will ask about the chances of reproducing that deformity in offspring. Referral to a knowledgeable expert, usually a geneticist, for information and advice is mandatory. The patient or the parents may predicate the rest of their lives on the answer.

Vulcan, whom Carey mentioned as having fathered the deformed Ericthonius, was also deformed; he was lame. Vulcan compensated for his handicap by becoming the supreme artist. Those of us who treat patients with congenital or acquired deformities see numerous examples of this compensatory behavior: the little boy who has but one thumb and a single digit on one hand learning to play the piano like a virtuoso.

One should distinguish between deformity that is present from birth or developmental, and deformity that is acquired. While in both instances the deformity is not easy to accommodate, the person who suddenly suffers extensive facial malformation—for example, from an auto accident—may be devastated, at least, temporarily, by the abrupt change from normalcy to abnormality, from being singled out perhaps for good looks to being avoided because of ugliness. In these situations, the plastic surgeon and every physician, nurse, or medical worker concerned with the patient's care can influence enormously that individual's emotional, as well as physical recovery. Not only does this process require interest, skill and compassion, but it also demands time—much more time than some, unfortunately, are willing to give the patient. Too seldom we, who are normal in mind and body (or approximately so), ponder what it would be like to have fate change that which we have taken for granted. Many patients whom I have reconstructed after cancer ablation are ostensibly concerned more with their altered appearance than with their cancer prognosis. They are justifiably mindful of how they will live and relate to loved ones. They are concerned with the quality of their life and not just its length.

I would like to call attention to another category of deformity, one that many might not consider as such. I am referring to the aging process, a condition that leads to a person feeling unwanted and out of place. Many, maybe most, elderly people feel discarded by a society that idolizes youth, energy, athletics, thinness, and good looks—"good" to be synonymous with "youthful." One patient, a man in his eighties, complained, "I go to a store and the salesperson looks not at me—not at my face—but through me as if I didn't really exist, as if I really didn't count." The elderly are a distressing reminder to those younger that our fate will be the same. The disfigured are an unpleasant reminder of fate's capriciousness and cruelty, and of our human fragility and vulnerability.

Finally, I wish to register my concern that today, when the emphasis in our thinking about medical care is the "bottom line," perceived fiscal expediency might dictate an action that will overcome the traditional humane ideals of medicine. I fear that we might descend to the point of denying medical care to the disfigured. Already we are hearing talk of restricting access of care to the elderly. In our zeal to save money (to spend elsewhere, such as on munitions for maiming and killing), will we eliminate by inattention or design the deformed and the "tainted"? Carey has alluded to the kind of behavior that characterized the Third Reich. Human bestiality, however, is not purely a Nazi phenomenon. It has occurred before, is happening now, and will happen again. Those whom the majority in any culture consider different in a pejorative sense have seldom fared well. How society treats its disfigured is frequently a reliable index of its behavior in other spheres. The physically and emotionally less fortunate among us should represent not just a burden or a bother, but an opportunity to exert and reinforce our humanity.

NOTE

1. R. Lansdown, "Psychological Problems of Patients with Cleft Lip and Palate: Discussion Paper," *Journal of the Royal Society of Medicine* 83 (July 1990): 448.

From Shame and Body Image:
Culture and the Compulsive Eater

BARBARA McFARLAND, ED.D., AND TYEIS BAKER-BAUMANN, M.S.

GUILT AND SHAME: WHAT'S THE DIFFERENCE?

GUILT AND SHAME are often confused. Shame is more closely related to an inherent sense of the self being flawed or defective. It is linked to one's self-image. Karen Horney proposed a triple concept of the self: the actual self, derived from the sum total of our actual experiences; the real self, a force that lies dormant within us and can be reached if we establish a harmonious wholeness; and the ideal self, which Horney viewed as neurotic and the source of grandiose aspects of the self (*Neurosis and Human Growth,* 1950). The ideal self is based on feedback from others. The ideal self doesn't always have to be, as Horney says, neurotic, a negative factor in self-image. Actually when viewed in the context of healthy shame, it can be a motivating force to continue striving to reach our potential. Whenever we fall short of our ideal self-image, we may experience shame.

With guilt, we do not use an ideal image as a measure but rather we use ideal actions. Guilt results from actually having done something wrong. The behavior that activates guilt violates a moral or ethical code. Generally, people experience guilt when they have broken a rule or in some way violated their own beliefs or standards. Not accepting or carrying out responsibility can also activate guilt feelings. However, since guilt is associated with behaviors within a broad range of ethics and religion, the activators of guilt vary considerably from individual to individual, from culture to culture and ethnic group to ethnic group.

Guilt is activated in situations where the individual feels personally responsible as a result of his own acts or failure to act. Consequently, with guilt, restitution is possible. With shame, however, there is no restitution. With shame, it's not whether you have *done* anything bad, it's that you *are* bad.

The phenomenology of guilt stimulates a great deal of thought on the part of the person who experiences the guilt. That person not only spends a lot of mental energy preoccupied by the wrongdoing but also conjuring up schemes to make things right. Guilt is often followed by imageries of making amends, facing the person wronged, etc.

Shame, on the other hand, leaves a person speechless; it temporarily befuddles thinking. Shame is too difficult to tolerate so the individual tends to repress or deny the shaming experience. Since restitution is impossible, the individual's sense of self is deeply diminished and the self-image affected.

Another way of examining the differences between guilt and shame is to look at the difference in the meaning of the words "guiltless" and "shameless." Being guiltless is a desired state since it connotes innocence or freedom from blame. Being shameless, on the other hand, refers to a deficit in one's character. To be shameless is considered equal to having no sense of values or morals. . . .

SHAME AND BODY IMAGE

Just as everyone has a self-image and a sense of self-esteem so, too, we have a body image. Simply defined, body image is the mental representation or internal picture we have of our physical body, an inner view of our outer selves.

Body image, like self-esteem, can be positive and accurate or it can be negative, critical and vague. While built on our physical characteristics, it can remain quite independent of the reality of these characteristics. Since it is a product of our imagination, body image can easily be distorted. In spite of its changeability, for body image may be in a state of frequent flux, it *feels* very real and can be a source of pride or a source of great pain and dissatisfaction.[1]

Body image is very vulnerable to outside feedback. A flirtatious whistle can make us smile with pride while a critical comment or judgmental facial expression about our weight or body size from a significant person can make us cringe in shame.

BODY IMAGE AND PHYSICAL DEVELOPMENT

Most of us do not have an accurate image of our body. This is due to the fact that we learn about our bodies in a haphazard manner, partly because of the nature of physiological development and partly because it is impossible to see all dimensions of our bodies without the aid of several mirrors.[2]

James O. Lugo and Gerald L. Hershey in their text, *Human Development,* state, "The body is the single most significant avenue for expression of the child's total self. . . . Children actually construct varying physical self-images depending on their stage of development. The total of these self-images includes both ideal images of what could be and realistic images based on past experiences. Together, these images make up an integrated physical self-concept, which is but one component of the total self-concept."[3]

Human beings and the human body are perpetually changing and growing in the physical, emotional and cognitive realms. These three realms are continuously interrelating and influencing each other. For the purposes of our discussion, we will focus first on the physical or biological developmental process.

Physical Development

"Mass activity" is typical of infancy. As the infant receives physical and emotional nurturance, this mass activity becomes more specific and is then integrated into the child's behaviors, interactions and concept of self and others.

Lugo and Hershey use the example of hunger. When an infant experiences hunger, her whole body seems to quiver with this experience. As she grows, she will develop more specific feelings and responses to her hunger. Instead of quivering all over, she may develop a special sound or reaching movement to communicate her need.

It is also believed that physical coordination and concept occurs from the head to the toes (the cephalocaudal sequence) and from the center of the body outward (proximal-distal sequence). Again, referring to Lugo and Hershey, "Examples of cephalocaudal development are that at birth 25 percent of the infant's focal control resides in his head movements and the first step toward walking begins in head and neck control. A proximal-distal sequence is seen in the development of reaching. At first, the major activity centers around the torso and shoulders and then gradually moves to the arms, hands, and fingers."[4]

The way we learn about our bodies depends on two general types of physical development: sensory and perceptual development and motor development.

Sensory and Perceptual Development and Motor Development

Sensory and perceptual development includes both the internal and the external realms. Lugo and Hershey state that there are three major ways an individual receives information regarding the body through inner and outer experiences.[5]

The first way is by proprioceptors. These are the senses of smell, taste and the cutaneous (skin) senses of touch, pressure, pain and sensitivity to temperature.

Another avenue of sensory and perceptual development involves interoceptors. These include the sense of active movement through the muscles, tendons and joints; receptors in the inner ear which provide information about the body's reference to space, and receptors in the inner organs which provide information regarding bodily functions.

Motor development is the process of the development of physical movement and skills. As indicated earlier, this process through which learning and understanding of the human body takes place begins with gross or large muscle movement. As maturation occurs, the more refined or fine motor actions and skills develop. For example, a gross motor skill is walking; a fine motor skill is putting on shoes and socks.

Of course, sensory and perceptual development and motor development are influenced by neurological development—the growth of the nervous system whose organization controls the sending and receiving of messages throughout the entire body.

Generally, we can say that our concept of our body changes as our ability to sense, perceive and move matures. As human beings, we are not and cannot be born with a concept of our whole bodies. We learn about our bodies through its natural growth process and the experiences into which this process draws us to participate.

Activities which facilitate our body awareness include proper nutrition, interaction between child and others, which involves cooperative and imitative movements, and the encouragement of autonomous movement. These can be given by the caretaker by providing suitable space for the youngster to move around in; appropriate physical contact and play; toys and games to promote the development of various physical skills and competencies and encouragement, not force, from significant adults so the child can explore the environment and the body itself.[6]

BODY IMAGE AND SELF-ESTEEM

There is a relationship between body image and self-esteem, although the dynamics of the relationship vary from person to person. Research indicates that a high degree of satisfaction with one's body is strongly associated with a high self-concept.[7] Body image, body satisfaction and self-image are positively related. In one study, women who perceived themselves as thin had a better self-image than those who felt they were average weight.[8] Perception of body is an important factor in the perception that individuals have of themselves.

Many of our group members frequently report that when they were thinner, they liked themselves better, had more self-confidence and got along better with others. This, of course, is also part of the addictive cycle of dieting. The chronic dieter tries to recapture the feeling of success—*I am good when I am in control of my eating*—that she had when she was restricting her food intake and losing weight—*I look good when I am thinner.*

When she deviates from her diet regimen, however, she swings into a shame cycle in which she begins to hate herself—*I am bad because I am out of control*—and feels fat—*I look bad when I'm fat.* Her body image and self-image can dramatically change from acceptable to awful with just a few cookies. Consequently, shame may become a dominant theme in her body image and her self-image.

Body Image Disturbance

Body image disturbance is experienced by most women in Western culture and can be a serious problem. It occurs when an individual has distorted thoughts, feelings and perceptions with regard to her body; usually the individual's perception is different from her actual size, shape and appearance. Body image disturbance is a multifaceted phenomenon which includes the following issues: body size distortion, body size dissatisfaction, insensitivity to interoceptive cues and concern with body shape.[9]

Body image disturbance can also include distortions of certain body parts—thighs, arms, breasts, legs—which individuals see as fat, ugly, too big, too small, shriveled, etc. These defective body parts seem to dominate the entire physical self and influence the overall feelings these individuals have about themselves.

Miriam, a 32-year-old bulimic, entered our treatment program with a disparaging view of herself and her body. Though she was at an average weight for her height and bone structure, Miriam saw herself as fat. Her fat image focused on her hips, which she felt were much wider (and therefore fatter) than they should be. When other group members commented on her attractiveness, Miriam would look at them in shock and reply incredulously, "How can you say that? I'm so fat and I feel so big, especially in my hips." She pounded her hips with her fists as she spoke. "They are so big. You know, I can't stand to look at myself in the mirror when I'm undressed." As she averted her gaze from the group, tears spilled onto her lap.

Despite the fact that others objectively saw her as attractive, Miriam saw herself as defective and her body as proof of her inferiority. She was unable to move beyond what she perceived as defective and to focus on her personal and physical strengths.

Body image disturbance influences the individual's eating patterns and greatly affects self-esteem in a negative feedback loop. For example, a woman who feels fat may eat or binge in response to her anxiety about her body. This eating or binging behavior deepens her sense of failure thereby lowering her self-esteem.

Body image disturbance is one of the more common and accepted symptoms of anorexia, bulimia and compulsive eating. In our experience, we have noted that women of average weight and those who are slightly overweight tend to see themselves as bigger than they are, while our more overweight patients tend to see themselves as smaller than they are. Some of our obese patients report not having a sense of their bodies below the head and neck.

INFLUENTIAL FACTORS IN BODY IMAGE FORMATION

There are several influential factors that affect a person's body image either positively or negatively.

Interactions and Attitudes of Primary Caregivers

Much like psychological development, body image formation is highly influenced by the interactions and attitudes of the primary caregivers. However, adolescence is a particularly critical time for body image formation since this image is the one we typically carry throughout our adult lives.

Early Childhood Influences

In early childhood, body awareness and body image development is strongly influenced by the identification process[10] as well as by how significant adults deal with the child's feelings about her body (the interest in exploring it), the child's drive states and the child's needs as they relate to the body.

Prebirth Expectations

Ann Kearney-Cook, an expert in body image disturbances,[11] states that body image development begins prior to birth. When a woman becomes pregnant, the couple has an image of the way they would like their baby to look. Their idealized image of this baby is influenced by their own body image history.

If the child's physical appearance is acceptable to the parents, then its emotional needs will be met within the context of an accepting and loving relational environment which contributes to the infant's feelings of self-worth—the basis for a healthy body image.[12]

Body Awareness

The basic foundation of the psychological self is the awareness of the body. Body concept emerges from an awareness of internal and external kinesthetic sensations, somatic movements, mental representations and maturation. Body awareness is connected to the process of separation/individuation starting at approximately six months and continuing until individuation is achieved at about 23 months. At 1 to 14 months of age, as the infant's motor activity increases, the primary caretaker begins to identify the various body parts for the infant. In mirroring the infant's interest in its body, the mother assists the child in developing a body awareness. From 14 to 24 months the infant's body becomes more differentiated from the mother and it will actually resist being put in various positions.[13] As psychological separateness occurs so too does the body engage in more independent activity.

Psychological and physical development depend on the relationship that develops between mother and infant. Initially, the relationship between mother and infant is basically a tactile one involving feeding, changing, hugging, rocking, dressing, cooing and gazing.

The body reminds the infant of its vulnerability—the hunger pangs it feels when it has not been fed, the temperature fluctuations of heat or cold while not being able to remove or pull up its own blankets, the diaper pin that jabs its flesh and cannot be removed. All of these physical pains and sensations are a vivid reminder to the infant of its dependency upon the caretaker.

The mother is responsible for assisting the child in its physical development. The mother helps the child to sit or to stand, she holds her arms out to reach for the child, she offers praise and applause as the child accomplishes new physical tasks. The mother encourages exploratory and reaching behaviors. This interchange is essential to the child as it gains a greater awareness of its physical self and its increasing mobility.

The mother attempts to anticipate the child's need for sleep, for food or for attention. She dresses the child so that it will be comfortable. In all of these ways, the relationship between mother and child is the basis for the baby's capacity to understand its physical and psychological self.

Dysfunctional Families

The dysfunctional family is typically characterized as having boundary issues, communication problems, rigid rules, perfectionistic standards and difficulty with change or transition. These families have difficulty recognizing their children as separate individuals, as having a distinct body and a range of feelings. The children are perceived as an extension of the parents or of their feelings, bodily experience or desires. The parents are unable to let the child experience autonomous and internally directed actions.

The children's emotions and bodies are not seen by their parents as separate entities. The parents are incapable of effective mirroring, of affirming the child's uniqueness and psychic boundaries. Consequently they often do not experience the distinctness of their body boundaries. These individuals do not have a coherent, cohesive, organized body image. For them, there has been a failure in the early months of life to acknowledge and arrive at a body self that is separate from the caregiver.

They are estranged from their bodies. They do not have a sense of internal bodily sensations, so they starve or binge in order to feel something inside. They do not have a sense of external bodily sensations, so they exercise frenetically or wear clothing that will stimulate their skin—anything to help them *feel.*

Heidi, a 39-year-old compulsive eater and exerciser who entered treatment saying she felt "nothing, inside or out," recalls that her mother always answered for her. In one of their family therapy sessions when Heidi was 16 years old, she recalls that the therapist asked Heidi when she first started to binge. "My mother didn't miss a beat and responded, 'We didn't start binging until last year.' I remember feeling such rage! But all I did was nod my head in agreement. The therapist asked me how I felt about my body. My mother replied, 'Oh, we don't really like our hips. We have the same hips. They really are big.'"

In these families, the children are used as objects to verify the success of the family. Problems occur if any of the children are less than perfect. These parents, as a result of their own low self-esteem and early birth family dysfunction, look to their children as image makers.

When Ashley was a teenager, she had tremendous weight fluctuations. In a fat period, she recalls, "It was my parents' 25th anniversary and they were having a huge party. They invited relatives and friends from all over the country. A few weeks before the party, my mom and I went shopping for a dress for me. Nothing fit well and every time I tried on another dress, my mother would just heave a deep sigh of despair. She looked as though she were just disgusted with me.

"Finally, I said to her, 'Maybe I shouldn't go to the party. You could just tell everyone I was sick.' Suddenly, my mother's face lit up and, to my great shock, she said, 'That's a wonderful idea! Then you won't embarrass your father and me.'"

As she describes this scene, Ashley stares into space, far removed from her feelings, and says, "I just can't believe that she didn't want me there."

These children have a difficult time proving their sense of individuality and often their one area of control revolves around food and weight.

As we have discussed, the mutual responsiveness that infants and children need to develop a positive self-image and body image is both emotional and physical in nature. If the child's actual appearance measures up to the parents' ideal image, the parents will have a more accepting attitude toward the child and consequently will be more responsive emotionally and physically. This attitude will be reflected in the way the parents hold the child, the kind of touch felt by the child, and the way the parents talk to and about the child.

In a dysfunctional family, the child may experience rejection from the parents if she does not measure up to the idealized image that the parents have or does not have positively valued family characteristics or has marked birth defects. This rejection occurs because the family is fearful of exposing its shame and may see the child's "defect" as putting the family at higher risk for exposure as a failure.

One of our primary ways of expressing rejection is through withdrawal. This withdrawal is generally both emotional and physical. It is easy to see how a young child may construe a caretaker's inability to respond to its needs or avoidance of physical and emotional contact as rejection, and this can be the basis for the development of bodyshame and selfshame in the growing child.

Parents' Attitude About the Body

Another factor that can cause bodyshame in the developing child is the parents' level of acceptance or shame regarding the human body generally and his or her own body image specifically. We have discussed how this shaming of the human body makes the desire to explore, understand and experience pleasure through the body an evil, repulsive act. Yet all children are naturally curious and the desire to explore and experience pleasure through the body is part of learning and developing a solid body image.

The caretaker's response to this curiosity will strongly influence the child's later feelings about the body. If the child explores her body and finds delight in the experience, the mother who has her own bodyshame may grab the child's hand and slap it, letting the youngster know that the body is not only something you don't touch but, more important, something you don't get pleasure from. This is a particular problem for mothers and their daughters, given our cultural expectations.

IDENTIFICATION AND GENDER EXPECTATIONS

Because of the social ramifications of gender, mothers and daughters have a particularly complicated relationship which can greatly affect the development of bodyshame and selfshame in the daughter.

In mothering a girl, the mother is raising her daughter to be like her. In mothering a boy, the mother is raising him to be an "other." Due to the socialization differences of gender, mothers relate very differently to their female children than to their male children. Much of the difference is intentional and adheres to the sex role stereotyping required by our culture. Other differences are very subtle and promoted through the mother's unconscious feelings about what is feminine and what is masculine.

The feelings a woman has about her femininity are an essential part of what she brings to her role as a mother. When a mother looks at her daughter, she often identifies with her, based on their shared gender identity, social roles and social expectations. She transmits the process of her own physical and psychological feminine experience. Consequently, she may pass along the negative feelings about her own feminine side.

When a mother looks at a son, she sees someone who is different. This difference in gender helps the mother to be more cognizant of her boundaries. Not so with a daughter. Boundaries with a daughter are easily blurred.

Femininity, Beauty and Thinness

Being female is associated with beauty and softness from the earliest days of a child's life and being male is associated with aggressiveness and toughness.[14]

Research in early childhood development demonstrates that parents of girls described their infant daughters as beautiful, soft, pretty, cute and delicate while they rated their sons as strong, larger featured, better coordinated and hardier.[15] In another study, when asked what kind of person they wanted their children to become, parents mentioned being attractive and having a good marriage far more often for daughters than for sons.[16]

Parents felt that one of a little girl's major jobs is to look pretty. Little girls learn very early that being attractive is connected with pleasing and serving others, which will, in turn, secure love and acceptance. Research indicates that mothers treat their infant daughters with more caution and fear, curtailing their exploratory behaviors when it exceeds a certain physical distance from the mother. However, when it comes to sons, mothers are more apt to let boys explore the environment and will allow for a greater physical distance.[17]

Mother's Influence

A little girl looks to her mother in admiration when she dresses up in high heels, fusses with make-up, jewelry, etc. She gazes in utter amazement at the transformation of her mom. She sits for what seems like hours as her mother pokes at her eyes, pats her face, picks at her eyebrows and rouges her cheeks.

When mommy complains about her weight or shrieks as she gets on the scale, the little girl learns quite emphatically that the female body is not acceptable as it is.

At mealtimes, the little girl observes her mother weighing food or sometimes not eating at all. She hears her recite a litany of calories for each item on the table. These memories will permeate her idea of what it means to be a *girl.*

The mother transmits the cultural definition of femininity to her daughter in some very direct and some very subtle ways. Through identifying with a mother whom the child perceives as powerless and dissatisfied with her body, the child may grow up disliking her own body. Daughters often associate the bodily flaws of their mothers as evidence of inferiority and assume they are the basis for the mother's discontent and unhappiness.

Since mothers were little girls once too, they have their own feelings about their bodies, influenced by their own mothers. The mother is the major force in shaping the daughter's feelings about her body and her sexuality.

In dealing with her daughter's body, the mother has to teach a daughter how to deal with the many changes her body will undergo in her lifetime. These changes are not only related to menstruation and breast development but also to fluctuating body weight. A woman's body image changes constantly since her weight fluctuates in tandem with her menstrual/ovulation cycle. Some days she feels *fat,* while on other days she feels *normal.* These bodily changes have a direct impact on her self-image. As a role model, the way that the mother deals with her own bodily changes has a critical impact on the daughter's body image.

Girls experience shame as their interest and curiosity is met with contempt, fear or anger. Whether it's environmental exploration or bodily exploration, the little girl learns that this feeling of interest and initiative is shameful. As a result, females feel cautious about their need to initiate, to explore, to go beyond. They look to others for approval and validation and only when they receive it do they feel free to move.

Through parental feedback, verbal and nonverbal, children learn that a boy's body is to be strengthened and actively developed through athletic activities whereas a girl's body is to be protected and made attractive.

Marlene, a 43-year-old compulsive eater, was the only girl in a family of four children. She remembers clearly that Saturdays were the worst day of the week for her. Every Saturday morning her brothers would go out and shoot baskets. She desperately wanted to go out and play with them. However, her mother continually reprimanded her for wanting to play with the boys. She was likely to get hurt and be "scarred for life," her mother said. "Who would want to marry you if you were scarred or deformed? Look at me, your father left me 'cause I'm big and fat. That's how men are. If you're not perfect, they don't want you." She could never understand why Marlene didn't want to stay home with her and clean house (including her brothers' bedrooms). Her reward for helping her mother houseclean was to go shopping, when they would spend time perusing the clothing departments and make-up counters.

Adolescence

The physical changes that occur in adolescence do not take place in a linear fashion. They interact within the context and culture of a society. The adolescent growth spurt, the body shape and weight changes, the onset of sexual maturation and hormonal fluctuations have a tremendous impact on the adolescent's personality and behavior. Concurrently, the attitudes and values acquired from the culture and the family have an effect on the adolescent's reaction to bodily changes. Developing a comfortable body image is a major task of adolescence.

Even more difficult for the adolescent to cope with is that these physical changes are not a uniform process. There is an unevenness in the growth rates of the adolescent's various body parts and functions which can make the young person feel awkward and self-conscious. Preoccupied with their looks and appearance, adolescents are painfully sensitive to any physical differences they may have from their peer group. Consequently they may have a difficult time coping with the sudden and intense physical changes that take place both inside and outside their bodies.

Coming to terms with the critical adolescent question, *Who Am I?* means forming a new body image and integrating the new physical self into one's self-concept. This integration is critical since the body image formed in adolescence is the one we carry throughout our adult lives.

Due to the many bodily changes of puberty, adolescence is an extremely fertile time for the emergence and formation of bodyshame. Several factors contribute to the development of bodyshame at this critical stage of human development.

FACTOR ONE: PARENTAL ATTITUDE TOWARD THE CHANGING BODY

As we have indicated, dysfunctional families are characterized by their lack of communication, inability to deal with feelings and with overinvolvement or underinvolvement among family members. They also have difficulty with changes and transitions. The bodily changes of the adolescent signal a major developmental change for the family as a whole, particularly for the parents.

If it is difficult for the parents to accept their own bodies or natural bodily functions, it will be particularly tough to understand and be supportive of the adolescent's ever mercurial feelings about bodily changes.

If a daughter is prematurely developing secondary sexual characteristics (pelvic bone enlargement, fat deposits in the pelvic area, breast development), mother may react with anxiety, wondering if her daughter will be ridiculed. Dad may suddenly withdraw his attention and physical touching of his daughter, uncertain how to deal with her emerging womanhood. This is particularly true for dads who have distorted views of femininity and female sexuality.

Mother may feel uncomfortable with her son's changing body, testicular and penile growth and his first ejaculation or wet dreams. Dad may be concerned about his son's sexual adequacy and fear his son's sexual curiosity.

Changing bodies and raging hormones signal the emerging sexual needs and drives of the adolescent. Parents become frightened about bodily changes and equate them with sexual activity. They do not view the sexual activity of their daughters in the same light as that of their sons. Although the women's movement has done much to equalize and recognize women's sexual drives and needs as healthy and normal, there is still a tendency to treat the adolescent female's emerging sexuality with more caution and fear. The threat of pregnancy often contributes to the parents' anxiety—another shame bind for the adolescent female.

How sympathetic is the parent to the child's bodily changes? The manner in which the onset of menarche is dealt with has an impact on a young girl's feelings about this bodily function. A sudden growth spurt for a young boy coupled with an ever changing and cracking voice needs support and understanding from parents and siblings rather than ridicule and teasing. These bodily changes can precipitate a shame response if parents and siblings ridicule or exhibit a sense of shame over developing sexuality.

Bodily changes also signal emerging independence and autonomy. The ability of mothers and fathers to respond to their sons' and daughters' bodily and emotional changes at adolescence is a chief contributor in the development of selfshame and bodyshame. If mother and dad share joy in their child's emerging self, embrace the natural alterations arising in the parent-child relationship—the affectional bond moving toward the adult-to-adult level of mutuality versus the caregiver-care receiver level of interaction—then the child will experience herself as affirmed both physically and emotionally and will integrate a healthy self-image and body image.

FACTOR TWO: CULTURALLY DETERMINED STANDARDS OF PHYSICAL ACCEPTABILITY

Before we examine this factor more closely, we must remember that adolescent development poses a particular dilemma for girls.

As mentioned earlier, before puberty, girls have 10-15 percent more body fat than boys but, after puberty, girls have almost twice as much fat as boys. Boys' weight spurt is due to an increase in muscle and lean tissue. Given the cultural expectations for females to be thin—and for males to be muscular—it is no wonder that girls express lower body esteem than adolescent boys.[18] Their bodily changes move them away from the cultural ideal while bodily changes for boys move them much closer to what's acceptable.

According to the research,[19] adolescent girls are very concerned with their looks and are aware of the great value that society places on physical attractiveness for women. Girls listed weight as their leading concern about their appearance.

Falling short of the cultural ideal generates shame for the adolescent female. Resolving the conflict between one's real and ideal body image is another nearly impossible task of adolescence. In comparing herself to the ideal, the adolescent girl will always fall short, particularly the adolescent who is unable to see her body realistically (disturbed body image).

Research[20] has demonstrated that the feedback boys receive from their teachers centers around their intellectual achievements whereas girls were more often praised for things unrelated to intellectual achievement, such as neatness, good grooming, etc.

The importance of appearance to girls is also promoted through the mass media and children's books. *Women on Words and Images* revealed that the girls in these primers focused their attention on their looks whereas boys never did. Attending to one's appearance was a major activity for the female characters whereas male characters were more likely to be playing hard or solving problems. Television also promotes the cultural ideal of femininity and girls tend to internalize these standards. Developmental studies reveal that girls are more concerned than boys about their physical attractiveness.[21]

Even though menstruation and ovulation play a key role in the physiological functions of the female, the secondary sex characteristics play a greater social role in the way in which peers interact with adolescent girls. Breast, hip and thigh size can be a major source of shame or pride for girls. For adolescent boys, shame can result from a high-pitched cracking voice or a sudden erection. Shameful events, however, are more closely related to the shame of bodily functions than to the shame of falling short of the ideal and of what's considered beautiful and acceptable.

An additional complication in physical and psychological maturation for girls revolves around the notion that the self-image of a girl is more interpersonally oriented than a boy's. Girls seem to worry more about what other people think of them, are more concerned about being liked and try harder to avoid negative reactions from others. Girls are focused more on affiliation and interpersonal relationships.[22] They are concerned about being accepted by others whereas boys' adolescent issues seem to center on achievement, autonomy and control. Consequently, the adolescent girl becomes particularly sensitive to and compliant with social demands and appropriate sex role standards. This can exacerbate her shame feelings about her bodily fat and her need to control her body and appetites so that she can be better liked and valued.

Another shame-related bind that the adolescent girl becomes vulnerable to is her relational orientation. Gilligan[23] reported that adolescent girls conceptualize dependence as a positive attribute, with isolation as its polar opposite. This creates confusion and self-doubt in a culture that highly values independence and individualism and devalues dependence, viewing the latter as a serious flaw.

In gravitating toward others, the young girl tends to deny, ignore or suppress many of her needs and initiatives. Young girls learn that their ability to form relationships, especially with males, often depends on the acceptability of their bodies.

The young girl begins to feel a sense of shame over her need for others, sadness when a relationship is somehow in turmoil, anxiety when there is conflict in a relationship. She is taught that these feelings are a form of weakness rather than learning to appreciate them as part of her unique female psychological development.

Research indicates[24] that when other aspects of life seem out of control, weight and eating may be the one area where the female adolescent can feel some self-control, some sense of strength and power. Weight and dieting can be tied to the adolescent's struggle for what the culture defines as independence. Dieting may reflect a girl's desire to show others as well as herself that she is growing up and independent.[25] This is something that she does not innately feel. She resists her relational needs and views them as bad.

Losing weight may symbolize an attempt to defy her body's changes and help her maintain a more childlike body, keeping her feeling safe in her dependency needs.

The culture in which an individual takes pride in being independent, in control, thin and powerful, also creates a shame-laden spirit for the emerging female who needs and values relationships and whose body fails to conform to the culture's body ideal.

FACTOR THREE: ATTITUDES OF THE PEER GROUP

The peer group assumes the central role in the life of the adolescent. The family is replaced. The peer group serves as a buffer between the family and the wider community that is not yet ready to accept the adolescent.[26]

The peer group holds up standards regarding attitudes toward authority figures, dress codes, sexual mores, social and academic performance, drug and alcohol use and appearance. All of the research indicates that there is a correlation between physical attractiveness and popularity among adolescent peer groups.[27] This makes the need to be thin even more of a consuming passion for the female adolescent.

If the peer group centers around an activity which requires a certain weight or body type such as dancing, diving, swimming, wrestling or modeling then the adolescent will feel additional pressure to maintain a certain body type and weight.

Terri, an 18-year-old bulimic, had been a diver since she was seven years old. She showed great promise and her parents were extremely proud of her many diving accomplishments. At 13, however, her body started to change. Her coach began to pressure her about her weight. Terri wasn't the only one on the team, though, with a changing and growing body. She struggled with her diet and tried to maintain her weight. One day a group of her teammates asked her to go along with them for a pizza. She was surprised. "Well," she said, "I'd rather go somewhere else because I don't think I can withstand the temptation to eat pizza. Anyway, we have weigh-ins tomorrow." They all giggled and told her not to worry about the weigh-in. A teammate assured her she could eat pizza as much as she wanted and still make weight. "How can I do that?" Terri asked with great curiosity. Her teammate said, "You can eat as much pizza as you want and then you can vomit or take laxatives. We've been doing it for weeks now and it works! We can have our cake and eat it too!" When she hesitated, they continued to assure her that this was a great way to eat whatever she wanted and still maintain her diving weight. She finally agreed to go. They had frequent binge/vomit parties throughout high school. Her bulimia increasingly became a problem. Finally out of control, she sought treatment.

An individual's body changes constantly throughout life. However, these changes are not immediately incorporated into the body image. Research has demonstrated that a time lag exists between the actual body change and its integration into the person's body image.[28] This explains why an overweight person, who loses a great deal of weight, still sees herself as fat.

Ideals and Expectations of the Culture

A person's self-esteem is partly her assessment of herself against an ideal model. In earliest life, this model is typically a parent or significant adult—even a media star. As we mature, our ideal self image becomes less dependent upon a specific model and more on an image of the way we would like to be. This image is a synthesis of the individuals we admired in the earlier stages of our development.

As we have discussed, shame theorists postulate that shame can be generated when the individual falls short of her idealized version of herself. The ideal versus the real image goes beyond the inner self and includes the body. Consequently, our ideal self image includes a mental representation of the body type we wish for.

The cultural standards promote a woman's tendency to have an idealized body image based on these standards. Whenever a woman becomes acutely aware that her real body falls far short of her ideal, she may experience deep feelings of shame. Many of our patients cite painful bodyshame experiences.

Alyssa, who weighed 375 pounds, did not see herself as that large. When she arrived at a party, she tried to sit down in an armchair and was shocked to discover that she did not fit in it. The hostess, noticing that she might even break the chair since it was made of wicker, ran to Alyssa and quickly escorted her to another chair. Alyssa reported feeling a deep sense of shame as other guests saw what was happening. She was so ashamed that she left the party early, feigning illness. When she shared this experience in group, she sobbed uncontrollably, castigating herself for not realizing she was so large.

Faye, a bulimic whose real body size was about a size 10, had been rigidly dieting for several weeks. She felt certain that she had lost a lot of weight because her clothes were feeling quite loose. Since her closet contained what she called "fat clothes" and "thin clothes," she grabbed a pair of her thin jeans to change into at her boyfriend's apartment. When she got there, she began to change and as she was putting on her jeans, which refused to zip up, her boyfriend walked into the bedroom. When she caught his gaze, she reported feeling a profound sense of shame about her body. "I couldn't believe it," she sobbed. "He must think I'm a fat slob!"

Bodyshame is experienced not only in relation to falling short of the ideal but it is exacerbated by the shame-drive bind of hunger. The body is a visible source of shame that reveals a failure to keep our appetites in check. For women, the appetite encompasses more than just a hunger for food. It represents our inability to control our emotions and needs. We have examined this earlier.

The feelings of bodyshame are often related to early childhood and adolescent experiences which focused on the body or specific body parts. Once again, research strongly supports the notion that the body image formed in adolescence may be a major component of the adult's body image.[29]

Physical Trauma and Physical Boundary Violations

Body image can be deeply affected by traumatic experiences such as sexual abuse, surgery and physical deformity. Ann Kearney-Cook[30] postulates that a disturbance in body image could result from a sexual victimization experience, since the body is where the original trauma took place. The shameful feelings do not subside once the abuse ends.

Problems that survivors of sexual abuse may experience with their bodies include splitting, numbing, addictions and self-mutilation.[31] Initially, these are defenses developed by the sexual abuse survivor to cope and survive psychologically and emotionally. Because it was the body that was abused, survivors tend to blame their bodies. If this blaming (and shaming) continues, however, it will be hard for the survivor to heal from the sexual abuse and she may be further hurt emotionally, psychologically and physically by a defense system which is no longer useful. One of the defenses that a sexual abuse survivor may use is compulsive eating behavior. The specific reasons to use food compulsively may vary but initially it is for protection. Some sexual abuse survivors compulsively overeat, undereat or binge and purge as a sedative—a way to numb feelings of anger, hurt and shame. For others, eating compulsively is a way to be nurtured because the sexual abuse has either kept them from learning or too fearful to engage in any other forms of nurturance.

Some women who are survivors of sexual abuse will compulsively overeat and become overweight as a way to try to protect themselves physically. They hope that by being "big" and by not fitting into the cultural ideal of beautiful, no sexual attraction and consequently no sexual assault can occur. Conversely, the anorexic hopes that by starving she can keep her body from developing or showing any physical characteristics—for example, breasts—which would be seen as sexual and therefore risk promoting sexual contact.

Compulsive overeating which results in overweight, anorexia and bulimia are all efforts by the sexual abuse survivor to control her body and, in effect, try to get back the power she felt robbed of by the sexual abuse. It is important to note that individuals who have been physically and emotionally abused in ways other than sexual ones will experience the same sense of violation, shame and need for protection as the sexual abuse survivor. It is also important to note that sexual abuse is not confined to rape and incest. Sexual abuse includes any physical or emotional violation which takes place through coercion and intimidation. Women who have been the objects of inappropriate sexual kissing, caressing, staring, grabbing or conversation have experienced a form of sexual abuse and will often respond emotionally and physically just like the survivor of incest or childhood beatings.

Physical Disability and Deformity Trauma

Due to our society's emphasis on physical perfection and bodily control, individuals who are physically disabled or physically deformed through injury, illness or heredity quickly become aware that they are looked upon by others as inadequate and consequently inferior. The body image and self-concept of the individual who is physically different because of a deformity or disability is deeply affected by the attitudes and interactions of others and by what she is encouraged to learn and do.

Involvement in physical activity such as wheelchair sports is important to help the individual realize that she is more physically capable than she, and possibly others, have realized. Those with neurological disorders such as cerebral palsy need to become acquainted with their bodies through visual stimulation—looking at pictures, examination and conscious movement of the body and body parts. Beyond physical therapy, occupational therapy and psychotherapy, dance therapy is often used to allow these people to identify, explore and express feelings of anger, love, grief and guilt. It is useful in increasing body awareness and promotes mind/body integration.

As with physical, emotional and sexual abuse survivors, the individual trying to cope with a physical deformity or disability may use eating as a way to numb the hurt, the anger and the sense of isolation or to provide herself with nurturance. This is particularly needed because many people fail to or avoid making any physical contact with someone who has a physical deformity or disability.

A woman who has had a mastectomy may be angry with her body for "betraying" her as she tries to cope with the feelings of now, somehow, being "less of a woman." She is questioning her general physical and sexual attractiveness. Children with developmental disabilities which retard the development of motor skills or general physical signs of maturation may become frustrated with themselves and with their bodies for being different in an alienating way. Burn victims and other individuals with distinctly visible deformities are frequently stared at and experience a shame response in the wake of a sense of exposure and fear of judgment by others.[32]

NOTES

1. R. M. Lerner, S. A. Karabenick, and J. L. Stuart, "Relations among physical attractiveness, body attitudes and self-concept in male and female college students," *Journal of Psychology* 85 (1973): 119–29; P. F. Secord and S. M. Jourard, "The appraisal of body-cathexis: Body-cathexis and the self," *Journal of Consulting Psychology* 17 (1953): 343–47.

2. Pamela Powers and Marilyn Erickson, "Body image in women and its relationship to self-image and body satisfaction," *The Journal of Obesity & Weight Regulation* 5 (Spring 1986): 37–50.

3. James Lugo and Gerald Hershey, *Human Development* (New York: Macmillan, 1974), 125–27.

4. Ibid., 276.

5. Ibid., 125–27.

6. Ibid.

7. Lerner, Karabenick, and Stuart, "Relations among physical attractiveness," 119–29; Secord and Jourard, "Appraisal of body-cathexis," 343–47.

8. Powers and Erickson, "Body image in women," 37–50.

9. D. M. Garner and P. E. Garfinkel, "Body image in anorexia nervosa: measurement, theory and clinical implications," *International Journal of Psychiatry in Medicine* 11 (1981): 263–84.

10. P. Shilder, *The Image and Appearance of the Human Body* (New York: International University Press, 1950–51).

11. Ann Kearney-Cook, "Decoding the obsession: using guided imagery in the treatment of body image disturbance among bulimic women" from draft of chapter prepared for L. Hornyak and E. Baker, *Experiential Therapies for Eating Disorders* (New York: Guilford Press, 1989).

12. S. Fisher, *Development and Structure of Body Image* (Hillsdale, N.J.: Erlbaum, 1986).

13. M. Mahler, F. Pine, and A. Bergman, *The Psychological Birth of the Human Infant* (New York: Norton, 1975).

14. E. Tronick, H. Als, L. Adamson, S. Wise, and T. Brazelton, "The infant's response to entrapment between contradictory messages in face-to-face interaction," *Journal of Child Psychiatry* 17 (1978): 1–13.

15. J. Rubin, F. Provenzano, and Z. Luria, "The eye of the beholder: Parents' views on sex of newborns," *American Journal of Orthopsychiatry* 44 (1974): 512–19.

16. A. M. Henschel-Ambert, *Sex Structure* (Don Mills, Ont.: Longman Canada, 1973).

17. I. Broverman, D. Broverman, F. Clarkson, P. Rosencrantz, and S. Vogel, "Sex role stereotypes and clinical judgements of mental health," *Journal of Consulting and Clinical Psychology* 34 (1970): 1–7.

18. R. Striegel-Moore, L. Silberstein, and J. Rodin, "Toward an understanding of risk factors for bulimia," *American Psychologists* 41 (1986): 246–63.

19. A. H. Crisp and R. S. Kalucy, "Aspects of the perceptual disorder in anorexia females," *Journal of Psychopathology and Behavioral Assessment* 7 (1974): 289–301; M. Rosenbaum, "The changing body image of the adolescent girl" in *Female Adolescent Development*, ed. M. Sugar (New York: Brunner/Mazel, 1979), 234–52.

20. C. Dweck, W. Davidson, S. Nelson, E. Bradley, "Sex differences in learned helplessness: II The contingencies of evaluative feedback in the classroom and III: An experimental analysis,"

Developmental Psychology 14, no. 3 (May 1978): 268–76.

21. Striegel-Moore, Silberstein, and Rodin, "Risk factors for bulimia," 246–63.

22. N. Chodorow, *The Reproduction of Mothering: Psychoanalysis and the Sociology of Gender* (Berkeley: University of California Press, 1978); R. G. Simmons and F. Rosenberg, "Sex, sex roles and self-image," *Journal of Youth and Adolescence* 4 (1975): 229–58; E. Douvan and J. Adelson, *The Adolescent Experience* (New York: Wiley, 1966).

23. Carol Gilligan, *In A Different Voice: Psychological Theory and Women's Development* (Cambridge, Mass.: Harvard University Press, 1982).

24. J. Hood, T. Moore, and D. Garner, "Locus of control as a measure of ineffectiveness in anorexia nervosa," *Journal of Consulting and Clinical Psychology,* 50, no. 1 (1982): 3–13.

25. C. I. Steele, "Weight loss among teenage girls: An adolescent crisis," *Adolescence* 15 (1980): 823–29.

26. Striegel-Moore, Silberstein, and Rodin, "Toward an understanding of risk factors for bulimia," 246–63.

27. Dweck et al., "Sex differences," 268–76.

28. Powers and Erickson, "Body image in women," 37–50.

29. Ann Kearney-Cooke, "Group treatment of sexual abuse among women with eating disorders," *Women and Therapy* 71, no. 1 (1988): 5–21.

30. Ibid.

31. E. Bass and L. Davis, *The Courage to Heal* (New York: Harper & Row, 1988).

32. Robert Goldenson, ed., *Disability and Rehabilitation Handbook* (New York: McGraw-Hill, 1978).

Introduction to The Mismeasure of Woman

CAROL TAVRIS

THE UNIVERSAL MALE

Man is the measure of all things.

—Protagoras (c. 485–410 B.C.)

JOIN ME, IF you will, in a brief flight of fancy. George Jones, age thirty-four, visits the "psychology and health" section of his local bookstore. There he finds an assortment of books designed to solve his problems with love, sex, work, stress, and children:

- *Women Who Hate Men and the Men Who Love Them* explains why he remains in a self-defeating relationship with Jane.
- *The X Spot and other new findings about male sexuality* tells him exactly how to have the right kind of multiple orgasm that women have.
- *The Male Manager* shows why his typically male habits of competitiveness and individualism prevent him from advancing in the female-dominated, cooperative corporate world.
- *Cooperation Training* offers practical instructions for overcoming his early competitive socialization as a man, showing him how to get along more smoothly with others.
- *The Superman Syndrome* explains that because men are physically less hardy than women throughout their lives, men find it difficult to combine work and family. They would live as long as women do if they would scale down their efforts to seek power and success.
- *The Father Knot* and *The Reproduction of Fathering* explore the reasons that George feels so guilty about the way he is raising his children. Women feel comfortable with motherhood, these books argue, because they bear and nurse their offspring. But men for basic anatomical reasons are doomed to feel insecure and guilty in their role as fathers because unconsciously they never quite believe the child is theirs.

• *Erratic Testosterone Syndrome (ETS)—What it is and how to live with it* provides medical and psychological information to help George cope with his hormonal ups and downs. Because men do not have a visible monthly reminder of hormonal changes, they fail to realize that their moodiness and aggressive outbursts are hormonally based. A special concluding chapter helps the wives of men with ETS learn to live with their husbands' unpredictable mood swings.

Lucky George. He will never feel obliged to read books like these, were anyone ever to write them; but of course women feel obliged to read the comparable volumes directed to them. It's a puzzle that they do, actually, because most of these books imply that women aren't doing anything right. Women are irrational and moody because of their hormones. They cry too much. They love too much. They talk too much. They think differently. They are too dependent on unworthy men, but if they leave the men to fend for themselves, they are too independent, and if they stay with the men they are codependent. They are too emotional, except when the emotion in question is anger, in which case they aren't emotional enough. They don't have correct orgasms, the correct way, with the correct frequency. They pay too much attention to their children, or not enough, or the wrong kind. They are forever subject to syndromes: the Superwoman Syndrome causes the Stress Syndrome, which is exacerbated by Premenstrual Syndrome, which is followed by a Menopausal Deficiency Syndrome.

Why do women buy so many self-help books every year to improve their sex lives, moods, relationships, and mental health? Simone de Beauvoir gave us one answer in 1949: because women are the second sex, the other sex, the sex to be explained. Men and women are not simply considered different from one another, as we speak of people differing in eye color, movie tastes, or preferences for ice cream. In almost every domain, men are considered the normal human being, and women are "ab-normal," deficient because they are different from men. Therefore, women constantly worry about measuring up, doing the right thing, being the right way. It is normal for women to worry about being abnormal, because male behavior, male heroes, male psychology, and even male physiology continue to be the standard of normalcy against which women are measured and found wanting.

Despite women's gains in many fields in the last twenty years, the fundamental belief in the normalcy of men, and the corresponding abnormality of women, has remained virtually untouched. Now even this entrenched way of thinking is being scrutinized and the reverberations are echoing across the land. Everywhere we look, it seems, teachers, courses, theories, and books are being challenged to examine their implicit assumption that man is the measure of all things.

Thus, in politics, we have "important issues" (drugs, economics, war) and then "women's issues" (day care, birth control, peace), as if these matters could or should be divided at the gender line. Congress and the United Nations worry about international violations of "human rights," but these rarely include violations of women's rights such as denial of suffrage, wife-beating, genital mutilation, forced prostitution, or sweatshops that run on underpaid female labor. Somehow, these are "women's issues," not "human rights" issues. We worry, as well we should, about the feminization of poverty, but we do not see its connection to the masculinization of wealth. The phrase "unfit mother" rolls trippingly off judicial tongues, but "unfit father" is nowhere to be heard. We ponder the problem of unwed, "sexually irresponsible" teenage mothers, not the problem of unwed, sexually irresponsible teenage fathers. Boys will be boys, we say, but girls better not be mothers. Indeed, reproductive freedom in general is a "woman's issue," as if men were merely disinterested bystanders on the matter of sexuality and its consequences.

The perception of female otherness occurs in every field, as we are learning from critical observers in science, law, medicine, history, economics, social science, literature, and art.[1] In medicine, students learn anatomy and physiology and, separately, female anatomy and physiology; the male body is anatomy-itself. In art, we have works of general excellence and, separately, works by women artists, generally regarded as different and lesser; male painters represent art-itself. In literature, a college course on "black female writers of the twentieth century" is considered a specialized seminar; yet when an English instructor at Georgetown University called her course "white male writers," it was news—because the works of white male writers are regarded as literature-itself.[2] In psychoanalysis, Freud took the male as the developmental norm for humanity, regarding female development as a pale and puny deviation from it.

In history, the implicit use of men as the norm pervades much of what schoolchildren learn about American and Western civilization. Was Greece the cradle of democracy? It was no democracy for women and slaves. Was the Renaissance a time of intellectual and artistic rebirth? There was no renaissance for women—"at least," wrote historian Joan Kelly, "not during the Renaissance."[3] Did the Enlightenment expand "the rights of man" in education, politics, and work? Yes, but it narrowed the rights of women, who were denied control of their property and earnings and barred from higher education and professional training. Was the American frontier "conquered" by single scouts, brave men "taming" the wilderness and founding a culture based on self-reliance? This mythic vision excludes the women who struggled to establish homes, survive childbirth, care for families, and contribute with men to the community that was essential to survival.

In economics, supposedly the study of pure market forces and the "Rational Man" (in comparison to the irrational—whom?), the field relies on measures of gross national product as the main gauge of a nation's economic performance, overlooking the value of women's unpaid labor in the home and the invisible work they do that lies outside market economies. For example, as political economist Marilyn Waring has shown, the work of women farmers in underdeveloped nations is not computed in economic formulas that are the basis for agricultural assistance programs.[4] The result is that women farmers lose government aid, with devastating results for food production and the nutritional health of their families. "Economics-itself" does not concern itself with such matters. Students of economics are left with the impression that women's unpaid labor and the systematic underpayment of women's labor in the work force do not matter, or that they are aberrations in an otherwise rational system, or that women are to blame for allowing themselves to become trapped in low-paying or nonpaying jobs.

In philosophy, the centrality in thought and language of the universal male affects the ability to reason about humanity. The philosopher Elizabeth Minnich reminds us of the famous syllogism:

> All men are mortal.
> Socrates is a man.
> Therefore, Socrates is mortal.

But, Minnich suggests, try this one:

> All men are mortal.
> Alice is ———

Alice is—what? We can't say "Alice is a man." So we say she is a woman. Therefore—what? Alice is immortal? Alice, being female, is in a category that is neither masculine nor mortal:

Alice ends up in the peculiar position of being a somewhat mortal, some-what immortal, creature. Or, we must admit, we cannot thus reason about Alice while thinking of her as a female at all. We can think of Socrates as a man without derailing the syllogism; we cannot think of Alice as a woman. Reason flounders; the center holds, with Man in it, but it is an exclusive, not a universal or neutral, center. Alice disappears through the looking glass.[5]

Many people, Minnich adds, find it odd, uncomfortable, or threatening to suggest that it is appropriate to expand a field's horizons to include all humankind. "What does it mean for democracy," she asks, "that only some few kinds of humans can be imagined as our representatives? What does it mean for all of us on this shrinking globe?"[6]

My inquiry in this book is motivated by the spirit of Minnich's question: I wish to examine the consequences for us all, male and female, when only some few of us set the standards of normalcy and universality. My goal is to expand our visions of normalcy, not to replace a male-centered view with a female-centered one. But to do so we must first unmask the three most popu-lar disguises of the universal male. Each of these currently popular ways of thinking about men and women has its adherents and detractors, and each leads to different consequences for how we live our lives:

- *Men are normal; women, being "opposite," are deficient.* This us-them, yin-yang, masculine-is-good, feminine-is-bad view of the sexes is the oldest tradition in civilization. It regards men and women as polar opposites, with males as the repository of culture, intellectuality, and strength, and females the repository of nature, intuition, and weakness.
- *Men are normal; women are opposite from men, but superior to them.* Pro-ponents of this view emphasize aspects of female experience or female "nature"—such as menstruation, childbirth, compassion, spirituality, cooperation, pacifism, and harmony with the environment—and cel-ebrate them as being morally superior to men's experiences and quali-ties. In this view, nevertheless, man is still the standard against which woman's behavior is judged, even if the judgments are kinder.
- *Men are normal, and women are or should be like them.* Proponents of this approach, which would seem to be the antidote to the fundamental-difference schools, actually commit an intrinsic error of their own. By ignoring the differences that *do* exist between men and women—in life experiences, resources, power, and reproductive processes—the basically-

alike school assumes that it is safe to generalize from the male standard to all women.

These three errors, in their various incarnations, have done serious harm to women's feelings about themselves, to their relationships, and to their position in society. They are responsible for the guilt-inducing analyses that leave women feeling that once again they lack the right stuff and aren't doing the right thing. They have made sicknesses and syndromes of women's normal bodily processes, and "diseases" of women's normal experiences. They have framed the debate over solutions to social problems, and led reformers down unproductive paths. They have excluded men from the language of love, intimacy, and connection, perpetuating unhappiness and outright warfare in the family, where many men and women remain baffled by the mysterious opposite sex.

The confusion over whether women are the "same" as men, and whether they can be "different but equal," is at the heart of the current debates between (and about) the sexes. In contrast, I take as my basic premise that there is nothing *essential*—that is, universal and unvarying—in the natures of women and men. Personality traits, abilities, values, motivations, roles, dreams, and desires: all vary across culture and history, and depend on time and place, context and situation. Of course, if you photograph the behavior of women and men at a particular time in history, in a particular situation, you will capture differences. But the error lies in inferring that a snapshot is a lasting picture. What women and men *do* at a moment in time tells us nothing about what women and men *are* in some unvarying sense—or about what they can be.

THE MISMEASURE OF WOMAN

Not long ago the firm of Price Waterhouse was charged with discrimination in not granting partnership status to a woman named Ann Hopkins. Everyone agreed that Hopkins did her job well. She brought in over $40 million in new business to the firm, far more than any of the eighty-seven other nominees, all of whom were male, and forty-seven of whom were invited to become partners. Most of the opposition to Hopkins came from brief comments from the partners who had had limited contact with her and were unaware of her track record. They described her as "macho," harsh, and aggressive, and one speculated that she "may have overcompensated for being a woman." One man, trying to be helpful, advised her to "walk more femininely, talk more femininely, dress more femininely, wear make-up, have her hair styled, and wear jewelry."

Hopkins's supporters described her behavior as outspoken, independent, self-confident, assertive, and courageous. Her detractors interpreted the same behavior as overbearing, arrogant, self-centered, and abrasive. "Why is it," asked Lynn Hecht Schafran, an attorney on Hopkins's case, "that men can be bastards and women must wear pearls and smile?"[7]

At the same time that the Hopkins case was wending its way to the Supreme Court (where she eventually won), an attorney named Brenda Taylor lost her job because she was too feminine: she favored short skirts, designer blouses, ornate jewelry, and spike heels. Her boss told her that she looked like a "bimbo," and she was fired after she complained about his remarks to the Equal Employment Opportunity Commission.

Ann Hopkins and Brenda Taylor illustrate the pressures on modern women to be feminine *and* masculine, to be different from men but also the same. How is a woman supposed to behave: like an ideal male, in which case her male colleagues will accuse her of not being feminine enough, or like an ideal female, in which case her male colleagues will accuse her of not being masculine enough?

We will never know the truth about Ann Hopkins—whether she is outspoken or overbearing, confident or arrogant—because both sets of perceptions are true, from the beholder's standpoint. But by framing the problem as one of her personality, her colleagues deflected attention from the systematic practices of their company and from their own behavior. Suppose, instead, we ask: *Under what conditions* is the negative stereotype of women like Hopkins more likely to occur? The answer, according to research summarized in a brief prepared by the American Psychological Association on behalf of Hopkins, is that men are likely to behave like the Price Waterhouse partners under three conditions: when the woman (or other minority) is a token member of the organization; when the criteria used to evaluate the woman are ambiguous; and when observers lack necessary information to evaluate the woman's work.[8] All three conditions were met in Hopkins's situation. She could have read 435 books on how to behave, and they would have failed her. She could have gone to work dressed in a muu-muu or Saran Wrap, and she still would have lost that promotion. In this case, her personality had nothing to do with it.

Ann Hopkins's dilemma—whether a woman is supposed to behave like a man or a woman—is played out a thousand times a day, in the varied domains of women's lives. A woman who leaves her child in day care worries that she is failing as a mother; but if she leaves her job temporarily to stay home with her child, she worries that she will fail in her career. A woman who cries at work worries whether crying is good, since she is a woman, or wrong, since she is a professional. A woman who spends endless hours taking care of her husband and ailing parents feels that she is doing the right thing as a woman, but the wrong thing as an independent person. A woman who cannot penetrate her husband's emotional coolness alternates between trying to turn him into one of her expressive girlfriends and trying to cure her "dependency" on him.

Of the countless self-help books on the market that address these dilemmas, most direct the reader's attention to women's alleged inner flaws and psychological deficiencies. Women's unhappiness, in many of these accounts, is a result of their fear of independence, fear of codependence, fear of success, fear of failure, or fear of fear. Women are told to be more masculine in some ways and more feminine in others. Each of these explanations has a brief moment in the sun. And each eventually fades from sight, to be replaced by similar explanations that flourish briefly and die, because they do not touch the basic reasons for women's dilemmas: Inequities and ambiguities about "woman's place" are built into the structure of our lives and society. These dilemmas are normal for women. They will persist as long as women look exclusively inward to their psyches and biology instead of outward to their circumstances, and as long as women blame themselves for not measuring up.

It may seem, after two decades of the modern women's movement, that issues of difference and equality have been talked into the ground, that equality has been won. Unquestionably, women have made great progress. But our society continues to fight a war over the proper place of women, and the battleground is the female body. Once again we are in the midst of a pronatalist revival that praises motherhood as women's basic need and talent, and that persists in trying to limit and control women's reproductive choices. Once again we are hearing arguments about women's nature, their unreliable physiology, their unmasculine hormones and brains. And once again we are hearing about the problems that face women who wish to combine careers and families, as experts warn of the dangers of day care, the stresses of being superwomen, the empty satisfactions of being corporate executives.

Researchers in the fields of science, medicine, and psychology all celebrate a renewed emphasis on biological explanations of women's behavior and a medical approach to women's problems and their cures. They enthusiastically seek physiological differences in brain structure and function, biochemical reasons that more women than men suffer from depression, and hormonal changes that supposedly account for women's (but not men's) moods and abilities. Their assertions are more likely to make the news than is the evidence that contradicts them. Similarly, women hear much less these days about the psychological benefits of having many roles and sources of esteem, let alone the benefits of having a personal income.

In *The Mismeasure of Man*, the scientist Stephen Jay Gould showed how science has been used and abused in the study of intelligence to serve a larger social and political agenda: to confirm the prejudice that some groups are assigned to their subordinate roles "by the harsh dictates of nature."[9] The mismeasure of woman persists because it, too, reflects and serves society's prejudices. Views of woman's "natural" differences from man justify a status quo that divides work, psychological qualities, and family responsibilities into "his" and "hers." Those who are dominant have an interest in maintaining their difference from others, attributing those differences to "the harsh dictates of nature," and obscuring the unequal arrangements that benefit them.

Throughout this book, I will be examining the stories behind the headlines and popular theories of sex differences, traveling the trail of the universal male, showing how the belief in male normalcy and female deficiency guides scientific inquiry, shapes its results, and determines which findings make the news and which findings we live by. The following chapters will offer some new ways of looking at the old dilemmas that women and men confront daily. My goal is not to analyze, let alone solve, all the problems that women and men face in their complex lives. But by bringing hidden assumptions into the light, I hope to show how our ways of thinking about women and men lead to certain predictable results for all of us: in law and medicine, in social reforms, in standards of mental health, in the intimacies of sex and love, and in our private reveries of what is possible.

NOTES

1. Elizabeth K. Minnich, *Transforming Knowledge* (Philadelphia: Temple University Press, 1990). See also Dale T. Miller, Brian Taylor, and Michelle L. Buck, "Gender Gaps: Who Needs to be Explained?" *Journal of Personality and Social Psychology* 61 (1991): 5–12.

2. The assistant professor of English is Valerie Babb. The story was reported in *The New York Times*, March 4, 1991, p. B4.

3. Quoted in Bonnie S. Anderson and Judith P. Zinsser, *A History of Their Own: Women in Europe from Prehistory to the Present, Vols. I and II* (New York: Harper & Row, 1988).

4. Marilyn Waring, *If Women Counted: A New Feminist Economics* (San Francisco: Harper &

Row, 1989). See also Gayle Kirshenbaum, "Why Aren't Human Rights Women's Rights?" *Ms.*, July–August 1991, 12–14.

5. Minnich, *Transforming Knowledge*, 39. Minnich observes that many students "do not see the men represented and discussed in their courses *as men* but, rather, as philosophers, writers, painters, significant historical figures, important composers. But they do see the women *as women* because they have learned from the use of prefixes in course titles and the omissions in their courses that women are oddities in the dominant tradition, that women are always a kind of human, a kind of writer or whatever, and never the thing-itself" (p. 79).

6. Ibid., 79.

7. Schafran quoted in *Ms.*, January–February 1989, 137.

8. American Psychological Association, brief for *amicus curiae* in support of respondent Ann B. Hopkins (Washington, D.C.: American Psychological Association, 1988).

9. Stephen J. Gould, *The Mismeasure of Man* (New York: W. W. Norton & Co., 1981), 74.

To Be or Not Be A Woman:
Anorexia Nervosa, Normative Gender Roles, and Feminism

MARY BRIODY MAHOWALD

INTRODUCTION

ANOREXIA NERVOSA has been called an epidemic in our day (Brumberg, 1988, p. 31; Gordon, 1988, p. 151). Although historical precedents abound, its apparent prevalence among affluent white teenage girls is a relatively recent phenomenon (Leichner and Gertler, 1988, pp. 131–47). Clearly, it is a disease whose causes and treatment are psychosocial as well as psychological (Gordon, 1988, p. 161). Feminists and nonfeminists alike have recognized its association with an ideal of thinness as essential to feminine beauty (Brumberg, 1988, pp. 31–38; Leon and Finn, 1984, p. 326). Some have attributed its rising incidence to the impact of the women's movement (Brumberg, 1988, p. 38).

Throughout history, feminine beauty has had different models, some associated with ample body size rather than thinness. Nowadays, however, only slender models, with whom the majority of women can scarcely identify, are presented as ideal. These are the models that sell cars, clothes, perfumes and various other consumer goods, while also selling their image as a stereotypic interpretation of feminine beauty. The term "beauty" is itself gendered: it is rarely associated with what is "masculine", and in fact it may be used derogatorily in that connection. If thinness is an essential component of feminine beauty, it is not typically related to a comparable masculine ideal. The closest parallel for men is an ideal of tallness, musculature, strength, and physical fitness, positive traits that contrast with the unhealthy reality and appearance to which the anorexic aspires. Although the premorbid characteristics, illness features, and prognosis of anorexia nervosa are similar for both sexes, its occurrence in men is relatively rare (Crisp and Burns, 1990, p. 92). Some of the views developed in this article are applicable to men also. In what follows, however, I focus on women without attempting to address the implications of my critique for men who suffer from anorexia nervosa.

In recent years, women have increasingly participated in aerobic and body building programs in pursuit of their own health and fitness. While such efforts may also be associated with a "fear of fatness" or preference for slenderness, they are not necessarily associated with excessive thinness as an ideal of feminine beauty. Nonetheless, clinical reports and autobiographical statements from anorexics indicate a tendency to exercise with ritualistic intensity. As Brumberg puts it, "How much one runs and how little one eats is the prevailing moral calculus in present-day anorexia nervosa" (1988, p. 255). Ironically, since fitness requires attention to proper nutrition as well as exercise, the anorexic's practice of refusing to eat is incompatible with the goal of fitness.

Because anorexia nervosa occurs mainly in young women who are influenced by a socially induced concept of feminine beauty, it is particularly significant to those concerned about the injustice of gender stereotypes, and their impact on women. As "one of those," I propose in this paper to review the salient characteristics of anorexia nervosa, examine its relationship to normative gender roles, and critique those roles on feminist grounds. Much of what I argue is also applicable to bulimia nervosa, another disease associated with "fear of being fat," which occurs even more rarely in men than anorexia nervosa (Pyle and Mitchell, 1988, p. 262).[1] However, because differences between the two diseases would need to be further explained and explored for their implications, I limit the discussion here to anorexia nervosa.

My critique of normative gender roles rests on their being interpreted stereotypically. I use the term "normative" as a standard against which behaviors are measured. The term "stereotype" refers to so rigid a normative categorization of human behaviors that the possibility of individual variation is ignored, overlooked, or disvalued. At times the categorization leads to the labeling of psychologically healthy individuals as "abnormal" (Goleman, 1990, pp. B1, B7). Various versions of feminism condemn these stereotypes as obstructing the development of women's potential as individuals and social beings.

Essential Features of Anorexia Nervosa

According to the diagnostic and statistical manual of mental disorders (DSM-III-R), the diagnostic criteria for anorexia nervosa are the following:

A. Refusal to maintain body weight over a minimal normal weight for age and height, e.g., weight loss leading to maintenance of body weight 15% lower that expected; or failure to make expected weight gain during period of growth, leading to body weight 15% below that expected.
B. Intense fear of gaining weight or becoming fat, even though underweight.
C. Disturbance in the way in which one's body weight, size, or shape is experienced, e.g., the person claims to "feel fat" even when emaciated, believes that one area of the body is "too fat" even when obviously underweight.
D. In females, absence of at least three consecutive menstrual cycles when otherwise expected to occur (*DSM-III-R*, 1987, p. 67).[2]

Note that these criteria do not allude to the fact that the great majority of anorexics are young women; nor do they suggest that the anorexic's behavior is related to a culturally, temporally defined ideal of feminine beauty. Yet these are circumstances that most diagnosticians recognize as associated with the disease. Whether they ought to be included among the *DSM-III-R*'s criteria is a question worth considering. The current formulation indicates no linkage between anorexia nervosa and gender identity disorders. (I will return to this point later.)

Although the term anorexia literally means lack of appetite, in fact anorexics usually crave food, but deny themselves because of their unfounded fear of fatness. Because concern about diet and weight gain is so widespread among relatively healthy people, the severity of the disease may be overlooked. Consider, however, this sobering statistic: mortality rates range between 5% and 18% (*DSM-III-R*, 1987, p. 66). Ironically, although anorexics deliberately starve away 20% or more of their body weight, the disease prevalently occurs in cultures where food is abundant—in white, affluent, well-educated, hard driving families, where parents are conscientiously protective of their daughters (Lawson, 1985, p. 93). Recently, as media images of women reach poorer communities, the incidence of the disease has spread to them as well.

Fully 95% of anorexics are women (*DSM-III-R*, 1987, p. 66). Ordinarily, its symptoms are first observable in early to late adolescence, when boys and girls alike are concerned about their developing sexuality and gender identity. Predisposing factors include stressful life situations and "perfectionism." The experience of adolescence is stressful for many teenagers (as well as their parents), but those who are perfectionist are driven to conform to unrealistic ideals. For the anorexic, this ideal is construed as essential to personal worthwhileness. As Paul Garfinkel and David Garner put it,

> The feeling of self-worth in anorexic patients is closely bound to external standards for appearance and performance. . . . Pressures on women to be thin and to achieve, and also conflicting role expectations which force women to be paradoxically competitive, yet passive, may partially explain why anorexia nervosa has increased so dramatically. Patients with anorexia nervosa respond to these pressures by equating weight control with self-control and this in turn is equated with beauty and " success." (Garfinkel and Garner, 1982, p. 10)

What is missing in the above quotation is an explanation of the link between self-control and beauty. That link is represented by another equation, namely, that thinness *is* beautiful. The anorexic has clearly been socialized to believe this equation, but unlike equations that represent universally true statements, this one is seldom applied to men. Since the average fat mass of a normal teenage girl is about twice that of her male counterpart (Crisp and Burns, 1990, p. 78), the situation should be the opposite. Whether the ideal applies to women or men, however, equating thinness with beauty ignores the actual differences among individuals that make thinness unhealthy or abnormal for many people, male or female. In other words, the extreme thinness that the anorexic seeks is healthy for no one.

Because some anorexics cannot control their appetite to their own satisfaction, they may binge from time to time, or have bulimic episodes followed by vomiting (*DSM-III-R*, 1987, p. 66). Other behavioral characteristics of anorexia nervosa include a tendency to spend considerable time around food, preparing elaborate meals for others, while ensuring that one's own intake includes only a narrow selection of low-calorie foods. Anorexics often hoard or conceal food, and break it into small pieces before eating or throwing it away (*DSM-III-R*, 1987, p. 66). Their preoccupation with food and its preparation is reinforced by an image of women as more nurturant than men. Whether or not this image is supportable by biological or social scientific data, it is often perceived prescriptively as well as descriptively. Its stereotypic imposition belies the fact that some women are not as nurturant as some men.

Cultural expectations have long exerted unhealthy influences on women, presenting them with a forced option between conformity to an ideal of the feminine and physical normality. In prerevolutionary China, for example, the footbinding of women was not only considered beautiful, but a status symbol for their husbands, indicating that their wealth was sufficient for their wives to stay at home. Obviously, this practice limited women's mobility, severely restricting their social involvement (Garfinkel and Garner, 1982, p. 105). In the nineteenth century, the wearing of tight corsets was a way of promoting the thin appearance expected of women. These not only induced discomfort and interference with digestion, but sometimes caused serious injury. Even when their harmful effects were recognized, the impetus to wear corsets continued because of their association with beauty and "purity" (Garfinkel and Garner, 1982, p. 105).

Men have also been affected by expectations that impose health risks. Tattooing, scarification, and cranial deformation are historical examples of this (Garfinkel and Garner, 1982, p. 105). Susan Sontag describes "the tubercular appearance" among upper classes of the last century as an "index of being genteel, delicate and sensitive" (Sontag, 1978, p. 28). Such attributes were mainly esteemed in artists and in women. Note, however, that the characteristics generally attributed to artists conform with feminine rather than masculine stereotypes. The weakness and fragility associated with extreme thinness hardly reflected the strength and robustness attributed to men in general.

Several authors cite consumption as the precursor of anorexia nervosa (Garfinkel and Garner, 1982, p. 106; Brumberg, 1988, pp. 43–44). Pallor was a fashionable attribute which women used whitening powders to promote. The consumptive appearance pursued by women gave rise to the anorexic look currently glamorized by the media as an ideal of feminine beauty. In a study of dieting behavior among adolescents in Sweden, Nylander found that the "feeling of fatness" increased with age among females: 50% at 14 years of age, and 70% among 18-year-olds. Boys of comparable ages seldom reported feeling fat or dieting. Nylander observed a 10% prevalence of "mild cases" of anorexia among girls, and one "serious case" out of every 155 of those considered (Crisp et al., 1976, p. 549). Crisp and Toms studied a relatively large school population in London, and found a prevalence rate of 1 in 100 girls aged 16–18 years (Crisp et al., 1976, p. 549).

Most anorexics deny or minimize the severity of their illness, and are therefore resistant to therapy. They avoid expressions of sexuality, and their psychosexual development is usually delayed. Other types of compulsive behavior, such as excessive handwashing, are often associated with anorexia. Compulsiveness and rigidity reinforce the decision to forego normal food intake. They also reinforce the tendency to conform to gender stereotypes.

Although the *DSM-III-R* categorizes anorexia nervosa as an eating disorder rather than a gender identity disorder, its definitions of gender identity and gender role suggest that components of this diagnosis are importantly relevant to anorexics. Gender identity, according to the *DSM-III-R*,

> is the private experience of gender role, and gender role is the public expression of gender identity. Gender role can be defined as everything that one says and does to indicate to others or to oneself the degree to which one is male or female. (1987, p.71)

Attempts to reveal one's degree of femininity or masculinity are influenced by one's understanding of societal expectations in that regard. In either of two apparently contradictory ways, anorexia may illustrate a gender role disorder as defined above. First, the anorexic's obsessive pursuit of a feminine ideal of thinness indicates that she is insecure in her gender identity but fiercely wants to fulfill her perceived gender role. Second, the actual look promoted through her refusal of food is more masculine (boylike) than feminine, and amenorrhea is a means of avoiding the monthly reminder of her femininity; in other words, she fiercely wants *not* to fulfill her perceived gender role.

As already remarked, the *DSM-III-R* fails to indicate a linkage between anorexia nervosa and gender identity disorders, despite the fact that the principal symptom of anorexia, obsessive pursuit of extreme thinness, is associated with a feminine ideal. The section on gender identity disorders lists four subsets of disorders: (a) those that occur in childhood (302.60); (b) transsexualism (302.50); (c) nontranssexual disorder of adolescence or adulthood (302.85); and (d) "gender identity disorder not otherwise specified" (302.85). Anorexics seldom if ever meet one of the diagnostic criteria included in (c) and (d), viz., cross-dressing in the role of the other sex. But they definitely meet one criterion for Gender Identity Disorder of Adolescence or Adulthood: "persistent or recurrent discomfort and sense of inappropriateness about one's assigned sex," and usually meet a second criterion: "the person has reached puberty" (p. 77). The third criterion present in (b) but not in other listed gender identity disorders may also be viewed as fulfilled in anorexics, at least if one interprets pursuit of thinness as an attempt to appear masculine rather than feminine: "persistent preoccupation for at least two years with getting rid of one's primary and secondary sex characteristics and acquiring the sex characteristics of the other sex" (p. 77).

Because gender identity issues are so prevalently linked with anorexia nervosa, it seems appropriate to indicate this association among diagnostic criteria for the disease. Alternatively, the disease could be included in the list of gender identity disorders, thus accenting the connection between an obsession with thinness, and the obsessive embracing or rejecting of a socially induced stereotype of femininity, both traits that occur in the majority of anorexics. Either revision would also suggest the limitations of the *DSM-III-R*'s consideration of gender identity and gender role as normative standards. In the next section, I will discuss the content of these standards and their impact on adolescents.

NORMATIVE GENDER ROLES AND ADOLESCENTS

While there is general agreement about the content of gender-based behaviors, they have different formulations by different authors. Alfred Heilbrun, for example, begins a discussion of "Sex-role Identity in Adolescent Females" by defining the sex-role identity of the child as "the degree to which his or her behavior and attitudes coincide with cultural stereotypes of masculinity and femininity." He then distinguishes between behaviors:

> Typical of the behavior subsumed under the adult masculine sex-role are: achievement, autonomy, dominance, and endurance; feminine adult sex-role behavior would include deference, abasement, succorance, nurturance, and affiliation. (Heilbrun, 1968, p. 80)

After thus linking sex-role identity with gender stereotypes, Heilbrun goes on to define adjustment as "the degree to which the individual is capable of maintaining herself interpersonally without seeking professional help for personal problems." He describes the "best adjusted girls" as those who are in "better psychological health" in comparison with others; these need not seek professional help (pp. 80–81). Some obvious problems arise from identifying health with social adjustment. By such an account, for example, those who adapt to regimes that perpetuate atrocities may be considered healthy, while those who persist in resisting a manifestly evil *status quo*, or seek help in resisting it, are not. Surely, this is not the type of adjustment that Heilbrun had in mind.

Nonetheless, adjustment to one's gender role is often construed as an essential component of healthy maturation. Although maternal identification is sometimes thought to facilitate such adjustment in daughters, research has not borne this out. In fact, when Heilbrun and Donald Fromme studied girls whose parents were atypical with regard to sex roles ("feminine father–masculine mother") they found no relationship between the daughters' parental-identification and their level of adjustment. When their parents represented sex-typical models ("masculine father–feminine mother"), the best-adjusted girls identified more strongly with their fathers than with their mothers. They thus diverged from conformity to gender stereotypes (Heilbrun and Fromme, 1965, pp. 52–54). Supporting this finding, Toby Sitnick and Jack Katz found that girls with eating disorders had lower ratings of masculine traits than their healthy counterparts. They concluded that "one characteristic of those women vulnerable to developing this syndrome may be a failure to develop adequately those 'masculine' traits that are also necessary for optimal adult female functioning in contemporary society" (Sitnick and Katz, 1984, p. 81).

Although some clinical studies reflect the widespread practice of measuring adolescent health and psychological maturation by gender specific behavior,[3] this view is troublesome, to say the least. It suggests that the feminine traits that have led to and maintained the oppression of women are crucial to their health, and that the masculine traits that have permitted men to pursue personal power unselfconsciously are healthy for them. To be healthy, therefore, girls should be compliant, while boys should be in charge. The developing capacity for autonomous decision making is thus more likely to be frustrated in girls than in boys. In either case, conformity to normative (stereotypic) gender roles belies the fact that sexuality does not entail a simple division of humanity into two disparate parts, but a continuum for each human trait, various assortments of which are necessary to the health of unique individuals of either sex. On one end of the spectrum are those that epitomize the stereotype of femininity, at the other those that epitomize the stereotype of masculinity. The gender type of individuals is determined by the proportion of masculine or feminine traits that each one embodies. For most, this does not represent conformity to normative gender roles. Accordingly, the health of adolescents should not be defined in terms of adjustment to stereotypically defined gender traits.

Jean Humphrey Block suggests a healthier and more egalitarian approach to adolescent socialization when she writes that the ultimate goal in development of sexual identity is *not* [my italics] the achievement of masculinity or femininity as popularly conceived. Rather, sexual identity means, or will mean, the earning of a sense of self in which there is a recognition of gender secure enough to permit the individual to manifest human qualities our society, until now, has labeled as unmanly or unwomanly. (Block, 1973, p. 512)

According to this view, a healthy adolescent is one who does not need professional help because she tends to be dominant rather than deferential in her interactions with others, or because affiliation is less important to her than autonomy. Nor would a male adolescent be construed as needing professional help solely because he is more oriented towards nurturance than self-interest, or more compliant than autocratic in his behavior. From a feminist perspective (as well as other perspectives), imposition of normative gender roles on individuals whose natural propensities lie in different directions should be resisted.

Resistance to imposition of normative gender roles is a particular challenge for teenagers because socialization based on gender distinctions reaches a high point during adolescence. Without settling the question of whether observed behavioral differences between boys and girls are triggered more by socialization than by the onset of puberty, many writers support a gender intensification hypothesis as the explanation for such changes. According to John Hill and Mary Ellen Lynch, adolescence is a period when new domains may become "the object of gender-differential socialization pressure," and increased demands for conformity to such pressure arise (Hill and Lynch, 1983, p. 201). The pressures intensify because of specific developmental tasks faced by teenagers: (a) establishment of a stable sense of self and self-worth, reflecting acceptance of the bodily changes that accompany puberty; (b) achievement of strong friendships, and comfortableness in relating to the opposite sex; (c) transition from physical and emotional dependence on parents to relative independence. Definitions of gender identity relate to each of these tasks, with different implications for boys and girls. The differences, unfortunately, have sexist consequences.

Consider, for example, the fact that early pubertal change tends to be an advantage for boys and a disadvantage for girls. Roberta Simmons and her colleagues suggest that the key difference is whether the changes lead one to approximate the cultural ideal or not. For the boy, the physical changes of puberty render him more muscular and athletic and thus more in line with the American physical ideal for males. For the girl, the changes at first lead her to be bigger than all her male and female peers and then on average to be shorter and heavier than the later-developing girls. The result is that she is less likely to approximate the female ideal of beauty than the late-developing tall and slim girl. (Simmons et al., 1983, p. 264)

When the "cultural ideal" is rigidly imposed on male and female adolescents it thus affects them not only differently but unequally. "Unequally" here refers to the ranking of differences as positive or negative traits (Mahowald, 1987, p. 21). Even if the cultural ideal perfectly reflected the natural propensities of boys and girls as they move towards adulthood, it would entail prejudicial consequences for those of either sex who don't or can't conform to their normative gender role. Moreover, since the role generally relegates women to secondary social status, its overall influence on female adolescents would impede rather than facilitate the development of their full potential.

As already suggested, the reinforcement of gender roles extends beyond physical differences. According to Hill and Lynch, parents are more likely to discourage aggressive behavior in girls than in boys, and this differentiation by parents may increase during adolescence. Standards for achievement become more sex-stereotyped with age, with boys demonstrating better spatial skills and girls better verbal skills during adolescence (Hill and Lynch, 1983, pp. 218–19). In contrast with teenage boys, girls tend to experience decreased self-esteem, increased self-consciousness, and instability of self-concept, but studies have not yet proved that this is related to reinforcement of gender roles (Hill and Lynch, 1983, pp. 218–20). Nonetheless, parents are often more tolerant of independence for their sons; they expect their daughters to be more concerned about their appearance, and most still expect their sons to be the initiators of opposite-sex interactions. The double standard thus evoked tends to become a self-fulfilling promise that has clinical as well as social repercussions. Anorexia nervosa may be a tragic example of these repercussions.

Social Causes of Anorexia

Despite the severity and apparent increase of anorexia nervosa, few authors have argued that normative gender roles should be targeted in pursuit of its cure. For the most part, they simply document the epidemiology of the disease, and some clearly delineate the concurrence of gender socialization and anorexia[4] (Garfinkel and Garner, 1982, pp. 105–19; Pettinati et al., 1987, p. 280; Gordon, 1988, pp. 160–61). From a feminist standpoint, however, preventive treatment is called for, and such treatment clearly requires not only rejection of gender stereotypes but positive efforts to thwart pervasive social tendencies in this regard. Moreover, in treating those who have already contracted the disease, a comparable critique is crucial. So long as girls "buy into" a feminine ideal of thinness that threatens their psychological and physical well being, their low self-esteem is bound to be reinforced, and with that a prolongation or exacerbation of their illness. Insofar as the disease is provoked by gender socialization, they will continue to fall prey to anorexia nervosa until the ideal itself is changed.

Few, however, would argue that anorexia nervosa is caused by gender socialization alone. In *Fasting Girls,* Joan Brumberg describes three types of factors that contribute to its development: biological, psychological, and cultural. Although different theoretical models have emerged for each of these sources, Brumberg maintains that none is adequately explicative of "the current rash of eating disorders and the place of anorexia nervosa in the long history of female food refusal" (Brumberg, 1988, p. 24). While she gives most weight to cultural influences, Brumberg clearly views biological vulnerability and psychological predisposition as the villains also. Among biomedical influences, a number of more specific causal candidates emerge: hormonal imbalance, dysfunction of the hypothalamus, lesions in the brain's limbic system, irregular output of vasopressin and gonadotropin, and excess cortisol production. Neither singly nor together do these features adequately explain the distinctive socioeconomic and gender status of anorexic patients, or why its incidence is so great at this time in history.

Psychological explanations interpret anorexia nervosa as "a pathological response to the developmental crisis of adolescence" (Brumberg, 1988, p. 28). The teenager's refusal of food is seen as an expression of a struggle for autonomy, individuation, and sexuality (Lawrence, 1979, p. 93). Following Freud, psychoanalysts have equated an unwillingness to eat with the desire to suppress one's libido or sexual drive, and resistance to the inexorable progress towards adulthood. Ironically, while repressing that drive, the anorexic nonetheless seeks to control the only thing she feels she can control, her body. Much of her behavior is obsessively compulsive. Family systems theory imputes the behavior traits of anorexics to other family members as well. The "psychosomatic family" is then viewed as "controlling, perfectionistic, and nonconfrontational," descriptives that apply equally to their anorexic daughter (Brumberg 1988, p. 29).

As with other psychiatric disorders, mothers are targeted as contributing to the disease. The mother of the anorexic is described as frustrated, depressed, perfectionistic, passive, dependent, and unable to see and reflect her daughter as an independent being (Brumberg, 1988, p. 30). Allegedly, preoedipal mother conflict arises from a young girl's identification with her kind, passive father, and suppressed hostility towards an aggressive, castrating mother (Boskins-Lodahl, 1976, pp. 344–45). The anorexic's intense, unconscious hatred of her mother leads to rejection of femininity in general. The straight-chested appearance and amenorrhea that anorexia involves are further signs of success in her avoidance of femininity.

The same problems found in the biological model of anorexia nervosa are present in the psychological model: incidence, gender, and socioeconomic features of the disease are not thereby explained. Which returns us to the socialization issue, and the cultural model as a limited response to those problems. In general, the incidence of anorexia nervosa has increased because society has intensified and extended the perception that thinness is a sign of fitness and attractiveness. Its message, like most new styles, has been "bought" most prevalently by those who have the time, energy and interest to buy it, i.e., affluent or moderately affluent white women.

Susan Bordo describes anorexia nervosa as a crystallization of the psychopathology of contemporary culture. It illustrates "the social manipulation of the female body" that has emerged "as an absolutely central strategy in the maintenance of power relations between the sexes over the last hundred years" (Bordo, 1985–86, pp. 76–77). The strategy has its roots in the metaphysical dualism that characterizes the writings of Plato, Augustine, and Descartes. It is a mind/body dualism that does not simply separate but prioritizes mind over body. To the extent that women are viewed (by themselves as well as by men) as sex objects valued solely or primarily for their bodies, sex inequality will inevitably prevail.

To Bordo the patriarchal Graeco-Christian tradition provides a "particularly fertile soil for the development of anorexia" (Bordo, 1985–86, p. 97). Popular American culture contributes to the development through its emphasis on control of the body, and the overcoming of its vulnerability through physical fitness. Paradoxically and tragically, although the will to conquer and subdue the body sometimes leads to an aesthetic or moral rebellion, "powerlessness is its most outstanding feature" (Bordo 1985–86, p. 85).

A sexual double standard is clearly to blame for the fact that anorexia so predominantly afflicts women more than men. According to Hilde Bruch, many anorexics are self-consciously aware of two selves that are in constant conflict: one a dominating male self that represents greater spirituality, intellectuality, and willpower; the other a female self that represents uncontrollable appetites and flaws (Bruch, 1979). It is the male self that the anorexic seeks to develop, precisely because it has been so ingrained in her that male is better. Presumably, the adolescent's sense of self-worth is most threatened by the fact that she knows she is female, and therefore a less valued or valuable human being than her male counterpart. Short of changing her social environment, improvement of her sense of self-worth requires helping her to see that worth independently of others' evaluations. This may be cognitively impossible.

FEMINIST CRITICISMS

Feminists are particularly prone to blame anorexia on gender socialization, and to propose socially corrective measures as preventive therapy, and feminist consciousness raising as individual therapy. For some feminists, however, anorexia nervosa is not only caused by a sexist culture, but constitutes a behavior that is antithetical to that culture. Construed in this way, anorexia nervosa does not involve enslavement to an unhealthy idea of the feminine, nor does it simply mean refusal to accept femininity. It means more than the latter: rebellion against patriarchy through rejection of one's own sexuality. Cases of anorexia nervosa in males may illustrate the same construal.

Liberal feminists[5] are likely to view sexism as a cause of anorexia, and to argue for elimination of the gender stereotyping that imposes so unequal a burden on women. In order to liberate women to develop their full potential as individuals, their options need to be expanded rather than restricted by an ideal of feminine behavior or appearance. Liberal feminism thus supports the right of individual women to pursue this or any ideal, even if it leads to unhealthy consequences for themselves, so long as the pursuit does not impede the liberty or welfare of others. In a capitalist society the means through which to fulfill the ideal of thinness are evident in the huge commercial success of diet, weight loss, and fitness programs that generally attract more women than men. Selling thinness has clearly become a profitable industry. The goal of liberal feminism is to preserve this social structure, but to rectify its sexist flaws. Given the embeddedness gender socialization within the structure, it is doubtful that so limited a critique could much reduce the impact of socialization as a cause of anorexia.

Radical feminism would extend its criticism of sexism as a cause of anorexia nervosa to a critique of the patriarchal structure that pervades society as a whole. The critique thus applies to women as a class rather than as individuals. Women become an exploited class in a system wherein men profit by the feminine ideal of thinness. As Susie Orbach put it, "Fat is a feminist issue" because it exemplifies resistance to that ideal. A cult that has enshrined "slimness" as "the new god" is blasphemously anti-feminist and anti-woman (Orbach, 1982, pp. 27–31). The goal, then, is to recognize the patriarchal nature of the new god, to topple it by substituting a goddess that embodies an ideal of femininity that takes account of the fact that healthy women come in all shapes and sizes, even as men do. In Orbach's words,

> Some of us are short, some of us are tall. We can have short legs, medium-length legs, long legs, big breasts, medium-size breasts, small breasts, . . . large, medium or small hips; we can be pear-shaped, broad or rounded, have flat stomachs, full stomachs, even teeth, crooked teeth, large eyes, dimpled cheeks. (Orbach, 1982, p. 27)

Men of course come in all shapes and sizes also. While tallness remains an advantage to them as well as to some women, society generally accepts a broader range of physical shapes and sizes for men than for women.

A socialist version of feminism would concur with the radical version, particularly targeting the inequality of a social system that creates needs out of desires provoked by a profit motive. Anorexia nervosa exemplifies the dehumanizing effects of such a system. If the feminine ideal were stripped of its debilitating impact on the development of women as individuals, and a masculine ideal were similarly cleansed of its impeding influence on men, then a socialist ideal of equality might be approximated. Socialist feminism would not eschew concern about obesity and health for women, but unlike radical feminism, it would have equal concern about such matters for men. In other words, equality, construed as respect for differences as well as potential among individuals of either gender, would be the criterion governing any ideal of body size or fitness.

Although socialism is in disrepute these days, socialist feminism represents an extension of the radical feminist critique to other social classes, and a critique of the excesses of individualism that liberalism permits. Socialist feminists oppose a free market system that allows affluence in the midst of poverty. Because anorexia nervosa occurs mainly among the affluent, a more equitable distribution of income might reduce its incidence. In other words, anorexia nervosa occurs in part because of the power of a free market system to define a profitable ideal of feminine beauty, and to persuade many women of the necessity of conforming to it. Adolescents, unfortunately, are especially vulnerable to this persuasion. While predisposing biological and psychological factors are also at work, the impact of the social environment fashioned by the marketeers is undeniable.

There is another factor that may contribute to the high incidence of anorexia nervosa among adolescent girls, in contrast with their male counterparts: the ambiguity that many women experience throughout their lives because of conflicts precipitated (in part at least) by gender socialization and social practices. Years ago Simone de Beauvoir defined ambiguity as characteristic of the female sex (de Beauvoir, 1972, p. 133). Despite the progress of the women's movement, ambiguity remains a common experience of women who struggle to maintain a healthy balance between home and work responsibilities, while their male counterparts are rarely expected or inclined to devote comparable energies to both sets of tasks. When daughters observe the conflicts their mothers confront and the discrepancy between their and their brothers' future prospects, they experience similar ambiguity. To the extent that pressures exerted by normative gender roles are reduced, the ambiguity may be resolved.

For anti-feminists, another means of resolving ambiguity, and thus reducing the incidence of anorexia nervosa among adolescents, is to revert to the days before "women's liberation," when gender stereotypes were generally unchallenged, and little ambiguity or conflict existed with regard to women's options (Brumberg, 1988, p. 38). This position ignores two facts: most women deal successfully and enthusiastically with a broader range of options; and the prevalence of anorexia nervosa in women predates the modern women's movement. Ambiguity is not a problem for most women or men if it simply represents a range of pursuable options. If it involves increased responsibilities with no corresponding increase in opportunities or support for their fulfillment, then the ambiguity has an overall negative impact. According to Carol Gilligan, such ambiguity is greater in girls because of their desire to maintain attachments while establishing their own identity. In *Mapping the Moral Domain*, she writes: "In resisting detachment and critiquing exclusion adolescent girls hold to the view that change can be negotiated through voice, and that voice is the way to sustain attachment across the leavings of adolescence" (Gilligan, 1988, p. 148).

Typically, the adolescent's "exit" from childhood leaves a problem of loyalty that she tries to negotiate through use of her own voice. The anorexic's voice is loud at first, but destined to be silenced by weakness, sickness, or even death from the disease. Her desire to be loyal to herself as well as to others inevitably leads to ambiguity. Bruch describes the ambiguity as a conflict between two selves. By dual accounts of anorexic behavior, feminists also suggest a conflict: one between conformity to a socially induced unhealthy stereotype, and refusal to accept the sexist connotations of being female. I believe the anorexic is in fact affirming both messages. Ironically, the messages converge in the reality of the anorexic's behavior, defining the content of her ambiguity: to be or not be a woman.

This returns us to the earlier point about the effect of gender socialization and the fact that anorexia nervosa is not linked with gender identity disorders in the *DSM-III-R*. So awful a disease deserves fuller critique of its social as well as biological and psychological causes. Physicians in various specialties have often defined their professional responsibilities as encompassing attempts to correct the social causes of illness—e.g., by lobbying against cigarette advertisements and by organizing other physicians to speak out against the development of nuclear weapons. Just as social behaviors need to be modified for therapeutic reasons in these cases, so also with gender socialization as a cause of anorexia nervosa. Therapeutic effectiveness calls for efforts to limit the health threatening effects of gender stereotypes.

NOTES

I wish to thank the following for their helpful comments and criticism in preparing this article: Regina C. Casper, Loretta M. Kopelman, François Primeau, Morton Silverman, and Nada Stotland.

1. Although both diseases occur in some individuals, bulimic anorectics, unlike restrictive anorectics, have been characterized as outgoing, articulate, socially confident, sexually experienced, and less optimistic before the onset of their illness (Casper, Eckert, Helmi et al., 1980, pp. 1030–40).

2. It is unlikely that the *DSM-IV*, now in preparation, will alter the classification or diagnostic criteria for anorexia nervosa. I base this observation on a talk on "*DSM-IV*—Work in Progress" by Allen J. Frances, M.D., who heads the Nomenclature Task Force of the American Psychiatric

Association, at the annual meeting of the American Orthopsychiatric Association in 1990 in Miami Beach, Florida. In order to align *DSM-IV* classifications as much as possible with the 10th edition of the International Classification of Diseases, which appeared in 1993, Dr. Frances indicated that controversial revisions will be avoided, with changes made only on the basis of compelling evidence.

3. Heilbrun cites studies by Emmerich, Bray, Helper Johnson, Mussen and Distler. In contrast to clear and consistent findings that father-identification in boys is consistent with good subsequent adjustment, Heilbrun considers the findings of studies regarding mother-identification in girls to be equivocal.

4. Exceptions to this trend include Marlene Boskind-Lodahl (1976), Toby Sitnick and Jack Katz (1984), Susan Bordo (1985–86), and Susie Orbach (1982).

5. Labels for the versions of feminism here described could be debated. My use, however, is consistent with Jaggar's account in *Feminist Politics and Human Nature* (1983), and with Tong's more recent *Feminist Thought* (1989).

BIBLIOGRAPHY

Block, J. H. "Conceptions of sex role: Some cross-cultural and longitudinal perspectives." *American Psychologist* 28 (1973): 64–78.

Bordo, S. "Anorexia nervosa: Psychopathology as the crystallization of culture." *Philosophical Forum* 17 (1985–86): 73–104.

Boskind-Lodahl, M. "Cinderella's stepsisters: A feminist perspective on anorexia nervosa and bulimia." *Signs: Journal of Women in Culture and Society* 1 (1976): 342–56.

Bruch, H. *The Golden Cage.* New York: Vintage, 1979.

Brumberg, J. J. *Fasting Girls.* Cambridge: Harvard University Press, 1988.

Crisp, A. H. and T. Burns. "Primary anorexia nervosa in the male and female: A comparison of clinical features and prognosis." In *Males with Eating Disorders,* edited by A. E. Andersen, 77–99. New York: Brurmer/Mazel, 1990.

de Beauvoir, S. *The Second Sex.* Translated by H. M. Parshley. New York: Alfred A. Knopf, 1972.

Diagnostic and Statistical Manual of Mental Disorders. 3d ed. revised *(DSM-III-R)*: 1987, American Psychiatric Association, Washington, D.C.

Garfinkel, P. E., and D. M. Garner. *Anorexia Nervosa.* New York: Brunner-Mazel, 1982.

Gilligan, C. "Exit-voice dilemmas in adolescent development." In *Mapping the Moral Domain,* edited by C. Gilligan et al., 141–57. Cambridge: Harvard University Press, 1988.

Goleman, D. "Stereotypes of the sexes said to persist in therapy." *New York Times,* 10 April 1990, pp. C1, C10.

Gordon, R. A. "A socio and cultural interpretation of the current epidemic of eating disorders," in *The Eating Disorders,* edited by B. J. Blinder, B. F. Chaitin, and R. S. Goldstein, 151–63. New York: PMA Publishing Company, 1988.

Heilbrun, A. B., Jr. "Sex-role identity in adolescent females: A theoretical paradox." *Adolescence* 3 (1968): 79–88.

Hill, J. P., and M. E. Lynch. "The intensification of gender-related role expectations during early adolescence," in *Girls at Puberty: Biological and Psychosocial Perspectives,* edited by J. Brook-Gunn and A. C. Peterson, 201–28. New York: Plenum, 1983.

Jaggar, A. M. *Feminist Politics and Human Nature.* Totowa, N.J.: Rowman and Allanheld, 1983.

Lawrence, M. "Anorexia nervosa—the control paradox," *Women's Studies International Quarterly* 2 (1979): 93–101.

Lawson, C. "Anorexia: It's not a new disease." *New York Times,* 8 December 1985, p. 93.

Leichner, P., and A. Gertler. "Prevalence and incidence studies of anorexia nervosa," in *The Eating Disorders,* edited by B. J. Blinder, B. F. Chaitin, and R. S. Goldstein, 131–49. New York: PMA Publishing Company, 1988.

Leon, G. R., and S. Finn. 1984, "Sex-role stereotypes and the development of eating disorders," *Sex Roles and Psychopathology,* edited by C. S. Widom, 317–37. New York: Plenum, 1984.

Mahowald, M. B. "Sex-role stereotypes in medicine," *Hypatia* 2 (1987): 21–38.

Nylander, I. "The feeling of being fat and dieting in a school population," *Acta Socio-Medica Scandinavia* 1 (1971): 17–26.

Orbach, S. *Fat is a Feminist Issue.* New York: Berkeley, 1982. 27–31.

Pettinati, H. M., J. H. Wade, V. Franks, L. G. Kogan. "Distinguishing the role of eating disturbance from depression in the sex role self-perceptions of anorexic and bulimic inpatients," *Journal of Abnormal Psychology* 96 (August 1987): 280–82.

Simmons, R. G., D. A. Blyth, K. L. McKinnery. "The social and psychological effects of puberty on white females," in *Girls at Puberty: Biological and Psychosocial Perspectives,* edited by J. Brooks-Gunn and A. C. Peterson, 229–72. New York: Plenum, 1983.

Sitnick, T., and J. L. Katz. "Sex role identity and anorexia nervosa," *International Journal of Eating Disorders* 3 (1984): 81–89.

Sontag, S. *Illness as Metaphor.* New York: Farrar, Straus and Giroux, 1978.

Tong, R. *Feminist Thought.* Boulder: Westview, 1989.

PART TWO

Fiction, Poetry, and Drama

SECTION A
Abnormal Weight and Eating Disorders

Washing Your Feet

JOHN CIARDI

Washing your feet is hard when you get fat.

*   *   *

In lither times the act was unstrained and pleasurable.

*   *   *

You spread the toes for signs of athlete's foot.

*   *   *

You used creams, and rubbing alcohol, and you powdered.

*   *   *

You bent over, all in order, and did everything.

*   *   *

Mary Magdalene made a prayer meeting of it.

*   *   *

She, of course, was washing not her feet but God's.

*   *   *

Degas painted ladies washing their own feet.

*   *   *

Somehow they also seem to be washing God's feet.

*   *   *

To touch any body anywhere should be ritual.

*   *   *

To touch one's own body anywhere should be ritual.

*   *   *

Fat makes the ritual wheezy and a bit ridiculous.

*   *   *

Ritual and its idea should breathe easy.

*   *   *

They are memorial, meditative, immortal.

*   *   *

Toenails keep growing after one is dead.

*   *   *

Washing my feet, I think of immortal toenails.

*   *   *

What are they doing on these ten crimped polyps?

*   *   *

I reach to wash them and begin to wheeze.

*   *   *

I wish I could paint like Degas or believe like Mary.

*   *   *

It is sad to be naked and to lack talent.

*   *   *

It is sad to be fat and to have dirty feet.

The Six Hundred Pound Man

JACK COULEHAN

Of the six hundred pound man on two beds,
nothing remains,
not the bleariness with which he moved his eyes
nor the warm oil curling in his beard.

Though the sheets and plastic bags are gone,
his grunts, his kind acceptance gone,
I see him now, rising in the distance,
an island, mountainous
and hooded with impenetrable vine.

When I awaken to the death
of the six hundred pound man
and cannot sleep again,
I paddle to his shore

in search of those flamboyant trees
that flame his flanks,
in search of bougainvillea
blossoming his thighs,
of women who rise to touch him
tenderly with ointment,

in search of healers, singers
who wrestle souls of old bodies
back to bones, back to dirt, and back back
to their beginnings.

As I enter for the first time
this medicine circle,
bearing chickens in honor of the god,
words dancing from my lips,

spirit like the plume of a child's volcano
rises

and then the medicine, the medicine is good
and the tongues, the tongues are dancing
and the fathers, oh! the fathers are dancing

and this worthless and alien body,
this six hundred pound man,
I discover him beautiful.

Fat

RAYMOND CARVER

I AM SITTING over coffee and cigarettes at my friend Rita's and I am telling her about it.

Here is what I tell her.

It is late of a slow Wednesday when Herb seats the fat man at my station.

This fat man is the fattest person I have ever seen, though he is neat-appearing and well dressed enough. Everything about him is big. But it is the fingers I remember best. When I stop at the table near his to see to the old couple, I first notice the fingers. They look three times the size of a normal person's fingers—long, thick, creamy fingers.

I see to my other tables, a party of four businessmen, very demanding, another party of four, three men and a woman, and this old couple. Leander has poured the fat man's water, and I give the fat man plenty of time to make up his mind before going over.

Good evening, I say. May I serve you? I say.

Rita, he was big, I mean big.

Good evening, he says. Hello. Yes, he says. I think we're ready to order now, he says.

He has this way of speaking—strange, don't you know. And he makes a little puffing sound every so often.

I think we will begin with a Caesar salad, he says. And then a bowl of soup with some extra bread and butter, if you please. The lamb chops, I believe, he says. And baked potato with sour cream. We'll see about dessert later. Thank you very much, he says, and hands me the menu.

God, Rita, but those were fingers.

I hurry away to the kitchen and turn in the order to Rudy, who takes it with a face. You know Rudy. Rudy is that way when he works.

As I come out of the kitchen, Margo—I've told you about Margo? The one who chases Rudy? Margo says to me, Who's your fat friend? He's really a fatty.

. . .

Now that's part of it. I think that is really part of it.

I make the Caesar salad there at his table, him watching my every move, meanwhile buttering pieces of bread and laying them off to one side, all the time making this puffing noise. Anyway, I am so keyed up or something, I knock over his glass of water.

I'm so sorry, I say. It always happens when you get into a hurry. I'm very sorry, I say. Are you all right? I'll get the boy to clean up right away, I say.

It's nothing, he says. It's all right, he says, and he puffs. Don't worry about it, we don't mind, he says. He smiles and waves as I go off to get Leander, and when I come back to serve the salad, I see the fat man has eaten all his bread and butter.

A little later, when I bring him more bread, he has finished his salad. You know the size of those Caesar salads?

You're very kind, he says. This bread is marvelous, he says.

Thank you, I say.

Well, it is very good, he says, and we mean that. We don't often enjoy bread like this, he says.

Where are you from? I ask him. I don't believe I've seen you before, I say.

He's not the kind of person you'd forget, Rita puts in with a snicker.

Denver, he says.

I don't say anything more on the subject, though I am curious.

Your soup will be along in a few minutes, sir, I say, and I go off to put the finishing touches to my party of four businessmen, very demanding.

When I serve his soup, I see the bread has disappeared again. He is just putting the last piece of bread into his mouth.

Believe me, he says, we don't eat like this all the time, he says. And puffs. You'll have to excuse us, he says.

Don't think a thing about it, please, I say. I like to see a man eat and enjoy himself, I say.

I don't know, he says. I guess that's what you'd call it. And puffs. He arranges the napkin. Then he picks up his spoon.

God, he's fat! says Leander.

He can't help it, I say, so shut up.

I put down another basket of bread and more butter. How was the soup? I say.

Thank you. Good, he says. Very good, he says. He wipes his lips and dabs his chin. Do you think it's warm in here, or is it just me? he says.

No, it is warm in here, I say.

Maybe we'll take off our coat, he says.

Go right ahead, I say. A person has to be comfortable, I say.

That's true, he says, that is very, very true, he says.

But I see a little later that he is still wearing his coat.

My large parties are gone now and also the old couple. The place is emptying out. By the time I serve the fat man his chops and baked potato, along with more bread and butter, he is the only one left.

I drop lots of sour cream onto his potato. I sprinkle bacon and chives over his sour cream. I bring him more bread and butter.

Is everything all right? I say.

Fine, he says, and he puffs. Excellent, thank you, he says, and puffs again.

Enjoy your dinner, I say. I raise the lid of his sugar bowl and look in. He nods and keeps looking at me until I move away.

I know now I was after something. But I don't know what.

How is old tub-of-guts doing? He's going to run your legs off, says Harriet. You know Harriet.

For dessert, I say to the fat man, there is the Green Lantern Special, which is a pudding cake with sauce, or there is cheesecake or vanilla ice cream or pineapple sherbet.

We're not making you late, are we? he says, puffing and looking concerned.

Not at all, I say. Of course not, I say. Take your time, I say. I'll bring you more coffee while you make up your mind.

We'll be honest with you, he says. And he moves in the seat. We would like the Special, but we may have a dish of vanilla ice cream as well. With just a drop of chocolate syrup, if you please. We told you we were hungry, he says.

I go off to the kitchen to see after his dessert myself, and Rudy says, Harriet says you got a fat man from the circus out there. That true?

Rudy has his apron and hat off now, if you see what I mean.

Rudy, he is fat, I say, but that is not the whole story.

Rudy just laughs.

Sounds to me like she's sweet on fat-stuff, he says.

Better watch out, Rudy, says Joanne, who just that minute comes into the kitchen.

I'm getting jealous, Rudy says to Joanne.

I put the Special in front of the fat man and a big bowl of vanilla ice cream with chocolate syrup to the side.

Thank you, he says.

You are very welcome, I say—and a feeling comes over me.

Believe it or not, he says, we have not always eaten like this.

Me, I eat and I eat and I can't gain, I say. I'd like to gain, I say.

No, he says. If we had our choice, no. But there is no choice.

Then he picks up his spoon and eats.

What else? Rita says, lighting one of my cigarettes and pulling her chair closer to the table. This story's getting interesting now, Rita says.

That's it. Nothing else. He eats his desserts, and then he leaves and then we go home, Rudy and me.

Some fatty, Rudy says, stretching like he does when he's tired. Then he just laughs and goes back to watching the TV.

I put the water on to boil for tea and take a shower. I put my hand on my middle and wonder what would happen if I had children and one of them turned out to look like that, so fat.

I pour the water in the pot, arrange the cups, the sugar bowl, carton of half and half, and take the tray in to Rudy. As if he's been thinking about it, Rudy says, I knew a fat guy once, a couple of fat guys, really fat guys, when I was a kid. They were tubbies, my God. I don't remember their names. Fat, that's the only name this one kid had. We called him Fat, the kid who lived next door to me. He was a neighbor. The other kid came along later. His name was Wobbly. Everybody called him Wobbly except the teachers. Wobbly and Fat. Wish I had their pictures, Rudy says.

I can't think of anything to say, so we drink our tea and pretty soon I get up to go to bed. Rudy gets up too, turns off the TV, locks the front door, and begins his unbuttoning.

I get into bed and move clear over to the edge and lie there on my stomach. But right away, as soon as he turns off the light and gets into bed, Rudy begins. I turn on my back and relax some, though it is against my will. But here is the thing. When he gets on me, I suddenly feel I am fat.

I feel I am terrifically fat, so fat that Rudy is a tiny thing and hardly there at all.

That's a funny story, Rita says, but I can see she doesn't know what to make of it.

I feel depressed. But I won't go into it with her. I've already told her too much.

She sits there waiting, her dainty fingers poking her hair.

Waiting for what? I'd like to know.

It is August.

My life is going to change. I feel it.

Weight Bearing

PATRICIA GOEDICKE

Opening the door to a fat person
Is like drowning, sometimes you think you can't stand it,

What are all those immense, painfully thick slabs

Of skin built up to hold out
Or in?

Poured into himself like concrete,
Like a candle big as an elephant that has gone out,

Sweat beads on the forehead
Of the young Kiowa sitting in my office.

With hair so black you'd think it came from a box,
In shirts fragrant with Tide,

With sides drooping all over my tiny chair
Like a grand piano in soft sculpture

He lets kids climb on him like puppies.

The murmur of his soft voice
Surrounds all sides of the subject like honey,

But if he is a messenger what has he got to say?

Wind passes its rough hand over the keyboard,
Then sighs.

In the vast folds of his body

First there is the hissing of warm breath,
Then there is all that flesh pressing against its own belt buckle.

How does he manage to sit, stand, breathe?
But he does, he tells me he's not had a drop to drink for months

And I believe him: self pity in liquid form
Is poison he doesn't need.

Besides, he has his own pupils to think of.

Back home on the reservation
The river is beginning to dry up.

The old stories disappear: whose grandmother
First spoke with Harvest Woman,

Whose uncle thought he could trick Coyote...

Next door a gang of white sociologists discusses the matter loudly,
Quarreling like magpies.

But who has time nowadays to listen?

The traffic ticket for speeding, the pain
Visiting his parents in a Home,

These things sink into the ground like blood,
Like antelope oil into earth

That has absorbed too much.

Expanding into the room like a balloon
Hotter and hotter, it is about to burst

And the young man knows it, he tries to say something,
Anything, at the center of himself he is starving,

He thinks he is a wild leaf snapping against the sky
And then folding, when there is no breeze

What food should he take to soothe him?

Heavy with lard, with the children heaped up on his back
He bows to suffering like a gentleman.

Out there on the mesa he is a lone cottonwood
Muttering to itself in the wind.

Anxious as a smoke signal looking left right left right
Finally there is no comforting the dry purplish lips

That shape words out of the air like waterless clouds
Scouring the land for sustenance.

Skanks

RENNIE SPARKS

DAWN AND ME eat scrambled eggs with tomato juice because we're on a diet. Dawn knows how to make herself throw up so she eats toast and butter too. I eat only English muffins because my fingers go so far down my throat, but nothing comes up. I'm a fat cow.

Dawn and me are best friends. I sleep over Dawn's house since my stepfather called me a pig for eating all his cocktail onions. I'm waiting for my mother to call and beg me back home, but it's been two weeks.

Every night we share Dawn's single bed with the quilted pink covers. We stay up late smoking cigarettes, the ashtray balanced between us on the sheets. We talk about love. Dawn loves guys who give long wet kisses. I love bites that last like red splashes on my neck for weeks. But, we both agree, we want to fall in love. Tonight, we're going to the Mall to fall in love.

Dawn's mother is divorced. Dawn calls her Lorraine instead of Mom. We smoke Lorraine's Marlboro Lights at the kitchen table with a green ashtray. Lorraine is in the shower. She's getting ready to go out with an optometrist she met at work. Lorraine works behind the counter at the U-Haul center on Motor parkway. The optometrist came in to rent a car-top to move his things out of his wife's house.

Lorraine models new underwear for us when she comes out of the shower. Her hair is slicked back and wet. The underwear is red lace with a fishnet heart in the bottom that shows her hair. Lorraine has bags under her eyes and chin. The shower has washed away her makeup. There is a long purple scar up Lorraine's stomach from where they had to pull Dawn out to get her born, but Lorraine's stomach is flat and tight. She must know how to throw up too.

Lorraine says, "Ta Da!"

"You look fox, Lorraine," Dawn says.

"You look really fox," I say.

. . .

The optometrist pulls up in a Pinto. He wears a blue jacket with suede patches on the elbows. Lorraine wears a red satin dress she bought at Shoes and Things at the Mall.

Lorraine says, "Dawn, I'll be home late or not at all." Dawn looks at me and says, "Skank."

Lorraine says, "Watch your mouth, lady."

The optometrist says, "Okay, Lorraine, is Seafood okay?"

"Okay, Mel," Lorraine says. They drive away.

Dawn and me work at the bakery after school. We mix raisins into cookie dough and squeeze frosting in swirls on birthday cakes. We eat only raw cookie dough at work because we're on a diet. Tonight, we have off and we're going to the Mall to look for babes. Dawn says if she falls in love at the Mall tonight she'll go out to the Pit.

"And leave me hanging out at the fountain!"

"No," Dawn says. She plugs in her curling iron. "There'll be a babe for you too. We'll find two babes and fall in love and make them take us to the Pit. And," she says as she puts the curling iron to her bangs, "They won't be named Mel. They'll be named Luke or Dougie."

Dawn's in love with Luke from General Hospital. We stare at his picture taped to Dawn's wall over her bed. Dawn says she'd wear crotchless panties to go to bed with him. I say I'd wear crotchless, edible panties to go to bed with him. Dawn says crotchless edible panties with strawberry flavor and we fall off the bed laughing until Dawn's brother screams, "Shut up" from the next room.

It's 7:30 and Dawn has to brush her teeth three times before we go out. I sit on her bed and listen to Pink Floyd coming through from her brother's room. Her brother goes to college. We don't talk to him. Dawn says college guys are skanks. Dawn's going to be a stewardess when she graduates or work at the U-Haul with her mother. I'm going to Wilfred Beauty Academy to learn how to do nails. I have two months until I graduate high school. Soon I'll be able to work full time at the bakery and save up for an apartment and tuition to Wilfred. When I get out of Wilfred, no one will call me a fat cow, they'll call me a beauty stylist.

Dawn says I'm her best friend for life. I can stay here as long as I want. My stepfather's a skank for hoarding cocktail onions anyway.

I have a new makeup stick in dark coral pink. I put it above my eyes like I saw in Beauty Digest. Dawn puts it on her cheeks and outlines her lips in

Burnt Sienna. She rubs a stick of musk behind her ears and under her arms and the room smells like a jungle.

We lie down flat on the bed next to each other to zip our jeans. When I stand there's a roll of fat over the waist band so I borrow a loose sweater with draw strings at the bottom. Dawn is straight and thin and wears padded bras that make tiny puff breasts in her tight tube top. I wish I could throw up like Dawn.

Dawn and me each swallow four of Lorraine's Dexitrims. We fluff our hair with rat tail combs. We grind up Lorraine's No-Doz on Dawn's compact mirror with a razor blade and pretend it's coke. We do three lines each with a cut-off Sweetheart straw. We steal only two of Lorraine's Valiums because those she counts.

Dawn calls the cab and we wrap Maxi Pads in tin foil and put them in our purses. Since I've been sleeping over, we get our periods at the same time. With tin foil around the pads we can open our purses in public and not have some skank scream, "Look, she's on the rag."

The cab lets us off at the Sears entrance and we go straight in through luggage to the Ladies bathroom. Dawn doesn't like the way her hair turned out so she wets it in the sink and kneels under the hand dryer, one knee on the tile floor, to do it over. I look at myself in the mirror. My hair and nails are perfect. I know how to copy the looks, but my cheeks are full and red, not hollow and sharp like Dawn's. Tomorrow I will eat nothing but cocktail onions.

We walk out to the benches around the fountain and see Carol and Gail. Carol's face looks thin and white and I'm instantly jealous. Carol was always a fat cow like me even though she won Miss Teen Angel last summer. Her picture was in the Smithtown News and she got two free tanning sessions at TanFastic. But, I was never jealous because I've seen her stomach roll to fat when she bends over in a bikini. But, Carol had to go to the Clinic last week for an abortion and threw up for two days after the anesthetic.

Two weeks before Carol went to the clinic she said, "Janine, walk with me to the Deli." So I walked with her to the Deli and got a Chef's Salad in a styrofoam bowl and Carol got change for the pay phone.

She called the Clinic. She said, "I got raped and I need the morning-after pill." The Clinic said she had to tell the police first or else pay for an abortion. Carol said, "Skank," and hung up the phone. She cried against gallon jars of dill pickles. I tried to put my arm around her and she said, "You smell like ham, Janine." I didn't care. Dawn's my best friend, not Carol.

Dawn and me sit down next to Gail and Carol by the fountain. Everybody likes Gail because she's beautiful and goes out with Joey Cosmo the absolute total babe of the school. Joey has a roll bar on his truck and four-wheel drive and even had his hair permed to look like a rock star.

Tonight Gail has made Chinese eyes with blue eyeliner. She has a tiny white pimple over one eye that never goes away. She has frosted hair that curls up at her shoulders. She looks long and lean in pink cords and a black sweater that shows white bra under her arm when she lifts a hand to flip her hair back from her face.

"What's up?" Gail says. She throws her cigarette into the fountain.

"Nothin'," I say.

"Carol and me are going to Rocky IV."

"You seen that five times."

"Yeah, but Carol likes the usher."

"The one with the blond hair?" Dawn says. "I seen him at school."

"Yeah," Carol says. "He's a babe. He gave me free popcorn last week. I'm in love."

"How you feelin' anyway, Carol?" I say. "You doin' all right?"

"Sure," Carol says. "I'm all right. I'm sleeping over Gail's till I feel better."

"That's cool," Dawn says. "Janine is staying over my house."

"How come?" Gail asks.

"My stepfather's a skank," I say.

"All stepfathers are skanks," Gail says. "My stepfather stole ten bucks from my purse last week."

Dawn and me lean back with our toes stretched out in high heels. I can feel the water spray across my back, but I don't move. The waist of my jeans feels like an iron band and I can hardly breathe.

I see three guys come walking out of McCrory's. Two in bomber jackets and one in a red leather.

Dawn nudges me. "Babes."

"They're all right."

"Babes," Dawn says. "Come on, Janine."

"Come on, Dawn. We just sat down. I'm tired."

"Look at the babe in the red leather, Janine. You saw him looking at me."

"We could get a pretzel at Sears and just hang out for awhile."

"Janine, do you want to be a fat cow all your life? Come on. The blond one isn't so bad. He's got long hair. Let's go for it."

"All right." I follow Dawn as she goes after the babes. They strut around the corner with long pink combs sticking out of their back pockets. Dawn's right. I have to do something if I don't want to be a fat cow all my life.

They go into Orange Julius and Dawn clicks fast on high heels behind them. The two bomber jackets buy chili dogs, but the red leather buys fries. He turns as he squirts ketchup. He has sea green eyes. I feel a butterfly flapping its wings in my stomach, but I try and look at the blond one like Dawn wants. She's my best friend.

"What's up?" the red leather says to Dawn. He smiles and I see his teeth are white and clean. He has dyed black hair with brown roots.

"Nothin'," Dawn says. They both laugh. I try and give a look at the blond one. His hair is long, but hangs flat against the sides of his face. His body is round and short and reminds me of Barney Rubble, but I'm a fat cow, so I give him a smile.

I order cheese fries and me and Dawn get a booth. We suck cheese off the fries and put them back on the plate. I eat only five. Dawn sucks down all the cheese. She can. She's already thrown up twice today.

The red leather babe comes over to our table. The other two stay back at the booth playing football with the ashtray.

Red leather says, "Hey, I'm Markie."

"Hey," Dawn says.

Markie says, "What's up?"

"Nothin'," Dawn says.

"You into hangin' out?"

"Sure," Dawn says. "I'm Dawn and this is my best friend Janine."

"Hey, Janine," Markie says. He's a definite babe. Tall and thin with hollow cheekbones.

"Hey," I say. I suck in my cheeks and grab the loose skin inside my mouth with my back teeth.

"Listen," Dawn says. She gives a look—perfect, all eyes and lips. "Janine was checking out your friend with the blond hair. She's in love with him." Dawn flips back her hair and pulls down her tube top.

Markie says, "Oh, that's Stevie. He's cool. He's my best friend. He'd be into hangin' out." He presses a hip into the edge of our table. Dawn's fingers stroke the table top.

"Cool," Dawn says. She stands up, brushes against Markie. "We gotta go to the bathroom. We'll meet you by the Macy's exit."

In the Macy's bathroom, I open my eyes as wide as possible. I can feel the tears building up at the edge of my mascara. "I can't believe you, Dawn." My voice is heavy and scratched.

"What," Dawn says. She's putting on strawberry lip gloss with her fingertip. "What the fuck is wrong with you, Janine?"

"I don't wanna hang out with those guys is all." I press my index fingers to the corners of my eyes as hard as I can. The tips of my fingers turn black. There's a noise at the back of my throat that wants to come out, but I won't let it.

"Oh man," Dawn says. "You're copping out on me." She puts down the tube of lip gloss on the shelf under the mirror. She stares at me. "Look," she says. "Are you my best friend or not?"

"You know I'm your best friend." My voice cracks in half. I carefully wipe away the black line down my cheek with a twisted end of Kleenex. "I just don't feel like getting stuck with that blond guy. He's a skank. You know it, Dawn."

"That's bullshit, Janine. You're copping out on me." A lady comes in the bathroom carrying a big shopping bag. She goes into a stall. Dawn turns on the hand dryer so that lady won't hear us talk.

"Look," Dawn says. "If you're my best friend you'll do this for me. Besides, only my *best* friend can sleep over my house tonight."

"You're a skank, Dawn. I can't believe you." Two more black lines run down my cheeks. I bite down hard on the side of my tongue to keep my hand steady wiping away the black. I get out my compact and brush more powder across my cheekbones.

"Look," Dawn says, "You don't have to do anything. I just don't want to be alone with Markie the first time. You know. Just come hang out. We'll stay together. Nothing's gonna happen. Would you stop crying. God, are you in sixth grade or what?"

"All right," I say. My face is white and glowing again in the mirror. I open my eyes wide and put on a fresh coat of mascara. "Okay, Dawn, but, I'm only doing this 'cause you're my best friend." We head to the Macy's exit and they're waiting by the door. Markie sees us and pulls the wig crooked on a mannequin to show off. I smile the widest biggest smile I can manage and stretch my laugh as long as it'll go.

"Hey, what's up," Markie says. "Glad you could make it, girls. Janine, this is my best bud, Stevie. He's all right."

"Hi, Stevie," I say. I bend my lips up in a smile. Dawn is giggling with her hand over her mouth to hide her teeth.

"What's up," Stevie says. His eyes are crooked and small like they're the wrong size for his face.

We go out into the parking lot. It's dark out and the lights shine down on parked cars as we walk out to the strip of grass that separates the highway from Macy's parking lot. Thick green bushes are planted in a row to the ENTRANCE and EXIT signs lit up fluorescent to separate the two lanes in and out of the parking lot. Dawn and me lean against ENTER and Stevie and Markie stand across from us. Markie has a pint of Southern Comfort and he passes it around.

"So," Markie says. "What's up."

"I'm cold," Dawn says.

"Here," Markie says. He takes off his jacket and wraps it around Dawn. He leaves his arm on her shoulder and suddenly they're going at it. Dawn falls against the ENTER sign with a bang and I move away quick as Markie presses her into the sign with his hips and they're making out.

I look at Stevie and out at the cars streaming by on the highway. Stevie makes a noise in his throat and spits on the ground.

"What's up," Stevie says.

"Nothing," I say.

Stevie puts his arm around me. Markie has a hand up Dawn's shirt. I feel Stevie's hand pushing hard against the side of my breast. Markie says, "How 'bout we take this party down in the Pit?"

Dawn looks at me. "Come on, Janine." I shake my head, no.

Dawn says, "Markie, hang out, I gotta talk to Janine private."

Dawn and me go behind the EXIT sign. "Don't make me, Dawn." Dawn looks sweaty. Her makeup rises like a film over her face.

"Janine," she says. "You want a place to stay tonight?"

"But, Dawn!" It's dark enough outside that I let the mascara run down my face. It feels good like letting the plug out of the bathtub. Dawn shakes her head at me. She flips back her hair off her shoulders and steps back.

"Janine, look at yourself in a mirror sometime. You think you can do better than Stevie?"

We cross the highway and take a path down into the woods we call the Pit. It's just dug-up land from where they took the dirt to make the cement for the mall. Thin pine trees planted along the highway block out the street lights and sticker bushes divide the pit into tiny pathways and openings. Stevie has a hand on my ass. He whispers in my ear.

"You got a nice ass," he says. "That's like the first thing I noticed." Markie and Dawn have disappeared into the woods around us.

I call, "Dawn," but there's no answer. Stevie says, "Ssssh, relax, baby. Don't worry about your friend. She's with Markie. He's cool."

We walk a ways and find an overturned shopping cart. He sits down. I go to sit down next to him but he grabs my head tight over my ears so everything sounds like an ocean and behind the roar from far away I can hear him.

He says, "I love you. I love you. I love you."

He pushes my face into his zipper and I smell sex through his jeans. I open my eyes, and the darkness is the same. For a second I think I've gone blind, but then the gold thread along the zipper of his jeans appears. Tears are running into my mouth. The taste of salt mixed with that awful smell.

I try, I try so hard for Dawn, for my best friend, I try to keep my face pressed against the zipper, but I can't. I pull away and stand up.

"You're a skank," I say.

"Hey, come on, baby," Stevie says. "I really like you a lot. Help me out here."

"Dawn," I yell. There's no answer. "I'm going," I say.

"Hey, come on," Stevie says. "What are you on the rag or something?"

I turn and walk back up the path to the lights of the highway. I turn and yell once more for Dawn. There's no answer. I know if I walk back up to the Mall I will be doing something awful. I know as soon as I step out of the woods I won't have a best friend.

Stevie yells after me, "It's your loss, babe!"

I yell back, "Well, fuck yourself."

He yells back, "Fuck *yourself*, fat girl."

I run. I run through lines of parked cars and I run into Macy's and I run through lingerie and pantyhose and piles of scarves. I run through Macy's to the center of the mall and I have to stop as a burning cramp squeezes the side of my stomach.

The benches by the fountain are empty. I am all alone. Suddenly, I realize that I have nowhere to sleep tonight. I've gone over the edge. I'm not a fat cow anymore, I'm worse. I'm alone in the mall without a friend. I'm a skank.

I go in Anthony's and buy three slices with pepperoni. I eat the slices as fast as I can. My throat burns with swallowing so fast. I get up and run into Sears' bathroom. I turn on the hand dryer so no one will hear. I lean down over the bowl, one hand holding on to the toilet paper roll. The other hand turns into a knife and I stick it down into my throat until my stomach starts to shake and my mouth gags open wide and the pizza rushes back up my throat.

I lean against the wall of the stall, my head against the coat hook. My stomach feels thin and flat, empty. And just for one second I feel beautiful.

Fat People at the Amusement Park

RAWDON TOMLINSON

They are laughing like the rest of us,
amused at being here
among bright lights and whirling things

laughing, despite their particular knowledge
of gravity, which is why they ride
the fastest and highest rides,

a release from the demands of earth
between bouts with blue cotton candy,
stuffed bears and peanuts—

we watch them bounce along the midway
with their rosy-cheeked smiles and jouncing
asses, chattering as though they'd entered

the kingdom, they step into the cars
of the tilt-a-whirl, tilting, and take off
into a scream of weightlessness.

The Fat Girl

ANDRE DUBUS

HER NAME WAS Louise. Once when she was sixteen a boy kissed her at a barbecue; he was drunk and he jammed his tongue into her mouth and ran his hands up and down her hips. Her father kissed her often. He was thin and kind and she could see in his eyes when he looked at her the lights of love and pity.

It started when Louise was nine. You must start watching what you eat, her mother would say. I can see you have my metabolism. Louise also had her mother's pale blonde hair. Her mother was slim and pretty, carried herself erectly, and ate very little. The two of them would eat bare lunches, while her older brother ate sandwiches and potato chips, and then her mother would sit smoking while Louise eyed the bread box, the pantry, the refrigerator. Wasn't that good, her mother would say. In five years you'll be in high school and if you're fat the boys won't like you; they won't ask you out. Boys were as far away as five years, and she would go to her room and wait for nearly an hour until she knew her mother was no longer thinking of her, then she would creep into the kitchen and, listening to her mother talking on the phone, or her footsteps upstairs, she would open the bread box, the pantry, the jar of peanut butter. She would put the sandwich under her shirt and go outside or to the bathroom to eat it.

Her father was a lawyer and made a lot of money and came home looking pale and happy. Martinis put color back in his face, and at dinner he talked to his wife and two children. Oh give her a potato, he would say to Louise's mother. She's a growing girl. Her mother's voice then became tense: If she has a potato she shouldn't have dessert. She should have both, her father would say, and he would reach over and touch Louise's cheek or hand or arm.

In high school she had two girl friends and at night and on week-ends they rode in a car or went to movies. In movies she was fascinated by fat actresses. She wondered why they were fat. She knew why she was fat: she was fat because she was Louise. Because God had made her that way. Because she wasn't like her friends, Joan and Marjorie, who drank milk shakes after school and were all bones and tight skin. But what about those actresses, with their talents, with their broad and profound faces? Did they eat as heedlessly as Bishop Humphries and his wife who sometimes came to dinner and, as Louise's mother said, gorged between amenities? Or did they try to lose weight, did they go about hungry and angry and thinking of food? She thought of them eating lean meats and salads with friends, and then going home and building strange large sandwiches with French bread. But mostly she believed they did not go through these failures; they were fat because they chose to be. And she was certain of something else too: she could see it in their faces: they did not eat secretly. Which she did: her creeping to the kitchen when she was nine became, in high school, a ritual of deceit and pleasure. She was a furtive eater of sweets. Even her two friends did not know her secret.

Joan was thin, gangling, and flat-chested; she was attractive enough and all she needed was someone to take a second look at her face, but the school was large and there were pretty girls in every classroom and walking all the corridors, so no one ever needed to take a second look at Joan. Marjorie was thin too, an intense, heavy-smoking girl with brittle laughter. She was very intelligent, and with boys she was shy because she knew she made them uncomfortable, and because she was smarter than they were and so could not understand or could not believe the levels they lived on. She was to have a nervous breakdown before earning her Ph.D. in philosophy at the University of California, where she met and married a physicist and discovered within herself an untrammelled passion: she made love with her husband on the couch, the carpet, in the bathtub, and on the washing machine. By that time much had happened to her and she never thought of Louise. Joan would finally stop growing and begin moving with grace and confidence. In college she would have two lovers and then several more during the six years she spent in Boston before marrying a middle-aged editor who had two sons in their early teens, who drank too much, who was tenderly, boyishly grateful for her love, and whose wife had been killed while rock-climbing in New Hampshire with her lover. She would not think of Louise either, except in an earlier time, when lovers were still new to her and she was ecstatically surprised each time one of them loved her and, sometimes at night, lying in a man's arms, she would tell how in high school no one dated her, she had been thin and plain (she would still believe that: that she had been plain; it had never been true) and so had been forced into the week-end and night-time company of a neurotic smart girl and a shy fat girl. She would say this with self-pity exaggerated by Scotch and her need to be more deeply loved by the man who held her.

She never eats, Joan and Marjorie said of Louise. They ate lunch with her at school, watched her refusing potatoes, ravioli, fried fish. Sometimes she got through the cafeteria line with only a salad. That is how they would remember her: a girl whose hapless body was destined to be fat. No one saw the sandwiches she made and took to her room when she came home from school. No one saw the store of Milky Ways, Butterfingers, Almond Joys, and Hersheys far back on her closet shelf, behind the stuffed animals of her childhood. She was not a hypocrite. When she was out of the house she truly believed she was dieting; she forgot about the candy, as a man speaking into his office dictaphone may forget the lewd photographs hidden in an old shoe in his closet. At other times, away from home, she thought of the waiting candy with near lust. One night driving home from a movie, Marjorie said: "You're lucky you don't smoke; it's in*cred*ible what I go through to hide it from my parents." Louise turned to her a smile which was elusive and mysterious; she yearned to be home in bed, eating chocolate in the dark. She did not need to smoke; she already had a vice that was insular and destructive.

She brought it with her to college. She thought she would leave it behind. A move from one place to another, a new room without the haunted closet shelf, would do for her what she could not do for herself. She packed her large dresses and went. For two weeks she was busy with registration, with shyness, with classes; then she began to feel at home. Her room was no longer like a motel. Its walls had stopped watching her, she felt they were her friends, and she gave them her secret. Away from her mother, she did not have to be as elaborate; she kept the candy in her drawer now.

The school was in Massachusetts, a girls' school. When she chose it, when she and her father and mother talked about it in the evenings, everyone so carefully avoided the word boys that sometimes the conversations seemed to be about nothing but boys. There are no boys there, the neuter words said; you will not have to contend with that. In her father's eyes were pity and encouragement; in her mother's was disappointment, and her voice was crisp. They spoke of courses, of small classes where Louise would get more attention. She imagined herself in those small classes; she saw herself as a teacher would see her, as the other girls would; she would get no attention.

The girls at the school were from wealthy families, but most of them wore the uniform of another class: blue jeans and work shirts, and many wore overalls. Louise bought some overalls, washed them until the dark blue faded, and wore them to classes. In the cafeteria she ate as she had in high school, not to lose weight nor even to sustain her lie, but because eating lightly in public had become as habitual as good manners. Everyone had to take gym, and in the locker room with the other girls, and wearing shorts on the volleyball and badminton courts, she hated her body. She liked her body most when she was unaware of it: in bed at night, as sleep gently took her out of her day, out of herself. And she liked parts of her body. She liked her brown eyes and sometimes looked at them in the mirror: they were not shallow eyes, she thought; they were indeed windows of a tender soul, a good heart. She liked her lips and nose, and her chin, finely shaped between her wide and sagging cheeks. Most of all she liked her long pale blonde hair, she liked washing and drying it and lying naked on her bed, smelling of shampoo, and feeling the soft hair at her neck and shoulders and back.

Her friend at college was Carrie, who was thin and wore thick glasses and often at night she cried in Louise's room. She did not know why she was crying. She was crying, she said, because she was unhappy. She could say no more. Louise said she was unhappy too, and Carrie moved in with her. One night Carrie talked for hours, sadly and bitterly, about her parents and what they did to each other. When she finished she hugged Louise and they went to bed. Then in the dark Carrie spoke across the room: "Louise? I just wanted to tell you. One night last week I woke up and smelled chocolate. You were eating chocolate, in your bed. I wish you'd eat it in front of me, Louise, whenever you feel like it."

Stiffened in her bed, Louise could think of nothing to say. In the silence she was afraid Carrie would think she was asleep and would tell her again in the morning or tomorrow night. Finally she said Okay. Then after a moment she told Carrie if she ever wanted any she could feel free to help herself; the candy was in the top drawer. Then she said thank you.

They were roommates for four years and in the summers they exchanged letters. Each fall they greeted with embraces, laughter, tears, and moved into their old room, which had been stripped and cleansed of them for the summer. Neither girl enjoyed summer. Carrie did not like being at home because her parents did not love each other. Louise lived in a small city in Louisiana. She did not like summer because she had lost touch with Joan and Marjorie;

they saw each other, but it was not the same. She liked being with her father but with no one else. The flicker of disappointment in her mother's eyes at the airport was a vanguard of the army of relatives and acquaintances who awaited her: they would see her on the streets, in stores, at the country club, in her home, and in theirs; in the first moments of greeting, their eyes would tell her she was still fat Louise, who had been fat as long as they could remember, who had gone to college and returned as fat as ever. Then their eyes dismissed her, and she longed for school and Carrie, and she wrote letters to her friend. But that saddened her too. It wasn't simply that Carrie was her only friend, and when they finished college they might never see each other again. It was that her existence in the world was so divided; it had begun when she was a child creeping to the kitchen; now that division was much sharper, and her friendship with Carrie seemed disproportionate and perilous. The world she was destined to live in had nothing to do with the intimate nights in their room at school.

In the summer before their senior year, Carrie fell in love. She wrote to Louise about him, but she did not write much, and this hurt Louise more than if Carrie had shown the joy her writing tried to conceal. That fall they returned to their room; they were still close and warm, Carrie still needed Louise's ears and heart at night as she spoke of her parents and her recurring malaise whose source the two friends never discovered. But on most weekends Carrie left, and caught a bus to Boston where her boy friend studied music. During the week she often spoke hesitantly of sex; she was not sure if she liked it. But Louise, eating candy and listening, did not know whether Carrie was telling the truth or whether, as in her letters of the past summer, Carrie was keeping from her those delights she may never experience.

Then one Sunday night when Carrie had just returned from Boston and was unpacking her overnight bag, she looked at Louise and said: "I was thinking about you on the bus coming home tonight." Looking at Carrie's concerned, determined face, Louise prepared herself for humiliation. "I was thinking about when we graduate. What you're going to do. What's to become of you. I want you to be loved the way I love you. Louise, if I help you, *really* help you, will you go on a diet?"

Louise entered a period of her life she would remember always, the way some people remember having endured poverty. Her diet did not begin the next day. Carrie told her to eat on Monday as though it were the last day of her life. So for the first time since grammar school Louise went into a school cafeteria and ate everything she wanted. At breakfast and lunch and dinner she glanced around the table to see if the other girls noticed the food on her tray. They did not. She felt there was a lesson in this, but it lay beyond her grasp. That night in their room she ate the four remaining candy bars. During the day Carrie rented a small refrigerator, bought an electric skillet, an electric broiler, and bathroom scales.

On Tuesday morning Louise stood on the scales, and Carrie wrote in her notebook: *October 14: 184 lbs.* Then she made Louise a cup of black coffee and scrambled one egg and sat with her while she ate. When Carrie went to the dining room for breakfast, Louise walked about the campus for thirty minutes. That was part of the plan. The campus was pretty, on its lawns grew at least one of every tree native to New England, and in the warm morning sun Louise felt a new hope. At noon they met in their room, and Carrie broiled her a piece of hamburger and served it with lettuce. Then while Carrie ate in the dining room Louise walked again. She was weak with hunger and she felt queasy. During her afternoon classes she was nervous and tense, and she chewed her pencil and tapped her heels on the floor and tightened her calves. When she returned to her room late that afternoon, she was so glad to see Carrie that she embraced her; she had felt she could not bear another minute of hunger, but now with Carrie she knew she could make it at least through tonight. Then she would sleep and face tomorrow when it came. Carrie broiled her a steak and served it with lettuce. Louise studied while Carrie ate dinner, then they went for a walk.

That was her ritual and her diet for the rest of the year, Carrie alternating fish and chicken breasts with the steaks for dinner, and every day was nearly as bad as the first. In the evenings she was irritable. In all her life she had never been afflicted by ill temper and she looked upon it now as a demon which, along with hunger, was taking possession of her soul. Often she spoke sharply to Carrie. One night during their after-dinner walk Carrie talked sadly of night, of how darkness made her more aware of herself, and at night she did not know why she was in college, why she studied, why she was walking the earth with other people. They were standing on a wooden foot bridge, looking down at a dark pond. Carrie kept talking; perhaps soon she would cry. Suddenly Louise said: "I'm sick of lettuce. I never want to see a piece of lettuce for the rest of my life. I hate it. We shouldn't even buy it, it's immoral."

Carrie was quiet. Louise glanced at her, and the pain and irritation in Carrie's face soothed her. Then she was ashamed. Before she could say she was sorry, Carrie turned to her and said gently: "I know. I know how terrible it is."

Carrie did all the shopping, telling Louise she knew how hard it was to go into a supermarket when you were hungry. And Louise was always hungry. She drank diet soft drinks and started smoking Carrie's cigarettes, learned to enjoy inhaling, thought of cancer and emphysema but they were as far away as those boys her mother had talked about when she was nine. By Thanksgiving she was smoking over a pack a day and her weight in Carrie's notebook was one hundred and sixty-two pounds. Carrie was afraid if Louise went home at Thanksgiving she would lapse from the diet, so Louise spent the vacation with Carrie, in Philadelphia. Carrie wrote her family about the diet, and told Louise that she had. On the phone to Philadelphia, Louise said: "I feel like a bedwetter. When I was a little girl I had a friend who used to come spend the night and Mother would put a rubber sheet on the bed and we all pretended there wasn't a rubber sheet and that she hadn't wet the bed. Even me, and I slept with her." At Thanksgiving dinner she lowered her eyes as Carrie's father put two slices of white meat on her plate and passed it to her over the bowls of steaming food.

When she went home at Christmas she weighed a hundred and fifty-five pounds; at the airport her mother marvelled. Her father laughed and hugged her and said: "But now there's less of you to love." He was troubled by her smoking but only mentioned it once; he told her she was beautiful and, as always, his eyes bathed her with love. During the long vacation her mother cooked for her as Carrie had, and Louise returned to school weighing a hundred and forty-six pounds.

Flying north on the plane she warmly recalled the surprised and congratulatory eyes of her relatives and acquaintances. She had not seen Joan or Marjorie. She thought of returning home in May, weighing the hundred and fifteen pounds which Carrie had in October set as their goal. Looking toward the stoic days ahead, she felt strong. She thought of those hungry days of fall and early winter (and now: she was hungry now: with almost a frown, almost a brusque shake of the head, she refused peanuts from the stewardess): those first weeks of the diet when she was the pawn of an irascibility which still, conditioned to her ritual as she was, could at any moment take command of her. She thought of the nights of trying to sleep while her stomach growled. She thought of her addiction to cigarettes. She thought of the people at school: not one teacher, not one girl, had spoken to her about her loss of weight, not even about her absence from meals. And without warning her spirit collapsed. She did not feel strong, she did not feel she was committed to and within reach of achieving a valuable goal. She felt that somehow she had lost more than pounds of fat; that some time during her dieting she had lost herself too. She tried to remember what it had felt like to be Louise before she had started living on meat and fish, as an unhappy adult may look sadly in the memory of childhood for lost virtues and hopes. She looked down at the earth far below, and it seemed to her that her soul, like her body aboard the plane, was in some rootless flight. She neither knew its destination nor where it had departed from; it was on some passage she could not even define.

During the next few weeks she lost weight more slowly and once for eight days Carrie's daily recording stayed at a hundred and thirty-six. Louise woke in the morning thinking of one hundred and thirty-six and then she stood on the scales and they echoed her. She became obsessed with that number, and there wasn't a day when she didn't say it aloud, and through the days and nights the number stayed in her mind, and if a teacher had spoken those digits in a classroom she would have opened her mouth to speak. What if that's me, she said to Carrie. I mean what if a hundred and thirty-six is my real weight and I just can't lose anymore. Walking hand-in-hand with her despair was a longing for this to be true, and that longing angered her and wearied her, and every day she was gloomy. On the ninth day she weighed a hundred and thirty-five and a half pounds. She was not relieved; she thought bitterly of the months ahead, the shedding of the last twenty and a half pounds.

On Easter Sunday, which she spent at Carrie's, she weighed one hundred and twenty pounds, and she ate one slice of glazed pineapple with her ham and lettuce. She did not enjoy it: she felt she was being friendly with a recalcitrant enemy who had once tried to destroy her. Carrie's parents were laudative. She liked them and she wished they would touch sometimes, and look at each other when they spoke. She guessed they would divorce when Carrie left home, and she vowed that her own marriage would be one of affection and tenderness. She could think about that now: marriage. At school she had read in a Boston paper that this summer the cicadas would come out of their seventeen year hibernation on Cape Cod, for a month they would mate and then die, leaving their young to burrow into the ground where they would stay for seventeen years. That's me, she had said to Carrie. Only my hibernation lasted twenty-one years.

Often her mother asked in letters and on the phone about the diet, but Louise answered vaguely. When she flew home in late May she weighed a hundred and thirteen pounds, and at the airport her mother cried and hugged her and said again and again: You're so *beautiful*. Her father blushed and bought her a martini. For days her relatives and acquaintances congratulated her, and the applause in their eyes lasted the entire summer, and she loved their eyes, and swam in the country club pool, the first time she had done this since she was a child.

She lived at home and ate the way her mother did and every morning she weighed herself on the scales in her bathroom. Her mother liked to take her shopping and buy her dresses and they put her old ones in the Goodwill box at the shopping center; Louise thought of them existing on the body of a poor woman whose cheap meals kept her fat. Louise's mother had a photographer come to the house, and Louise posed on the couch and standing beneath a live oak and sitting in a wicker lawn chair next to an azalea bush. The new clothes and the photographer made her feel she was going to another country or becoming a citizen of a new one. In the fall she took a job of no consequence, to give herself something to do.

Also in the fall a young lawyer joined her father's firm, he came one night to dinner, and they started seeing each other. He was the first man outside her family to kiss her since the barbecue when she was sixteen. Louise celebrated Thanksgiving not with rice dressing and candied sweet potatoes and mince meat and pumpkin pies, but by giving Richard her virginity which she realized, at the very last moment of its existence, she had embarked on giving him over thirteen months ago, on that Tuesday in October when Carrie had made her a cup of black coffee and scrambled one egg. She wrote this to Carrie, who replied happily by return mail. She also, through glance and smile and innuendo, tried to tell her mother too. But finally she controlled that impulse, because Richard felt guilty about making love with the daughter of his partner and friend. In the spring they married. The wedding was a large one, in the Episcopal church, and Carrie flew from Boston to be maid of honor. Her parents had recently separated and she was living with the musician and was still victim of her unpredictable malaise. It overcame her on the night before the wedding, so Louise was up with her until past three and woke next morning from a sleep so heavy that she did not want to leave it.

Richard was a lean, tall, energetic man with the metabolism of a pencil sharpener. Louise fed him everything he wanted. He liked Italian food and she got recipes from her mother and watched him eating spaghetti with the sauce she had only tasted, and ravioli and lasagna, while she ate antipasto with her chianti. He made a lot of money and borrowed more and they bought a house whose lawn sloped down to the shore of a lake; they had a wharf and a boathouse, and Richard bought a boat and they took friends waterskiing. Richard bought her a car and they spent his vacations in Mexico, Canada, the Bahamas, and in the fifth year of their marriage they went to Europe and, according to their plan, she conceived a child in Paris. On the plane back, as she looked out the window and beyond the sparkling sea and saw her country, she felt that it was waiting for her, as her home by the lake was, and her parents, and her good friends who rode in the boat and waterskied; she thought of the accumulated warmth and pelf of her marriage, and how by slimming her body she had bought into the pleasures of the nation. She felt cunning, and she smiled to herself, and took Richard's hand.

But these moments of triumph were sparse. On most days she went about her routine of leisure with a sense of certainty about herself that came merely from not thinking. But there were times, with her friends, or with Richard, or alone in the house, when she was suddenly assaulted by the feeling that she had taken the wrong train and arrived at a place where no one knew her, and where she ought not to be. Often, in bed with Richard, she talked of being fat: "I was the one who started the friendship with Carrie, I chose her, I started the conversations. When I understood that she was my friend I understood something else: I had chosen her for the same reason I'd chosen Joan and Marjorie. They were all thin. I was always thinking about what people saw when they looked at me and I didn't want them to see two fat girls. When I was alone I didn't mind being fat but then I'd have to leave the house again and then I didn't want to look like me. But at home I didn't mind except when I was getting dressed to go out of the house and when Mother looked at me. But I stopped looking at her when she looked at me. And in college I felt good with Carrie; there weren't any boys and I didn't have any other friends and so when I wasn't with Carrie I thought about her and I tried to ignore the other people around me, I tried to make them not exist. A lot of the time I could do that. It was strange, and I felt like a spy."

If Richard was bored by her repetition he pretended not to be. But she knew the story meant very little to him. She could have been telling him of a childhood illness, or wearing braces, or a broken heart at sixteen. He could not see her as she was when she was fat. She felt as though she were trying to tell a foreign lover about her life in the United States, and if only she could command the language he would know and love all of her and she would feel complete. Some of the acquaintances of her childhood were her friends now, and even they did not seem to remember her when she was fat.

Now her body was growing again, and when she put on a maternity dress for the first time she shivered with fear. Richard did not smoke and he asked her, in a voice just short of demand, to stop during her pregnancy. She did. She ate carrots and celery instead of smoking, and at cocktail parties she tried to eat nothing, but after her first drink she ate nuts and cheese and crackers and dips. Always at these parties Richard had talked with his friends and she had rarely spoken to him until they drove home. But now when he noticed her at the hors d'oeuvres table he crossed the room and, smiling, led her back to his group. His smile and his hand on her arm told her he was doing his clumsy, husbandly best to help her through a time of female mystery.

She was gaining weight but she told herself it was only the baby, and would leave with its birth. But at other times she knew quite clearly that she was losing the discipline she had fought so hard to gain during her last year with Carrie. She was hungry now as she had been in college, and she ate between meals and after dinner and tried to eat only carrots and celery, but she grew to hate them, and her desire for sweets was as vicious as it had been long ago. At home she ate bread and jam and when she shopped for groceries she bought a candy bar and ate it driving home and put the wrapper in her purse and then in the garbage can under the sink. Her cheeks had filled out, there was loose flesh under her chin, her arms and legs were plump, and her mother was concerned. So was Richard. One night when she brought pie and milk to the living room where they were watching television, he said: "You already had a piece. At dinner."

She did not look at him.

"You're gaining weight. It's not all water, either. It's fat. It'll be summertime. You'll want to get into your bathing suit."

The pie was cherry. She looked at it as her fork cut through it; she speared the piece and rubbed it in the red juice on the plate before lifting it to her mouth.

"You never used to eat pie," he said. "I just think you ought to watch it a bit. It's going to be tough on you this summer."

In her seventh month, with a delight reminiscent of climbing the stairs to Richard's apartment before they were married, she returned to her world of secret gratification. She began hiding candy in her underwear drawer. She ate it during the day and at night while Richard slept, and at breakfast she was distracted, waiting for him to leave.

She gave birth to a son, brought him home, and nursed both him and her appetites. During this time of celibacy she enjoyed her body through her son's mouth; while he suckled she stroked his small head and back. She was hiding candy but she did not conceal her other indulgences: she was smoking again but still she ate between meals, and at dinner she ate what Richard did, and coldly he watched her, he grew petulant, and when the date marking the end of their celibacy came they let it pass. Often in the afternoons her mother visited and scolded her and Louise sat looking at the baby and said nothing until finally, to end it, she promised to diet. When her mother and father came for dinners, her father kissed her and held the baby and her mother said nothing about Louise's body, and her voice was tense. Returning from work in the evenings Richard looked at a soiled plate and glass on the table beside her chair as if detecting traces of infidelity, and at every dinner they fought.

"Look at you," he said. "Lasagna, for God's sake. When are you going to start? It's not simply that you haven't lost any weight. You're gaining. I can see it. I can feel it when you get in bed. Pretty soon you'll weigh more than I do and I'll be sleeping on a trampoline."

"You never touch me anymore."

"I don't want to touch you. Why should I? Have you *looked* at yourself?"

"You're cruel," she said. "I never knew how cruel you were."

She ate, watching him. He did not look at her. Glaring at his plate, he worked with fork and knife like a hurried man at a lunch counter.

"I bet you didn't either," she said.

That night when he was asleep she took a Milky Way to the bathroom. For a while she stood eating in the dark, then she turned on the light. Chewing, she looked at herself in the mirror; she looked at her eyes and hair. Then she stood on the scales and looking at the numbers between her feet, one hundred and sixty-two, she remembered when she had weighed a hundred and thirty-six pounds for eight days. Her memory of those eight days was fond and amusing, as though she were recalling an Easter egg hunt when she was six. She stepped off the scales and pushed them under the lavatory and did not stand on them again.

It was summer and she bought loose dresses and when Richard took friends out on the boat she did not wear a bathing suit or shorts; her friend gave her mischievous glances, and Richard did not look at her. She stopped riding on the boat. She told them she wanted to stay with the baby, and she sat inside holding him until she heard the boat leave the wharf. Then she took him to the front lawn and walked with him in the shade of the trees and talked to him about the blue jays and mockingbirds and cardinals she saw on their branches. Sometimes she stopped and watched the boat out on the lake and the friend skiing behind it.

Every day Richard quarrelled, and because his rage went no further than her weight and shape, she felt excluded from it, and she remained calm within layers of flesh and spirit, and watched his frustration, his impotence. He truly believed they were arguing about her weight. She knew better: she knew that beneath the argument lay the question of who Richard was. She thought of him smiling at the wheel of his boat, and long ago courting his slender girl, the daughter of his partner and friend. She thought of Carrie telling her of smelling chocolate in the dark and, after that, watching her eat it night after night. She smiled at Richard, teasing his anger.

He is angry now. He stands in the center of the living room, raging at her, and he wakes the baby. Beneath Richard's voice she hears the soft crying, feels it in her heart, and quietly she rises from her chair and goes upstairs to the child's room and takes him from the crib. She brings him to the living room and sits holding him in her lap, pressing him gently against the folds of fat at her waist. Now Richard is pleading with her. Louise thinks tenderly of Carrie broiling meat and fish in their room, and walking with her in the evenings. She wonders if Carrie still has the malaise. Perhaps she will come for a visit. In Louise's arms now the boy sleeps.

"I'll help you," Richard says. "I'll eat the same things you eat."

But his face does not approach the compassion and determination and love she had seen in Carrie's during what she now recognizes as the worst year of her life. She can remember nothing about that year except hunger, and the meals in her room. She is hungry now. When she puts the boy to bed she will get a candy bar from her room. She will eat it here, in front of Richard. This room will be hers soon. She considers the possibilities: all these rooms and the lawn where she can do whatever she wishes. She knows he will leave soon. It has been in his eyes all summer. She stands, using one hand to pull herself out of the chair. She carries the boy to his crib, feels him against her large breasts, feels that his sleeping body touches her soul. With a surge of vindication and relief she holds him. Then she kisses his forehead and places him in the crib. She goes to the bedroom and in the dark takes a bar of candy from her drawer. Slowly she descends the stairs. She knows Richard is waiting but she feels his departure so happily that, when she enters the living room, unwrapping the candy, she is surprised to see him standing there.

The Traveler

ELLEN GILCHRIST

IT WAS JUNE in southern Indiana. I was locked in the upstairs bathroom studying the directions on a box of Tampax when the invitation came.

"LeLe," my father called, coming up the stairs with the letter in his hand. "Come out of there. Come hear the news. You're going to the Delta."

It seems my cousin Baby Gwen Barksdale's mother had died of a weak liver, and rather than leave the poor girl alone in a house with a grieving widower the family had invited me to Mississippi to spend the summer as her companion. There was even a suggestion that I might stay and go to school there in the fall.

What luck that the invitation came just as my own mother, giving in to a fit of jealous rage, left my father and fled to New Orleans to have a nervous breakdown.

"You'll love it in Clarksville," my father assured me. "Baby Gwen is just your age and just your speed. She'll be so glad to see you." And he pressed several more twenty-dollar bills into my hand and helped me pack my summer clothes.

"You try it for the summer, LeLe," he said. "We'll decide about school later on."

He might need to decide later on, but my mind was made up. I couldn't wait to leave Franklin, Indiana, where the students at Franklin Junior High had made the mistake of failing to elect me cheerleader. I wasn't unpopular or anything like that, just a little on the plump side.

Baby Gwen Barksdale, I whispered to myself as I arranged my things on the Pullman seat. I was sweating heavily in a pink linen suit, and my straw hat was making my head itch, but I sat up straight, trying to look like a lady. I had the latest edition of *Hit Parade Magazine* on my lap, and I was determined to learn every word of the Top Ten on the train ride.

Baby Gwen Barksdale, I said to myself, remembering the stories my father had told me. Baby Gwen, queen of the Delta subdeb dances, daughter of the famous Gwendolyn Montgomery Paine of Shaw, granddaughter of my grandmother's sainted sister, Frances Paine of Natchez. Baby Gwen Barksdale, daughter of Britain Barksdale who played halfback on the Ole Miss Sugar Bowl team.

It was all too good to be true. I marched myself down to the diner and ate several desserts to calm myself down.

By the time the Illinois Central made it all the way to Clarksville, Mississippi, my linen dress was helplessly wrinkled, my third pair of white gloves was damp and stained from the dye of the magazine, and my teeth were worn out from being brushed.

But there on the platform she waited, Baby Gwen Barksdale herself, five feet two inches of sultry dark-skinned, dark-eyed beauty. (The Barksdales have French blood.) She looked exactly like Ida Lupino. She was wearing a navy blue dotted Swiss sun dress and high-heeled shoes and her slip was showing, a thin line of ecru lace. Her dark pink lipstick exactly matched her fingernail polish, and she smelled divinely of Aprodisia perfume.

She was accompanied by a strong boy who smiled a lot and turned out to be the sheriff's son. He had come along to carry the luggage.

"I'm so glad you could come," she said, hugging me for the fourth time. "I can't believe you came all the way on the train by yourself."

"No one in Franklin believed I'd do it either," I said. "I just got elected cheerleader and practically the whole football team came to the station to tell me goodbye. They didn't believe I was leaving. Of course, they all know about Bob Aaron. That's the college boy I love. He's got cancer of the thyroid gland. My parents won't let me go out with him because he's Jewish. He's already had about five operations. He's having one right now in St. Louis. So I might as well be down here."

"Oh, LeLe, that's terrible. It's like my mother. I know just how you feel."

"Well, anyway, I'm here now and we can stick together," I said, taking a deep breath of the Aprodisia. "I love your perfume. It's wonderful."

"It's my signature," she said. "I wear Aprodisia in the summer and Tigress in the winter. There's a bottle in my purse. You can put some on if you want to."

We walked over to the Oldsmobile and Baby Gwen got behind the wheel. She was so short she had to sit on straw pillows to see over the dash, but she turned out to be a superb driver. The sheriff's son climbed into the back seat with my bags, and the three of us drove off down the streets of the town, past the gin and the post office and the Pontiac place, and on down the river road to a white frame house at the end of a street that dead-ended at the levee.

So I arrived in Clarksville, chattering away to a spellbound audience, spraying my neck and arms with Aprodisia perfume, happier than I had ever been in my life.

After her mother's funeral Baby Gwen had moved into the master bedroom as her father was too brokenhearted to ever enter that part of the house again.

I was led up the stairs and into a large sunny room with bay windows and a pale blue chaise lounge. There was a dressing room with a private bath and walk-in closets. Everything was just as Big Gwen had left it.

The closets were filled with unbelievable clothes. Navy blue and green and black silk dresses, gray and beige and brown gabardine suits, pastel evening dresses, house dresses, sun dresses, wool coats, skirts, jackets. There were twenty or thirty pairs of high-heeled shoes and a dozen hatboxes. There were drawers full of handmade underwear. There was a fur stole and several negligees and a real Japanese kimono.

It was all ours.

"You can wear anything you want to," Baby Gwen said. "Most of them are too long for me."

Best of all was the dressing table. It was three feet long with a padded stool and a large mirror surrounded by light bulbs.

On its surface, in a sea of spilled powder, were dozens of bottles and jars. Every product ever manufactured by Charles of the Ritz must have been there. There was foundation cream, astringent, eye shadow, rouge, clarifier, moisturizer, cleanser, refining oil, facial mask, night cream, hand cream, wrinkle cream, eye cream, all pervaded by the unforgettable smell of Revenescence, Charles of the Ritz's secret formula moisturizer.

There were hairpins, hand mirrors, tweezers, eyelash curlers, combs, hair rollers, mascara wands, cuticle sticks, nail polish, emery boards. There were numerous bottles of perfume and cologne and a cut-glass bowl filled with lipsticks.

I had never seen anything like it. I could hardly wait to sit down on the little padded stool and get started.

"You want a Coca-Cola?" Baby Gwen asked, growing bored with my inspection of her riches. "Some boys I know are coming over later this afternoon to meet you."

"Can we smoke?" I asked, pulling my Pall Malls out of my purse.

"We can do anything we want to do," she said, picking a Ronson lighter off the dressing table and handing it to me. She was smiling the famous Barksdale slow smile.

That night we lay awake until two or three in the morning telling each other our life stories. I told her about Bob Aaron's lymph node cancer, and she told me about her cousin Maurice, who taught French and hated Clarksville and was married to an unpleasant woman who sang in the choir. Maurice was secretly in love with Baby Gwen. He couldn't help himself. He had confessed his love at a spring wedding reception. Now they were waiting for Baby Gwen to grow up so they could run away together. In the meantime Baby Gwen was playing the field so no one would suspect.

Finally, exhausted by our passions, we fell asleep in each other's arms, with the night breezes blowing in the windows off the river, in our ironed sheets and our silk pajamas and our night cream, with the radio playing an all-night station from New Orleans. Oh, Bob, Bob, I whispered into Baby Gwen's soft black hair. Oh, Maurice, Maurice, she sighed into my hair rollers.

In the morning I woke early and wandered downstairs. I went into the kitchen, opened the freezer, found a carton of vanilla ice cream, and began to eat it with my fingers, standing with the freezer door open, letting the cool air blow on my face.

After a while I heard the back door slam and Sirena came in. She was the middle-aged black woman who turned out to be the only person in charge of us in any way. Baby Gwen's father disappeared before dawn to carry the mail and came home in the evenings and sank into his chair with his bourbon and his memories. Occasionally he would put in an appearance at the noon meal and ask us if we wanted anything.

I barely managed to close the freezer door before Sirena caught me. "You want me to make you some breakfast?" she said.

"No, thank you," I said. "I don't eat in the daytime. I'm on a diet."

I have always believed Sirena found my fingerprints in that ice cream. One way or the other I wasn't fooling her, she knew a Yankee when she saw one, even if I was Mr. Leland's daughter.

I wandered into the living room and read a *Coronet* for a while. Then I decided to go back upstairs and see if Baby Gwen was awake.

I found her in the bathroom sitting upright in a tub of soapy water while Sirena knelt beside it slowly and intently bathing her. I had never seen a grown person being bathed before.

Sirena was running her great black hand up and down Baby Gwen's white leg, soaping her with a terry-cloth washrag. The artesian well water was the color of urine and smelled of sulphur and sandalwood soap, and Sirena's dark hand was thick and strong moving along Baby Gwen's flawless skin. I sat down on the toilet and began to make conversation.

"You want to take a sunbath after a while," I said. "I'm afraid I'll lose my tan."

"Sure," she said. "We can do whatever you want to. Someone called a while ago and asked us to play bridge this afternoon. Do you like to play bridge?"

"I love it," I said. "That's practically all we do in Indiana. We play all the time. My mother plays duplicate. She's got about fifty silver ashtrays she won at tournaments."

"I bet you're really good," she said. She was squirming around while Sirena took her time finishing the other leg.

I lit a cigarette, trying not to look at Baby Gwen's black pubic hair. I had never seen anyone's pubic hair but my own, which was red. It had not occurred to me that there were different colors. "Want a drag?" I asked, handing her the cigarette. She nodded, wiped her hand on her terry-cloth turban, took a long luxurious drag, and French inhaled.

The smoke left her mouth in two little rivers, curled deliciously up over the dark hairs above her lips, and into her nostrils. She held it for a long moment, then exhaled slowly through her lips. The smoke mingled with the sunlight, and the steam coming from the bathwater rose in ragged circles and moved toward the open window.

Baby Gwen rose from the water, her flat body festooned with blossoms of sandalwood soap, and Sirena began to dry her with a towel.

So our life together took shape. In the mornings we sunbathed from 11:00 to 12:00. Thirty minutes on one side and thirty minutes on the other. There were two schools of thought concerning sunbathing. One, that it gave you wrinkles. The other, that it was worth it to look good while you were young.

Baby Gwen and I subscribed to the second theory. Still, we were careful to keep our faces oiled so we wouldn't ruin our complexions. There is no way you could believe how serious we were about such matters. The impenetrable mystery of physical beauty held us like a spell.

In the mornings we spread our blankets in the backyard where a patch of sunlight shone in through the high branches of the elm trees. We covered the blankets with white sheets and set out our supplies, bottles of baby oil, bottles

of iodine, alarm clock, eye pads, sunglasses, magazines. We carefully mixed
seven drops of iodine with seven ounces of baby oil, shook it for three minutes, then rubbed it on the uncovered parts of each other's bodies. How I
loved the feel of Baby Gwen's rib cage under my fingers, the smoothness of
her shaved legs. How I dreaded it when her fingers touched the baby fat on
my own ribs.

When we were covered with oil we would lie back and continue our discussion of our romances. I talked of nothing but the ill-fated Bob Aaron, of
the songs I would write and dedicate to his memory, of the trip I would take
to his deathbed, of the night he drove me home from a football game and let
me wear his gloves, of the child I would have by another man and name for
him, Robert or Roberta, Bob or Bobbie.

The other thing that fascinated me was the development of my "reputation." I was intensely interested in what people thought of me, in what was
being said about me. I set about to develop a reputation in Clarksville as a
"madcap," a "wild child," a girl who would do anything. A summer visitor
from Washington, D.C., said in my hearing that I reminded him of a young
Zelda Fitzgerald and, although I didn't know exactly who Zelda Fitzgerald
was, I knew that she had married a writer and drank like a fish and once
danced naked in a fountain in Rome. It seemed like a wonderful thing to
have said about myself, and I resolved to try to live up to it.

How wonderful it was to be "home," where people knew "who I was,"
where people thought I was "hilarious" and "crazy" and "just like Leland." I
did everything I could think of to feed my new image, becoming very outspoken, saying *damn* and *hell* at every opportunity, wearing dark glasses all
the time, even to church. I must have been the first person of normal vision
ever to attend the Clarksville Episcopal Church wearing dark glasses.

Baby Gwen's grandmother called every few days to see how we were getting along and once, in a burst of responsibility, came over bringing a dozen
pairs of new cotton underpants she had bought for us at the Chinaman's
store.

We never could figure out where she got the idea that we were in need of
cotton underpants, unless Sirena had mentioned it to her. Perhaps Sirena had
tired of hand washing the French lingerie we had taken to wearing every day.

The grandmother had outlived both her daughters and existed in a sort of
dreamy half-world with her servants and her religion.

Mostly we kept her satisfied by glowing telephone reports of our popularity and by stopping by occasionally to sit on her porch and have a Coca-Cola.

I fell in love nearly every day with one or the other of the seemingly endless supply of boys who came to call from Drew and Cleveland and Itta Bena and Tutweiler and Rosedale and Leland. Baby Gwen drew boys like honey, and there were always plenty left over to sit around the living room listening to my nonstop conversation.

Boys came by in the evenings, boys called on the telephone, boys invaded our daily bridge games, boys showed up after church, boys took us swimming at the Clarksville Country Club, boys drove us around the cotton fields and down to the river and out to the bootlegger's shack.

The boy I liked best was a good-natured football player named Fielding Reid. Fielding had eyes so blue and hair so blonde and shoulders so wide and teased me so unmercifully about my accent that I completely forgot he was the steady boyfriend of Clarice Fitzhugh, who was off on a trip to Mexico with her family. Fielding had taken to hanging around Baby Gwen and me while he waited for Clarice's return.

He loved to kibitz on our bridge games, eating all the mints and pecans from the little dishes and leaning over my shoulder cheering me on. In the afternoons we played endless polite bridge games, so different from the bitter hardfought bridge I had played in the forgotten state of Indiana.

Although I was an erratic and unpredictable bidder, I was a sought-after partner for I held good cards and nearly always won.

There was a girl from Drew named Sarah who came over several afternoons a week to play with us. She was Fielding's cousin and she had a wooden arm painted the color of her skin. It was not a particularly well made arm, and the paint was peeling in several places on the hand. She was pleasant enough looking otherwise and had nice clothes with loose sleeves that hid the place where the false arm joined the real one.

I made a great show of being nice to Sarah, lighting her cigarettes, asking her opinion about things, letting her be my bridge partner. She was delighted with the attention I gave her and was always telling someone how "wonderful" I was and how much it meant to her to have me in Clarksville.

The wrist and fingers of Sarah's false arm were hinged and she could move the joints with her good hand and lock them in place. She was in the habit of holding the wooden arm in front of her when she was seated at the bridge table. Then she would place her bridge hand in the wooden fingers and play out of it with her good hand.

Of course, anyone sitting on either side of her could see her cards by the slightest movement of their eyes. It took a lot of pressure off me when she was my partner.

Fielding thought I was "wonderful" too. He went around saying I was his "partner" and took me into his confidence, even telling me his fears that the absent Clarice Fitzhugh was being unfaithful to him in Mexico. That she might be "using" him.

Don't worry, I assured him. Clarice was a great girl. She wouldn't use anyone. He must trust her and not listen to idle gossip. Everything would be fine when she got home, and so forth. Part of my new reputation was that "LeLe never says a bad word about anyone," "LeLe always looks on the bright side," "everyone feels like they've known LeLe all their lives," "you can tell LeLe *anything.*"

I was beginning to believe my own publicity, that I was someone very special, that there might be some special destiny in store for me.

Several times that summer I was filled with an elation so powerful and overwhelming that it felt as though my body were leaving the earth. This always happened at night, when I was alone in the yard, caught in the shadow of the Nandina bushes which covered the side of the house like bright dark clouds. I remember standing in the starlight filled with some inexpressible joy. It would become very intense, like music. I was terribly excited by these feelings and could not bring myself to speak of them, even to Baby Gwen.

Often that summer I was given to seizures of abrupt excitement while I was dressing. I would catch a glimpse of myself in a mirror and burst into laughter, or, deciding for a moment that I was pretty, begin to tremble and jump up and go dancing around the room.

I had a recurrent dream that summer. I dreamed that I was walking through our old house in Indiana and I would notice that the dining room opened up into rooms and rooms I had not known existed, strange and oddly shaped rooms full of heavy furniture, expensive dusty dressers with drawers full of treasures, old gowns and sweaters and capes, jewels and letters and old documents, wills and deeds and diaries. These rooms opened onto patios and sun porches and solariums, and I saw that we were wealthy people. I wanted to run back and find my parents and tell them what I had found, but my curiosity drove me forward. I had to keep opening doors until I knew the extent of our riches, so I kept on moving through the strange rooms until I woke.

One morning Fielding came by unexpectedly and asked me to go with him to see about some repairs for his car. We left it with a mechanic at the filling station and walked to the Mayflower Café, a place on the square where farmers and merchants gathered in the mornings for coffee and gossip. I had never been alone in a restaurant with a boy, and I was excited and began talking very fast to cover my excitement. I ordered doughnuts and began turning my turquoise ring around on my finger so the waitress would think it was a wedding band.

"I've been wanting to talk to you alone," Fielding said.

"Sure," I said, choking on a powdered doughnut. It was all too wonderful, sitting in a booth so early in the morning with a really good-looking boy.

"LeLe," he said, smiling at me and reaching across the table to hold my hand. There was his garnet class ring, blazing at me from the tabletop. At any moment it might be mine. I could scarcely breathe. "LeLe," he repeated, "I don't want you to get me wrong when I say this. I don't want to hurt your feelings or anything, but, well, I really want to tell you something." He squeezed my hand tighter. "LeLe, you would be a really beautiful girl if you lost ten pounds, do you know that? Because you have a beautiful face. I'm only saying this because we've gotten to be such good friends and I thought I ought . . ."

I was stunned. But I recovered. "I'm not really this fat," I said. "At home I'm a cheerleader and I'm on the swimming team and I'm very thin. But last year the boy I love got cancer and I've been having a lot of trouble with my thyroid since then. The doctors think there may be something wrong with my thyroid or my metabolism. I may have to have an operation pretty soon."

"Oh, LeLe," he said. "I didn't know it was anything like that. I thought maybe you ate too much or something." He reached out and took my other hand. I was still holding part of a doughnut.

"Don't worry about it, Fielding. How could you know. You didn't hurt my feelings. Besides, I don't mind. The operation may not be so bad. It isn't like having polio or something they can't fix. At least I have something they can fix."

"Oh, LeLe."

"Don't worry about it. And don't tell anyone about it, even Baby Gwen. I don't want people feeling sorry for me. So it's a secret."

"Don't worry, LeLe. I'll never tell anyone. Are you sure it'll be all right? About the operation I mean?"

"Oh, sure. I might not even have to have it. My thyroid might get better all by itself."

After that Fielding and I were closer than ever. I began to halfway believe the part about the thyroid trouble. My mother was always talking about her thyroid and taking some sort of little white pill for it.

. . .

Late one afternoon Baby Gwen and I were sitting on the porch swing talking to Fielding. It was one of those days in August when you can smell autumn in the air, a feeling of change coming over the world. I had won at bridge that afternoon. I had made seven hearts doubled and redoubled with Fielding looking over my shoulder, and I was filled with a sense of power.

"Let's all go swimming tomorrow," I said. "They'll be closing the pool soon and I need to practice my strokes."

"Let's go to the lake," Fielding said. "I haven't made my summer swim across the lake. I was waiting for Russell to get home, but I don't guess he'll be back in time so I might as well go on and swim it myself."

"I'll swim it with you," I heard myself saying. "I'm a Junior Red Cross Lifesaver. I can swim forever."

"You couldn't swim this," he said. "It's five miles."

"I can swim a lot further than that," I said. "I practically taught swimming at camp. I never got tired."

"What about your . . . you know . . . your condition?"

"That's all right," I said. "Exercise is good for me. I'm supposed to go swimming all I can. The doctors said it was the best thing I could do."

Baby Gwen looked puzzled. "You can't swim all the way across the lake without a boat," she said. "Girls don't ever swim across the lake."

"I can swim it," I said, "I've been further than that at camp lots of times. What time you want to go, Fielding?"

By the time he came to pick us up the next morning I had calmed Baby Gwen down and convinced her there was nothing to worry about. I really was a good swimmer. Swimming was of no importance to me one way or the other. What mattered to me was that a boy of my own choosing, a first-rate boy, was coming to take me somewhere. Not coming for Baby Gwen and taking me along to be nice, but *coming for me.*

I had been awake since dawn deciding what to wear. I finally settled on my old green Jantzen and a white blouse from Big Gwen's wardrobe. The blouse had little shoulder pads and big chunky buttons and fell across my shoulders and arms in soft pleats. I wasn't worried at all about swimming the lake. The only thing that worried me was whether the blouse was long enough to cover my stomach.

Baby Gwen went with us. As soon as we left the shore she was supposed to drive around to the other side and watch for us. All the way out to the lake she sat beside me looking worried.

"You ought to have a boat going along beside you," she said.

"We don't need a boat," I said. "I'm a Junior Red Cross Lifesaver. I can swim all day if I want."

"It's O.K.," Fielding said. "Russell and I do it every summer."

By the time we got to the lake I felt like I could swim the Atlantic Ocean. The sun was brilliant on the blue water, and as soon as Fielding stopped the car I jumped out and ran down to the shore and looked out across the water to the pine trees on the far shore. It didn't look so far away, only very blue and deep and mysterious. I took off my blouse and shoes and waded out into the water. How clean it felt, how cool. I put my face down and touched my cheek to the water. I felt the water across my legs and stomach. My body felt wonderful and light in the water. I rose up on my toes and my legs felt strong and tall. I pulled in my stomach until my ribs stuck out. I was beautiful. I was perfect. I began to throw handfuls of water up into the air. The water caught in the sunlight and fell back all around me. I threw more into the air and it fell all around me, falling in pieces of steel and glass and diamonds, diamonds falling all around me. I called out, "Come on, Fielding. Either we're swimming across this lake or we aren't."

"Wait," he called back. "Wait up." Then he was beside me in the water and I felt his hands around my waist and the pressure of his knee against my thigh. "Let's go then," he said in a low sweet voice. "Let's do this together."

Then we began to swim out, headed for the stand of pine and oak and cypress on the far shore.

The time passed as if in a dream. My arms moved easily, taking turns pulling the soft yielding water alongside my body. I was counting out the strokes, one, two, three, four, five, six, seven, eight, one, two, three, four, five, six, seven, eight . . . over and over in the good old-fashioned Australian crawl. Every now and then Fielding would touch my arm and we would roll over on our backs and rest for a few minutes, checking our position. Then we would swim for a while on our sides, resting. There were long banks of clouds on the horizon and far overhead a great hawk circling like a black planet. Everytime I looked up he was there.

We swam for what seemed to be a long, long time, but whenever I looked ahead the trees on the shore never seemed to come any closer.

"Are you sure we're going in a straight line," I said, when we turned over to rest for a moment.

"I think so," Fielding said. "The current might be pulling us a little to the left. There's nothing we can do about it now anyway."

"Why," I said. "Why can't we do anything about it?"

"Well, we can't go back," he said. "We're past the point of no return."

The point of no return I said to myself. Maybe we would die out here and they would change the name of the lake in honor of us. Lake LeLe, Lake Leland Louise Arnold, Lover's Lake. "Don't worry about it then," I said. "Just keep on swimming."

Perhaps an hour went by, perhaps two. The sun was hot on the water, and every now and then a breeze blew up. Once a barge carrying logs to the saw-mill passed us without noticing us. We treaded water while it passed and then rocked in the wake for several minutes. They had passed us as though we didn't exist. After the barge went by we began to swim with more deter-mination. I was beginning to feel cold, but it didn't seem to really matter. Nothing mattered but this boy and the sun and the clouds and the great hawk circling and the water touching me everywhere. I put down my head and began to count with renewed vigor, one, two, three, four, five, six, seven, eight, one, two, three, four, . . .

"LeLe," Fielding called out. "LeLe, put your feet down. Put your feet down, LeLe." I looked up and he was standing a few feet away holding his hands up in the air. I let my feet drop and my toes touched the cool flat sand. We were on the sandbar. Then we were laughing and hugging and holding on to each other and moving toward the shore where Baby Gwen stood calling and call-ing to us. It was wonderful, wonderful, wonderful, wonderful. I was won-derful. I was dazzling. I was LeLe Arnold, the wildest girl in the Mississippi Delta, the girl who swam Lake Jefferson without a boat or a life vest. I was LeLe, the girl who would do anything.

All the way home in the car Fielding kept his arm around me while he drove and Baby Gwen fed me little pieces of the picnic lunch and I was happier than I had ever been in my life and I might have stayed that way forever but when we got home there was a message saying that my parents were on their way to Clarksville to take me home.

My parents. I had forgotten they existed. My father had gotten lonely and driven to New Orleans and talked my mother into coming home.

Later that afternoon they arrived. It seemed strange to see our Buick pull-ing up in Baby Gwen's driveway. My father got out looking very young and my mother was holding on to his arm. She looked like a stranger, thin and beautiful in a black cotton peasant dress with rows of colored rickrack around the hem and sleeves. Her hair was cut short and curled around her face in ringlets. I was almost afraid to touch her. Then she ran from my father's side and grabbed me in her arms and whirled me around and around and I smelled the delicate perfume on her skin and it made me feel like crying.

When she put me down I turned to my father. "I'm not going home," I said, putting my hands on my hips.

"Oh, yes you are," he said, so I went upstairs and began to pack my clothes.

Baby Gwen followed me up the stairs. "You can have the kimono," she said. "I want you to have it." She folded it carefully and packed it with tissue paper in a box from Nell's and Blum's and put it beside my suitcase.

"Come sit by me, Baby Gwen, and tell me the news," my mother said, and Baby Gwen went over and sat by her on the chaise. My mother put her arms around her and began to talk in a bright voice inviting her to spend Christmas with us in Indiana.

"It will snow for sure," my mother said. "And LeLe can show you the snow."

We left Clarksville early the next morning. Baby Gwen stood in the doorway waving good-bye. She was wearing a pink satin robe stained in places from where she had sweated in it during the hot nights of July, and her little nipples stuck out beneath the soft material.

I kept hoping maybe Fielding had gotten up early to come and tell me goodbye, but he didn't make it.

"I'll fix those hems when she comes to visit," my mother said, "and do something about that perfume."

I was too tired to argue. All the way to Indiana I slumped in the back seat eating potato chips and sneaking smokes in filling-station restrooms when we stopped for gas.

Then it was another morning and I woke up in my old room and put on my shorts and rode my bicycle over to Cynthia Carver's house. She was in the basement doing her Saturday morning ironing. Cynthia hated to iron. How many mornings had I sat on those basement steps watching the forlorn look on her face while she finished her seven blouses.

"So I might as well be dead," I said, taking a bite of a cookie. "So, anyway, I wish I was dead," I repeated, as Cynthia hung a blouse on a hanger and started on a dirndl skirt. "Here I am, practically engaged to this rich plantation owner's son . . . Fielding. Fielding Reid, LeLe Reid . . . so, anyway, my mother and father come and drag me home practically the same day we fell in love. I don't know how they got wind of it unless that damn Sirena called and told them. She was always watching everything I did. Anyway, they drag me home and I bet they won't even let him write to me."

"What's that perfume?" Cynthia said, lifting her eyes from the waistband of the skirt.

"That's my signature," I said. "That's what I wear now. Tigress in the winter and Aprodisia in the summer. That's what this writer's wife always wore. She got pneumonia or something from swimming in the winter and died when she was real young. Everyone in Clarksville thinks I'm just like her. She was from Mississippi or something. I think she's sort of my father's cousin."

Cynthia pulled the dirndl off the ironing board and began on a pair of pedal pushers. I leaned back on the stairs, watching the steam from the pedal pushers light up the space over Cynthia Carver's disgruntled Yankee head. I was dreaming of the lake, trying to remember how the water turned into diamonds in my hands.

To Make a Dragon Move:
From the Diary of an Anorexic

PAMELA WHITE HADAS

It would have starved a Gnat—
To live so small as I—
And yet I was a living Child—
With Food's necessity

Upon me—like a Claw—
I could no more remove
Than I could coax a Leech away—
Or make a Dragon—move—

—Emily Dickinson, No. 612

I have rules and plenty. Some things I don't touch.
I'm king of my body now. Who needs a mother—
a food machine, those miles and miles of guts?
Once upon a time, I confess, I was fat—
gross. Gross belly, gross ass, no bones
showing at all. Now I say, "No, thank you," a person
in my own right, and no poor loser. I smile
at her plate of brownies. "Make it disappear,"

she used to say, "Join the clean plate club." I disappear
into my room where I have forbidden her to touch
anything. I was a first grade princess once. I smile
to think how those chubby pinks used to please my mother.
And now that I am, Dear Diary, a sort of magical person,
she can't see. My rules. Even here I don't pour out my guts.
Rules. The writing's slow, but like picking a bone,
satisfying, and it doesn't make you fat.

Like, I mean, what would I want with a fat
Diary! Ha ha. But I don't want you to disappear
either. It's tricky . . . "Form in a poem is like the bones
in a body," my teacher says. (I wish he wouldn't touch
me—ugh!—he has B.O.—and if I had the guts
I'd send him a memo about it, and about his smile.
Sucking the chalk like he does, he's like a person
with leprosy.) I'm too sensitive, so says Mother.

She thinks Mr. Crapsie's Valentino. If my so-called mother
is getting it on with him behind my back, that fat
cow . . . What would he see in her? Maybe he likes a person
to have boobs like shivery jello. Does he want to disappear
between thighs like tapioca? His chalky smile
would put a frosting on her Iced Raspberry, his "bone"
(another word for IT, Sue said) would stick in her gut,
maybe, bitten right off! Now why did I have to touch

on that gross theme again, when I meant to touch
on "thoughts too deep for tears," and not my mother.
That Immortality thing, now—I just have a gut
reaction to poems like that—no "verbal fat"
in poems like that, or in "the foul rag and bone
shop of the heart." My God! How does a person
learn to write like that? Like they just open to smile
and heavy words come out. Like, I just *disappear*

beside that stuff. I guess that's what I want: to disappear.
That's pretty much what the doctor said, touching
me with his icy stethoscope, prying apart my smile
with that dry popsicle stick, and he said it to Mother.
And now all she says is "What kind of crazy person
would starve herself to death?" There I am, my gut
flipflopping at the smell of hot bread, my bone
marrow turning to hot mud as she eases the fat

glistening duck out of the microwave, the fat
swimming with sweet orange. I wish it would disappear,
that I . . . If I could just let myself suck a bone—
do bones have calories?—I wouldn't need to touch
a bite of anything else. I am so empty. My gut
must be loopy thin as spaghetti. I start to chew my smile.
Is lip-skin fattening? I know Hunger as a person
inside me, half toad, half dwarf. I try to mother

him: I rock and rock and rock him to sleep like a mother
by doing sit-ups. He leans his gargoyle head against the fat
pillow of my heart. But awake he raves, a crazy person,
turned on by my perpetual motion, by the disappearing
tricks of my body; his shaken fist tickles drool to my smile.
He nibbles at my vagus nerve for attention. Behind the bone
cage of my chest, he is bad enough. He's worse in my gut
where his stamped foot means binge and puke. Don't touch

me, Hunger, Mother . . . Don't you gut my brain.
Bones are my sovereign now, I can touch them here and here.
I am a pure person, magic, revealed as I disappear
into my final fat-free smile, where there is no pain.

When Fat Girls Dream

J. L. HADDAWAY

When fat girls dream
it is not of pies filled with cream,
and chocolate so sweet it would
make their mothers cry.
Nor do they dream in wishes
for Marilyn Monroe's waist
and Lana Turner's legs
hip bones, cheek bones, and short strapless dresses;
these would be easy,
the lottery wins of fat girls
that everyone would understand.

At night when round cheeks push eyes closed
and dimpled fingers tuck like prayer
under extra chins
their dreams are much smaller:
a dance with a man not blind drunk,
a folding chair that won't cringe,
one pair of non-stretch pants
and a mother/aunt/grandmother who doesn't say
"You could be such a pretty girl . . ."

They awaken with possibilities
that die in the bathroom mirror,
in the closet, in the refrigerator.
They wrap themselves up
in smiles and dark skirts

step out their door into the thin air of morning
and maybe
just maybe
into the arms of a man with Rubens' eyes.

The Meal

SHARON OLDS

Mama, I never stop seeing you there
at the breakfast table when I'd come home from school—
sitting with your excellent skeletal posture
facing that plate with the one scoop of cottage cheese on it,
forcing yourself to eat, though you did not want to live,
feeding yourself, small spoonful by
small spoonful, so you would not die and
leave us without a mother as you were
left without a mother. You'd sit
in front of that mound rounded as a breast and
giving off a cold moony light,
light of the life you did not want, you would
hold yourself there and stare down at it,
an orphan forty years old staring at the breast,
a freshly divorced woman down to 82 pounds
staring at the cock runny with milk gone sour,
a daughter who had always said
the best thing her mother ever did for her
was to die. I came home every day to
find you there, dry-eyed, unbent, that
hot control in the breakfast nook, your
delicate savage bones over the cheese
curdled like the breast of the mother twenty years in the
porous earth,

and yet what I remember is your
spoon moving like the cock moving in the
body of the girl waking to the power of her pleasure,
your spoon rising in courage, bite after bite, you
tilted rigid over that plate until you
polished it for my life.

The Pull

SHARON OLDS

As the flu goes on, I get thinner and thinner,
all winter, till my weight dips
to my college weight, and then drops below it,
drifts down through high school, and then
down into junior high,
down through the first blood,
heading for my childhood weight,
birth weight, conception. When I see myself naked
in the mirror, I see I am flirting with my father,
his cadaver the only body this thin
I have seen—I am walking around like his corpse
risen up and moving again, we
laugh about it a lot, my dead
dad and I. I do love being like him,
feeling my big joints slide
under the loose skin. My friends don't
think it's funny, this cake-walk
of the skeletons, and I can't explain it—
I wanted to lie down with him,
on the couch where he lay unconscious at night
and there on his death-bed, let myself down
beside him, and then, with my will, lift us both
up. Or maybe just lie with him
and never get up. Now that his dense
bones are in the ground, I am bringing
my body down. I'm not sure
how he felt about my life. Only twice

did he urge me to live—when the loop of his seed
roped me and drew me over into matter;
and once when I had the flu and he brought me
ten tiny Pyrex bowls
with ten leftovers down in the bottoms.
But when, in the last weeks of his life,
he let me feed him—slip the spoon
of heavy cream into his mouth
and pull it out through his closed lips,
I felt the suction of his tongue, his palate, his
head, his body, his death pulling at my hand.

Disappearing

Monica Wood

When he starts in, I don't look anymore, I know what it looks like, what he looks like, tobacco on his teeth. I just lie in the deep sheets and shut my eyes. I make noises that make it go faster and when he's done he's as far from me as he gets. He could be dead he's so far away.

Lettie says leave then stupid but who would want me. Three hundred pounds anyway but I never check. Skin like tapioca pudding, I wouldn't show anyone. A man.

So we go to the pool at the junior high, swimming lessons. First it's blow bubbles and breathe, blow and breathe. Awful, hot nosefuls of chlorine. My eyes stinging red and patches on my skin. I look worse. We'll get caps and goggles and earplugs and body cream Lettie says. It's better.

There are girls there, what bodies. Looking at me and Lettie out the side of their eyes. Gold hair, skin like milk, chlorine or no.

They thought when I first lowered into the pool, that fat one parting the Red Sea. I didn't care. Something happened when I floated. Good said the little instructor. A little redhead in an emerald suit, no stomach, a depression almost, and white wet skin. Good she said you float just great. Now we're getting somewhere. The whistle around her neck blinded my eyes. And the water under the fluorescent lights. I got scared and couldn't float again. The bottom of the pool was scarred, drops of gray shadow rippling. Without the water I would crack open my head, my dry flesh would sound like a splash on the tiles.

At home I ate a cake and a bottle of milk. No wonder you look like that he said. How can you stand yourself. You're no Cary Grant I told him and he laughed and laughed until I threw up.

When this happens I want to throw up again and again until my heart flops out wet and writhing on the kitchen floor. Then he would know I have one and it moves.

So I went back. And floated again. My arms came around and the groan of the water made the tight blondes smirk but I heard Good that's the crawl that's it in fragments from the redhead when I lifted my face. Through the earplugs I heard her skinny voice. She was happy that I was floating and moving too.

Lettie stopped the lessons and read to me things out of magazines. You have to swim a lot to lose weight. You have to stop eating too. Forget cake and ice cream. Doritos are out. I'm not doing it for that I told her but she wouldn't believe me. She couldn't imagine.

Looking down that shaft of water I know I won't fall. The water shimmers and eases up and down, the heft of me doesn't matter I float anyway.

He says it makes no difference I look the same. But I'm not the same. I can hold myself up in deep water. I can move my arms and feet and the water goes behind me, the wall comes closer. I can look down twelve feet to a cold slab of tile and not be afraid. It makes a difference I tell him. Better believe it mister.

Then this other part happens. Other men interest me. I look at them, real ones, not the ones on TV that's something else entirely. These are real. The one with the white milkweed hair who delivers the mail. The meter man from the light company, heavy thick feet in boots. A smile. Teeth. I drop something out of the cart in the supermarket to see who will pick it up. Sometimes a man. One had yellow short hair and called me ma'am. Young. Thin legs and an accent. One was older. Looked me in the eyes. Heavy, but not like me. My eyes are nice. I color the lids. In the pool it runs off in blue tears. When I come out my face is naked.

The lessons are over, I'm certified. A little certificate signed by the redhead. She says I can swim and I can. I'd do better with her body, thin calves hard as granite.

I get a lane to myself, no one shares. The blondes ignore me now that I don't splash the water, know how to lower myself silently. And when I swim I cut the water cleanly.

For one hour every day I am thin, thin as water, transparent, invisible, steam or smoke.

The redhead is gone, they put her at a different pool and I miss the glare of the whistle dangling between her emerald breasts. Lettie won't come over at all now that she is fatter than me. You're so uppity she says. All this talk about water and who do you think you are.

He says I'm looking all right, so at night it is worse but sometimes now when he starts in I say no. On Sundays the pool is closed I can't say no. I haven't been invisible. Even on days when I don't say no it's all right, he's better.

One night he says it won't last, what about the freezer full of low-cal dinners and that machine in the basement. I'm not doing it for that and he doesn't believe me either. But this time there is another part. There are other men in the water I tell him. Fish he says. Fish in the sea. Good luck.

Ma you've lost says my daughter-in-law, the one who didn't want me in the wedding pictures. One with the whole family, she couldn't help that. I learned how to swim I tell her. You should try it, it might help your ugly disposition.

They closed the pool for two weeks and I went crazy. Repairing the tiles. I went there anyway, drove by in the car. I drank water all day.

Then they opened again and I went every day, sometimes four times until the green paint and new stripes looked familiar as a face. At first the water was heavy as blood but I kept on until it was thinner and thinner, just enough to hold me up. That was when I stopped with the goggles and cap and plugs, things that kept the water out of me.

There was a time I went the day before a holiday and no one was there. It was echoey silence just me and the soundless empty pool and a lifeguard behind the glass. I lowered myself so slow it hurt every muscle but not a blip of water not a ripple not one sound and I was under in that other quiet, so quiet some tears got out, I saw their blue trail swirling.

The redhead is back and nods, she has seen me somewhere. I tell her I took lessons and she still doesn't remember.

This has gone too far he says I'm putting you in the hospital. He calls them at the pool and they pay no attention. He doesn't touch me and I smile into my pillow, a secret smile in my own square of the dark.

Oh my God Lettie says what the hell are you doing what the hell do you think you're doing. I'm disappearing I tell her and what can you do about it not a blessed thing.

For a long time in the middle of it people looked at me. Men. And I thought about it. Believe it, I thought. And now they don't look at me again. And it's better.

I'm almost there. Almost water.

The redhead taught me how to dive, how to tuck my head and vanish like a needle into skin, and every time it happens, my feet leaving the board, I think, this will be the time.

A *Hunger Artist*

Franz Kafka
Translated by Willa and Edwin Muir

DURING THESE LAST decades the interest in professional fasting has markedly diminished. It used to pay very well to stage such great performances under one's own management, but today that is quite impossible. We live in a different world now. At one time the whole town took a lively interest in the hunger artist; from day to day of his fast the excitement mounted; everybody wanted to see him at least once a day; there were people who bought season tickets for the last few days and sat from morning till night in front of his small barred cage; even in the nighttime there were visiting hours, when the whole effect was heightened by torch flares; on fine days the cage was set out in the open air, and then it was the children's special treat to see the hunger artist; for their elders he was often just a joke that happened to be in fashion, but the children stood open-mouthed, holding each other's hands for greater security, marveling at him as he sat there pallid in black tights, with his ribs sticking out so prominently, not even on a seat but down among straw on the ground, sometimes giving a courteous nod, answering questions with a constrained smile, or perhaps stretching an arm through the bars so that one might feel how thin it was, and then again withdrawing deep into himself, paying no attention to anyone or anything, not even to the all-important striking of the clock that was the only piece of furniture in his cage, but merely staring into vacancy with half-shut eyes, now and then taking a sip from a tiny glass of water to moisten his lips.

Besides casual onlookers there were also relays of permanent watchers selected by the public, usually butchers, strangely enough, and it was their task to watch the hunger artist day and night, three of them at a time, in case he should have some secret recourse to nourishment. This was nothing but a formality, instituted to reassure the masses, for the initiates knew well enough that during his fast the artist would never in any circumstances, not even under forcible compulsion, swallow the smallest morsel of food; the honor of his profession forbade it. Not every watcher, of course, was capable of understanding this, there were often groups of night watchers who were very lax in carrying our their duties and deliberately huddled together in a retired corner to play cards with great absorption, obviously intending to give the hunger artist the chance of a little refreshment, which they supposed he could draw from some private hoard. Nothing annoyed the artist more than such watchers; they made him miserable; they made his fast seem unendurable; sometimes he mastered his feebleness sufficiently to sing during their watch for as long as he could keep going, to show them how unjust their suspicions were. But that was of little use; they only wondered at his cleverness in being able to fill his mouth even while singing. Much more to his taste were the watchers who sat close up to the bars, who were not content with the dim night lighting of the hall but focused him in the full glare of the electric pocket torch given them by the impresario. The harsh light did not trouble him at all. In any case he could never sleep properly, and he could always drowse a little, whatever the light, at any hour, even when the hall was thronged with noisy onlookers. He was quite happy at the prospect of spending a sleepless night with such watchers; he was ready to exchange jokes with them, to tell them stories out of his nomadic life, anything at all to keep them awake and demonstrate to them again that he had no eatables in his cage and that he was fasting as not one of them could fast. But his happiest moment was when the morning came and an enormous breakfast was brought them, at his expense, on which they flung themselves with the keen appetite of healthy men after a weary night of wakefulness. Of course there were people who argued that this breakfast was an unfair attempt to bribe the watchers, but that was going rather too far, and when they were invited to take on a night's vigil without a breakfast, merely for the sake of the cause, they made themselves scarce, although they stuck stubbornly to their suspicions.

Such suspicions, anyhow, were a necessary accompaniment to the profession of fasting. No one could possibly watch the hunger artist continuously, day and night, and so no one could produce first-hand evidence that the fast had really been rigorous and continuous; only the artist himself could know that; he was therefore bound to be the sole completely satisfied spectator of his own fast. Yet for other reasons he was never satisfied; it was not perhaps mere fasting that had brought him to such skeleton thinness that many people had regretfully to keep away from such exhibitions, because the sight of him was too much for them, perhaps it was dissatisfaction with himself that had worn him down. For he alone knew, what no other initiate knew, how easy it was to fast. It was the easiest thing in the world. He made no secret of this, yet people did not believe him; at the best they set him down as modest, most of them, however, thought he was out for publicity or else was some kind of cheat who found it easy to fast because he had discovered a way of making it easy, and then had the impudence to admit the fact, more or less. He had to put up with all that, and in the course of time had got used to it, but his inner dissatisfaction always rankled, and never yet, after any term of fasting—this must be granted to his credit—had he left the cage of his own free will. The longest period of fasting was fixed by his impresario at forty days, beyond that term he was not allowed to go, not even in great cities, and there was good reason for it, too. Experience had proved that for about forty days the interest of the public could be stimulated by a steadily increasing pressure of advertisement, but after that the town began to lose interest, sympathetic support began notably to fall off; there were of course local variations as between one town and another or one country and another, but as a general rule forty days marked the limit. So on the fortieth day the flower-bedecked cage was opened, enthusiastic spectators filled the hall, a military band played, two doctors entered the cage to measure the results of the fast, which were announced through a megaphone, and finally two young ladies appeared, blissful at having been selected for the honor, to help the hunger artist down the few steps leading to a small table on which was spread a carefully chosen invalid repast. And at this very moment the artist always turned stubborn. True, he would entrust his bony arms to the outstretched helping hands of the ladies bending over him, but stand up he would not. Why stop fasting at this particular moment, after forty days of it? He had held out for a long time, an illimitably long time; why stop now, when he was in his best fasting form, or rather, not yet quite in his best fasting form? Why should he be cheated of the fame he would get for fasting longer, for being not only the record hunger artist of all time, which presumably he was already, but for beating his own record by a performance beyond human imagination, since he felt that there were no limits to his capacity for fasting? His public pretended to admire him so much, why should it have so little patience with him; if he could endure fasting longer, why shouldn't the public endure it? Besides, he was tired, he was comfortable sitting in the straw, and now he was supposed to lift himself to his full height and go down to a meal the very thought of which gave him a nausea that only the presence of the ladies kept him from betraying, and even that with an effort. And he looked up into the eyes of the ladies who were apparently so friendly and in reality so cruel, and shook his head, which felt too heavy on its strengthless neck. But then there happened yet again what always happened. The impresario came forward, without a word—for the band made speech impossible—lifted his arms in the air above the artist, as if inviting Heaven to look down upon its creature here in the straw, this suffering martyr, which indeed he was, although in quite another sense; grasped him around the emaciated waist, with exaggerated caution, so that the frail condition he was in might be appreciated; and committed him to the care of the blenching ladies, not without secretly giving him a shaking so that his legs and body tottered and swayed. The artist now submitted completely; his head lolled on his breast as if it had landed there by chance; his body was hollowed out; his legs in a spasm of self-preservation clung close to each other at the knees; yet scraped on the ground as if it were not really solid ground, as if they were only trying to find solid ground; and the whole weight of his body, a featherweight after all, relapsed onto one of the ladies, who looking round for help and panting a little—this post of honor was not at all what she had expected it to be—first stretched her neck as far as she could to keep her face at least free from contact with the artist, then finding this impossible, and her more fortunate companion not coming to her aid but merely holding extended on her own trembling hand the little bunch of knucklebones that was the artist's, to the great delight of the spectators burst into tears and had to be replaced by an attendant who had long been stationed in readiness. Then came the food, a little of which the impresario managed to get between the artist's lips, while he sat in a kind of half-fainting trance, to the accompaniment of cheerful patter designed to distract the public's attention from the artist's condition; after that, a toast was drunk to the public, supposedly prompted by a whisper from the artist in the impresario's ear; the band confirmed it with a mighty flourish, the spectators melted away, and no one had any cause to be dissatisfied with the proceedings, no one except the hunger artist himself, he only, as always.

So he lived for many years, with small regular intervals of recuperation, in visible glory, honored by the world, yet in spite of that troubled in spirit, and all the more troubled because no one would take his trouble seriously. What comfort could he possibly need? What more could he possibly wish for? And if some good-natured person, feeling sorry for him, tried to console him by pointing out that his melancholy was probably caused by fasting, it could happen, especially when he had been fasting for some time, that he reacted with an outburst of fury and to the general alarm began to shake the bars of his cage like a wild animal. Yet the impresario had a way of punishing these outbreaks which he rather enjoyed putting into operation. He would apologize publicly for the artist's behavior, which was only to be excused, he admitted, because of the irritability caused by fasting; a condition hardly to be understood by well-fed people; then by natural transition he went on to mention the artist's equally incomprehensible boast that he could fast for much longer than he was doing; he praised the high ambition, the good will, the great self-denial undoubtedly implicit in such a statement; and then quite simply countered it by bringing out photographs, which were also on sale to the public, showing the artist on the fortieth day of a fast lying in bed almost dead from exhaustion. This perversion of the truth, familiar to the artist though it was, always unnerved him afresh and proved too much for him. What was a consequence of the premature ending of his fast was here presented as the cause of it! To fight against this lack of understanding, against a whole world of non-understanding, was impossible. Time and again in good faith he stood by the bars listening to the impresario, but as soon as the photographs appeared he always let go and sank with a groan back on to his straw, and the reassured public could once more come close and gaze at him.

A few years later when the witnesses of such scenes called them to mind, they often failed to understand themselves at all. For meanwhile the aforementioned change in public interest had set in; it seemed to happen almost overnight; there may have been profound causes for it, but who was going to bother about that; at any rate the pampered hunger artist suddenly found himself deserted one fine day by the amusement seekers, who went streaming past him to other more favored attractions. For the last time the impresario hurried him over half of Europe to discover whether the old interest might still survive here and there; all in vain; everywhere, as if by secret agreement, a positive revulsion from professional fasting was in evidence. Of course it could not really have sprung up so suddenly as all that, and many premonitory symptoms which had not been sufficiently remarked or suppressed during the rush and glitter of success now came retrospectively to mind, but it was now too late to take any countermeasures. Fasting would surely come into fashion again at some future date, yet that was no comfort for those living in the present. What, then, was the hunger artist to do? He had been applauded by thousands in his time and could hardly come down to showing himself in a street booth at village fairs, and as for adopting another profession, he was not only too old for that but too fanatically devoted to fasting. So he took leave of the impresario, his partner in an unparalleled career, and hired himself to a large circus; in order to spare his own feelings he avoided reading the conditions of his contract.

A large circus with its enormous traffic in replacing and recruiting men, animals and apparatus can always find a use for people at any time, even for a hunger artist, provided of course that he does not ask too much, and in this particular case anyhow it was not only the artist who was taken on but his famous and long-known name as well; indeed considering the peculiar nature of his performance, which was not impaired by advancing age, it could not be objected that here was an artist past his prime, no longer at the height of his professional skill, seeking a refuge in some quiet corner of a circus; on the contrary, the hunger artist averred that he could fast as well as ever, which was entirely credible; he even alleged that if he were allowed to fast as he liked, and this was at once promised him without more ado, he could astound the world by establishing a record never yet achieved, a statement which certainly provoked a smile among the other professionals, since it left out of account the change in public opinion, which the hunger artist in his zeal conveniently forgot.

He had not, however, actually lost his sense of the real situation and took it as a matter of course that he and his cage should be stationed, not in the middle of the ring as a main attraction, but outside, near the animal cages, on a site that was after all easily accessible. Large and gaily painted placards made a frame for the cage and announced what was to be seen inside it. When the public came thronging out in the intervals to see the animals, they could hardly avoid passing the hunger artist's cage and stopping there for a moment; perhaps they might even have stayed longer had not those pressing behind them in the narrow gangway, who did not understand why they should be held up on their way towards the excitements of the menagerie, made it impossible for anyone to stand gazing quietly for any length of time. And that was the reason why the hunger artist, who had of course been looking forward to these visiting hours as the main achievement of his life, began instead to shrink from them. At first he could hardly wait for the intervals; it was exhilarating to watch the crowds come streaming his way, until only too soon—not even the most obstinate self-deception, clung to almost consciously, could hold out against the fact—the conviction was borne in upon him that these people, most of them, to judge from their actions, again and again, without exception, were all on their way to the menagerie. And the first sight of them from the distance remained the best. For when they reached his cage he was at once deafened by the storm of shouting and abuse that

arose from the two contending factions, which renewed themselves continuously, of those who wanted to stop and stare at him—he soon began to dislike them more than the others—not out of real interest but only out of
obstinate self-assertiveness, and those who wanted to go straight on to the
animals. When the first great rush was past, the stragglers came along, and
these, whom nothing could have prevented from stopping to look at him as
long as they had breath, raced past with long strides, hardly even glancing at
him, in their haste to get to the menagerie in time. And all too rarely did it
happen that he had a stroke of luck, when a father of a family fetched up
before him with his children, pointed a finger at the hunger artist and explained at length what the phenomenon meant, telling stories of earlier years
when he himself had watched similar but much more thrilling performances,
and the children, still rather uncomprehending, since neither inside nor outside school had they been sufficiently prepared for this lesson—what did
they care about fasting?—yet showed by the brightness of their intent eyes
that new and better times might be coming. Perhaps, said the hunger artist
to himself many a time, things would be a little better if his cage were set not
quite so near the menagerie. That made it too easy for people to make their
choice, to say nothing of what he suffered from the stench of the menagerie,
the animals' restlessness by night, the carrying past of raw lumps of flesh for
the beasts of prey, the roaring at feeding times, which depressed him continually. But he did not dare to lodge a complaint with the management;
after all, he had the animals to thank for the troops of people who passed his
cage, among whom there might always be one here and there to take an interest in him, and who could tell where they might seclude him if he called
attention to his existence and thereby to the fact that, strictly speaking, he
was only an impediment on the way to the menagerie.

A small impediment, to be sure, one that grew steadily less. People grew
familiar with the strange idea that they could be expected, in times like these,
to take an interest in a hunger artist, and with this familiarity the verdict
went out against him. He might fast as much as he could, and he did so; but
nothing could save him now, people passed him by. Just try to explain to
anyone the art of fasting! Anyone who has no feeling for it cannot be made to
understand it. The fine placards grew dirty and illegible, they were torn down;
the little notice board telling the number of fast days achieved, which at first
was changed carefully every day, had long stayed at the same figure, for after
the first few weeks even this small a task seemed pointless to the staff; and so
the artist simply fasted on and on, as he had once dreamed of doing, and it
was no trouble to him, just as he had always foretold, but no one counted the

days, no one, not even the artist himself, knew what records he was already breaking, and his heart grew heavy. And when once in a time some leisurely passer-by stopped, made merry over the old figure on the board and spoke of swindling, that was in its way the stupidest lie ever invented by indifference and inborn malice, since it was not the hunger artist who was cheating; he was working honestly, but the world was cheating him of his reward.

Many more days went by, however, and that too came to an end. An overseer's eye fell on the cage one day and he asked the attendants why this perfectly good cage should be left standing there unused with dirty straw inside it; nobody knew, until one man, helped out by the notice board, remembered about the hunger artist. They poked into the straw with sticks and found him in it. "Are you still fasting?" asked the overseer. "When on earth do you mean to stop?" "Forgive me, everybody," whispered the hunger artist; only the overseer, who had his ear to the bars, understood him. "Of course," said the overseer, and tapped his forehead with a finger to let the attendants know what state the man was in, "we forgive you." "I always wanted you to admire my fasting," said the hunger artist. "We do admire it," said the overseer, affably. "But you shouldn't admire it," said the hunger artist. "Well, then we don't admire it," said the overseer, "but why shouldn't we admire it?" "Because I have to fast, I can't help it," said the hunger artist. "What a fellow you are," said the overseer; "and why can't you help it?" "Because," said the hunger artist, lifting his head a little and speaking, with his lips pursed, as if for a kiss, right into the overseer's ear, so that no syllable might be lost, "because I couldn't find the food I liked. If I had found it, believe me, I should have made no fuss and stuffed myself like you or anyone else." These were his last words, but in his dimming eyes remained the firm though no longer proud persuasion that he was still continuing to fast.

"Well, clear this out now!" said the overseer, and they buried the hunger artist, straw and all. Into the cage they put a young panther. Even the most insensitive felt it refreshing to see this wild creature leaping around the cage that had so long been dreary. The panther was all right. The food he liked was brought him without hesitation by the attendants; he seemed not even to miss his freedom; his noble body, furnished almost to the bursting point with all that it needed, seemed to carry freedom around with it too; somewhere in his jaws it seemed to lurk; and the joy of life streamed with such ardent passion from his throat that for the onlookers it was not easy to stand the shock of it. But they braced themselves, crowded round the cage, and did not want ever to move away.

SECTION B
Abnormal Height—Dwarfism

Dwarf House

ANN BEATTIE

"ARE YOU HAPPY?" MacDonald says. "Because if you're happy I'll leave you alone."

MacDonald is sitting in a small gray chair, patterned with grayer leaves, talking to his brother, who is standing in a blue chair. MacDonald's brother is four feet, six and three-quarter inches tall, and when he stands in a chair he can look down on MacDonald. MacDonald is twenty-eight years old. His brother, James, is thirty-eight. There was a brother between them, Clem, who died of a rare disease in Panama. There was a sister also, Amy, who flew to Panama to be with her dying brother. She died in the same hospital, one month later, of the same disease. None of the family went to the funeral. Today MacDonald, at his mother's request, is visiting James to find out if he is happy. Of course James is not, but standing on the chair helps, and the twenty-dollar bill that MacDonald slipped into his tiny hand helps too.

"What do you want to live in a dwarf house for?"

"There's a giant here."

"Well it must just depress the hell out of the giant."

"He's pretty happy."

"Are you?"

"I'm as happy as the giant."

"What do you do all day?"

"Use up the family's money."

"You know I'm not here to accuse you. I'm here to see what I can do."

"She sent you again, didn't she?"

"Yes."

"Is this your lunch hour?"

"Yes."

"Have you eaten? I've got some candy bars in my room."

"Thank you. I'm not hungry."

"Place make you lose your appetite?"

"I do feel nervous. Do you like living here?"

"I like it better than the giant does. He's lost twenty-five pounds. Nobody's supposed to know about that—the official word is fifteen—but I overheard the doctors talking. He's lost twenty-five pounds."

"Is the food bad?"

"Sure. Why else would he lose twenty-five pounds?"

"Do you mind . . . if we don't talk about the giant right now? I'd like to take back some reassurance to Mother."

"Tell her I'm as happy as she is."

"You know she's not happy."

"She knows I'm not, too. Why does she keep sending you?"

"She's concerned about you. She'd like you to live at home. She'd come herself . . ."

"I know. But she gets nervous around freaks."

"I was going to say that she hasn't been going out much. She sent me, though, to see if you wouldn't reconsider."

"I'm not coming home, MacDonald."

"Well, is there anything you'd like from home?"

"They let you have pets here. I'd like a parakeet."

"A bird? Seriously?"

"Yeah. A green parakeet."

"I've never seen a green one."

"Pet stores will dye them any color you ask for."

"Isn't that harmful to them?"

"You want to please the parakeet or me?"

"How did it go?" MacDonald's wife asks.

"That place is a zoo. Well, it's worse than a zoo—it's what it is: a dwarf house."

"Is he happy?"

"I don't know. I didn't really get an answer out of him. There's a giant there who's starving to death, and he says he's happier than the giant. Or maybe he said he was as happy. I can't remember. Have we run out of vermouth?"

"Yes. I forgot to go to the liquor store. I'm sorry."

"That's all right. I don't think a drink would have much effect anyway."

"It might. If I had remembered to go to the liquor store."

"I'm just going to call Mother and get it over with."

"What's that in your pocket?"

"Candy bars. James gave them to me. He felt sorry for me because I'd given up my lunch hour to visit him."

"Your brother is really a very nice person."

"Yeah. He's a dwarf."

"What?"

"I mean that I think of him primarily as a dwarf. I've had to take care of him all my life."

"Your mother took care of him until he moved out of the house."

"Yeah, well it looks like he found a replacement for her. But you might need a drink before I tell you about it."

"Oh, tell me."

"He's got a little sweetie. He's in love with a woman who lives in the dwarf house. He introduced me. She's three feet eleven. She stood there smiling at my knees."

"That's wonderful that he has a friend."

"Not a friend—a fiancée. He claims that as soon as he's got enough money saved up he's going to marry this other dwarf."

"He is?"

"Isn't there some liquor store that delivers? I've seen liquor trucks in this neighborhood, I think."

His mother lives in a high-ceilinged old house on Newfield Street, in a neighborhood that is gradually being taken over by Puerto Ricans. Her phone has been busy for almost two hours, and MacDonald fears that she, too, may have been taken over by Puerto Ricans. He drives to his mother's house and knocks on the door. It is opened by a Puerto Rican woman, Mrs. Esposito.

"Is my mother all right?" he asks.

"Yes. She's okay."

"May I come in?"

"Oh, I'm sorry."

She steps aside—not that it does much good, because she's so wide that there's still not much room for passage. Mrs. Esposito is wearing a dress that looks like a jungle: tall streaks of green grass going every which way, brown stumps near the hem, flashes of red around her breasts.

"Who were you talking to?" he asks his mother.

"Carlotta was on the phone with her brother, seeing if he'll take her in. Her husband put her out again."

Mrs. Esposito, hearing her husband spoken of, rubs her hands in anguish.

"It took two hours?" MacDonald says good-naturedly, feeling sorry for her. "What was the verdict?"

"He won't," Mrs. Esposito answers.

"I told her she could stay here, but when she told him she was going to do that he went wild and said he didn't want her living just two doors down."

"I don't think he meant it," MacDonald says. "He was probably just drinking again."

"He had joined Alcoholics Anonymous," Mrs. Esposito says. "He didn't drink for two weeks, and he went to every meeting, and one night he came home and said he wanted me out."

MacDonald sits down, nodding nervously. The chair he sits in has a child's chair facing it, which is used as a footstool. When James lived with his mother it was his chair. His mother still keeps his furniture around—a tiny child's glider, a mirror in the hall that is knee-high.

"Did you see James?" his mother asks.

"Yes. He said that he's very happy."

"I know he didn't say that. If I can't rely on you I'll have to go myself, and you know how I cry for days after I see him."

"He said he was pretty happy. He said he didn't think you were."

"Of course I'm not happy. He never calls."

"He likes the place he lives in. He's got other people to talk to now."

"Dwarfs, not people," his mother says. "He's hiding from the real world."

"He didn't have anybody but you to talk to when he lived at home. He's got a new part-time job that he likes better, too, working in a billing department."

"Sending unhappiness to people in the mail," his mother says.

"How are you doing?" he asks.

"As James says, I'm not happy."

"What can I do?" MacDonald asks.

"Go to see him tomorrow and tell him to come home."

"He won't leave. He's in love with somebody there."

"Who? Who does he say he's in love with? Not another social worker?"

"Some woman. I met her. She seems very nice."

"What's her name?"

"I don't remember."

"How tall is she?"

"She's a little shorter than James."

"Shorter than James?"

"Yes. A little shorter."

"What does she want with him?"

"He said they were in love."

"I heard you. I'm asking what she wants with him."

"I don't know. I really don't know. Is that sherry in that bottle? Do you mind . . ."

"I'll get it for you," Mrs. Esposito says.

"Well, who knows what anybody wants from anybody," his mother says. "Real love comes to naught. I loved your father and we had a dwarf."

"You shouldn't blame yourself," MacDonald says. He takes the glass of sherry from Mrs. Esposito.

"I shouldn't? I have to raise a dwarf and take care of him for thirty-eight years and then in my old age he leaves me. Who should I blame for that?"

"James," MacDonald says. "But he didn't mean to offend you."

"I should blame your father," his mother says, as if he hasn't spoken. "But he's dead. Who should I blame for his early death? God?"

His mother does not believe in God. She has not believed in God for thirty-eight years.

"I had to have a dwarf. I wanted grandchildren, and I know you won't give me any because you're afraid you'll produce a dwarf. Clem is dead, and Amy is dead. Bring me some of that sherry, too, Carlotta."

At five o'clock MacDonald calls his wife. "Honey," he says, "I'm going to be tied up in this meeting until seven. I should have called you before."

"That's all right," she says. "Have you eaten?"

"No. I'm in a meeting."

"We can eat when you come home."

"I think I'll grab a sandwich, though. Okay?"

"Okay. I got the parakeet."

"Good. Thank you."

"It's awful. I'll be glad to have it out of here."

"What's so awful about a parakeet?"

"I don't know. The man at the pet store gave me a ferris wheel with it, and a bell on a chain of seeds."

"Oh yeah? Free?"

"Of course. You don't think I'd buy junk like that, do you?"

"I wonder why he gave it to you."

"Oh, who knows. I got gin and vermouth today."

"Good," he says. "Fine. Talk to you later."

MacDonald takes off his tie and puts it in his pocket. At least once a week he goes to a run-down bar across town, telling his wife that he's in a meeting, putting his tie in his pocket. And once a week his wife remarks that she doesn't understand how he can get his tie wrinkled. He takes off his shoes and puts on his sneakers and takes an old brown corduroy jacket off a coat hook behind his desk. His secretary is still in her office. Usually she leaves before five, but whenever he leaves looking like a slob she seems to be there to say goodnight to him.

"You wonder what's going on, don't you?" MacDonald says to his secretary.

She smiles. Her name is Betty, and she must be in her early thirties. All he really knows about his secretary is that she smiles a lot and that her name is Betty.

"Want to come along for some excitement?" he says.

"Where are you going?"

"I knew you were curious," he says.

Betty smiles.

"Want to come?" he says. "Like to see a little low life?"

"Sure," she says.

They go out to his car, a red Toyota. He hangs his jacket in the back and puts his shoes on the back seat.

"We're going to see a Japanese woman who beats people with figurines," he says.

Betty smiles. "Where are we really going?" she asks.

"You must know that businessmen are basically depraved," MacDonald says. "Don't you assume that I commit bizarre acts after hours?"

"No," Betty says.

"How old are you?" he asks.

"Thirty," she says.

"You're thirty years old and you're not a cynic yet?"

"How old are you?" she asks.

"Twenty-eight," MacDonald says.

"When you're thirty you'll be an optimist all the time," Betty says.

"What makes you optimistic?" he asks.

"I was just kidding. Actually, if I didn't take two kinds of pills, I couldn't smile every morning and evening for you. Remember the day I fell asleep at my desk? The day before I had had an abortion."

MacDonald's stomach feels strange—he wouldn't mind having a couple kinds of pills himself, to get rid of the strange feeling. Betty lights a cigarette, and the smoke doesn't help his stomach. But he had the strange feeling all day, even before Betty spoke. Maybe he has stomach cancer. Maybe he doesn't want to face James again. In the glove compartment there is a jar that Mrs. Esposito gave his mother and that his mother gave him to take to James. One of Mrs. Esposito's relatives sent it to her, at her request. It was made by a doctor in Puerto Rico. Supposedly, it can increase your height if rubbed regularly on the soles of the feet. He feels nervous, knowing that it's in the glove compartment. The way his wife must feel having the parakeet and the ferris wheel sitting around the house. The house. His wife. Betty.

They park in front of a bar with a blue neon sign in the window that says IDEAL CAF⁰. There is a larger neon sign above that that says SCHLITZ. He and Betty sit in a back booth. He orders a pitcher of beer and a double order of spiced shrimp. Tammy Wynette is singing "D-I-V-O-R-C-E" on the jukebox.

"Isn't this place awful?" he says. "But the spiced shrimp are great."

Betty smiles.

"If you don't feel like smiling, don't smile," he says.

"Then all the pills would be for nothing."

"Everything is for nothing," he says.

"If you weren't drinking you could take one of the pills," Betty says. "Then you wouldn't feel that way."

"Did you see *Esquire*?" James asks.

"No," MacDonald says. "Why?"

"Wait here," James says.

MacDonald waits. A dwarf comes into the room and looks under his chair. MacDonald raises his feet.

"Excuse me," the dwarf says. He turns cartwheels to leave the room.

"He used to be with the circus," James says, returning. "He leads us in exercises now."

MacDonald looks at *Esquire*. There has been a convention of dwarfs at the Oakland Hilton, and *Esquire* got pictures of it. Two male dwarfs are leading a delighted female dwarf down a runway. A baseball team of dwarfs. A group picture. Someone named Larry—MacDonald does not look back up at the picture to see which one he is—says, "I haven't had so much fun since I was born." MacDonald turns another page. An article on Daniel Ellsberg.

"Huh," MacDonald says.

"How come *Esquire* didn't know about our dwarf house?" James asks. "They could have come here."

"Listen," MacDonald says, "Mother asked me to bring this to you. I don't mean to insult you, but she made me promise I'd deliver it. You know she's very worried about you."

"What is it?" James asks.

MacDonald gives him the piece of paper that Mrs. Esposito wrote instructions on in English.

"Take it back," James says.

"No. Then I'll have to tell her you refused it."

"Tell her."

"No. She's miserable. I know it's crazy, but just keep it for her sake."

James turns and throws the jar. Bright yellow liquid runs down the wall.

"Tell her not to send you back here either," James says. MacDonald thinks that if James were his size he would have hit him instead of only speaking.

"Come back and hit me if you want," MacDonald hollers. "Stand on the arm of this chair and hit me in the face."

James does not come back. A dwarf in the hallway says to MacDonald, as he is leaving, "It was a good idea to be sarcastic to him."

MacDonald and his wife and mother and Mrs. Esposito stand amid a cluster of dwarfs and one giant waiting for the wedding to begin. James and his bride are being married on the lawn outside the church. They are still inside with the minister. His mother is already weeping. "I wish I had never married your father," she says, and borrows Mrs. Esposito's handkerchief to dry her eyes. Mrs. Esposito is wearing her jungle dress again. On the way over she told MacDonald's wife that her husband had locked her out of the house and that she only had one dress. "It's lucky it was such a pretty one," his wife said, and Mrs. Esposito shyly protested that it wasn't very fancy, though.

The minister and James and his bride come out of the church onto the lawn. The minister is a hippie, or something like a hippie: a tall, white-faced man with stringy blond hair and black motorcycle boots. "Friends," the minister says, "before the happy marriage of these two people, we will release this bird from its cage, symbolic of the new freedom of marriage, and of the ascension of the spirit."

The minister is holding the cage with the parakeet in it.

"MacDonald," his wife whispers, "that's the parakeet. You can't release a pet into the wild."

His mother disapproves of all this. Perhaps her tears are partly disapproval, and not all hatred of his father.

The bird is released: it flies shakily into a tree and disappears into the new spring foliage.

The dwarfs clap and cheer. The minister wraps his arms around himself and spins. In a second the wedding ceremony begins, and just a few minutes later it is over. James kisses the bride, and the dwarfs swarm around them. MacDonald thinks of a piece of Hershey bar he dropped in the woods once on a camping trip, and how the ants were all over it before he finished lacing his boot. He and his wife step forward, followed by his mother and Mrs. Esposito. MacDonald sees that the bride is smiling beautifully—a smile no pills could produce—and that the sun is shining on her hair so that it sparkles. She looks small, and bright, and so lovely that MacDonald, on his knees to kiss her, doesn't want to get up.

The Song the Dwarf Sings

Rainer Maria Rilke

It's possible my soul is upright and O.K.;
but it can't make my heart stand straight
or my crooked blood—it's from those things
that the pain comes.
My soul has no place to walk in, no place to lie,
it catches onto my sharp skeleton
with a terrified beating of wings.

My hands will never amount to anything either.
See how stunted they are?
They're moist, they hop around sluggishly
like toads after a rain
And everything else in me
is sad and old and worn out;
why does God hesitate to throw it all out
on the dump?

Is he angry with me, perhaps, for my face
with its sullen mouth?
It was ready, so often, to be full
of light and clear deep thought;
but nothing ever came as close to it
as the big dogs did.
And dogs don't have it.

The Dwarf

RAY BRADBURY

AIMEE WATCHED the sky, quietly.

Tonight was one of those motionless hot summer nights. The concrete pier empty, the strong red, white, yellow bulbs like insects in the air above the wooden emptiness. The managers of the various carnival pitches stood, like melting wax dummies, eyes staring blindly, not talking, all down the line.

Two customers had passed through an hour before. Those two lonely people were now in the roller coaster, screaming murderously as it plummeted down the blazing night, around one emptiness after another.

Aimee moved slowly across the strand, a few worn wooden hoopla rings sticking to her wet hands. She stopped behind the ticket booth that fronted the MIRROR MAZE. She saw herself grossly misrepresented in three rippled mirrors outside the Maze. A thousand tired replicas of herself dissolved in the corridor beyond, hot images among so much clear coolness.

She stepped inside the ticket booth and stood looking a long while at Ralph Banghart's thin neck. He clenched an unlit cigar between his long uneven yellow teeth as he laid out a battered game of solitaire on the ticket shelf.

When the roller coaster wailed and fell in its terrible avalanche again, she was reminded to speak.

"What kind of people go up in roller coasters?"

Ralph Banghart worked his cigar a full thirty seconds. "People wanna die. That rollie coaster's the handiest thing to dying there is." He sat listening to the faint sound of rifle shots from the shooting gallery. "This whole damn carny business's crazy. For instance, that dwarf. You seen him? Every night, pays his dime, runs in the Mirror Maze all the way back through to Screwy Louie's Room. You should see this little runt head back there. My God!"

"Oh, yes," said Aimee, remembering. "I always wonder what it's like to be a dwarf. I always feel sorry when I see him."

"I could play him like an accordion."

"Don't say that!"

"My Lord." Ralph patted her thigh with a free hand. "The way you carry on about guys you never even met." He shook his head and chuckled. "Him and his secret. Only he don't know I know, see? Boy howdy!"

"It's a hot night." She twitched the large wooden hoops nervously on her damp fingers.

"Don't change the subject. He'll be here, rain or shine."

Aimee shifted her weight.

Ralph seized her elbow. "Hey! You ain't mad? You wanna see that dwarf, don't you? Sh!" Ralph turned. "Here he comes now!"

The Dwarf's hand, hairy and dark, appeared all by itself reaching up into the booth window with a silver dime. An invisible person called, "One!" in a high, child's voice.

Involuntarily, Aimee bent forward.

The Dwarf looked up at her, resembling nothing more than a dark-eyed, dark-haired, ugly man who has been locked in a winepress, squeezed and wadded down and down, fold on fold, agony on agony, until a bleached, outraged mass is left, the face bloated shapelessly, a face you know must stare wide-eyed and awake at two and three and four o'clock in the morning, lying flat in bed, only the body asleep.

Ralph tore a yellow ticket in half. "One!"

The Dwarf, as if frightened by an approaching storm, pulled his black coat-lapels tightly about his throat and waddled swiftly. A moment later, ten thousand lost and wandering dwarfs wriggled between the mirror flats, like frantic dark beetles, and vanished.

"Quick!"

Ralph squeezed Aimee along a dark passage behind the mirrors. She felt him pat her all the way back through the tunnel to a thin partition with a peekhole.

"This is rich," he chuckled. "Go on—look."

Aimee hesitated, then put her face to the partition.

"You *see* him?" Ralph whispered.

Aimee felt her heart beating. A full minute passed.

There stood the Dwarf in the middle of the small blue room. His eyes were shut. He wasn't ready to open them yet. Now, now he opened his eyelids and looked at a large mirror set before him. And what he saw in the mirror made him smile. He winked, he pirouetted, he stood sidewise, he waved, he bowed, he did a little clumsy dance.

everyone wants a mirror

And the mirror repeated each motion with long, thin arms, with a tall, tall body, with a huge wink and an enormous repetition of the dance, ending in a gigantic bow!

"Every night the same thing," whispered Ralph in Aimee's ear. "Ain't that rich?"

Aimee turned her head and looked at Ralph steadily out of her motionless face, for a long time, and she said nothing. Then, as if she could not help herself, she moved her head slowly and very slowly back to stare once more through the opening. She held her breath. She felt her eyes begin to water.

Ralph nudged her, whispering.

"Hey, what's the little gink doin' *now?*"

They were drinking coffee and not looking at each other in the ticket booth half an hour later, when the Dwarf came out of the mirrors. He took his hat off and started to approach the booth, when he saw Aimee and hurried away.

"He wanted something," said Aimee.

"Yeah." Ralph squashed out his cigarette, idly. "I know what, too. But he hasn't got the nerve to ask. One night in this squeaky little voice he says, 'I bet those mirrors are expensive.' Well, I played dumb. I said yeah they were. He sort of looked at me, waiting, and when I didn't say any more, he went home, but next night he said, 'I bet those mirrors cost fifty, a hundred bucks.' I bet they do, I said. I laid me out a hand of solitaire."

"Ralph," she said.

He glanced up. "Why you look at me that way?"

"Ralph," she said, "why don't you sell him one of your extra ones?"

"Look, Aimee, do I tell you how to run your hoop circus?"

"How much do those mirrors cost?"

"I can get 'em secondhand for thirty-five bucks."

"Why don't you tell him where he can buy one, then?"

"Aimee, you're not smart." He laid his hand on her knee. She moved her knee away. "Even if I told him where to go, you think he'd buy one? Not on your life. And why? He's self-conscious. Why, if he even knew I knew he was flirtin' around in front of that mirror in Screwy Louie's Room, he'd never come back. He plays like he's goin' through the Maze to get lost, like everybody else. Pretends like he don't care about that special room. Always waits for business to turn bad, late nights, so he has that room to himself. What he does for entertainment on nights when business is good, God knows. No, sir, he wouldn't dare go buy a mirror anywhere. He ain't got no friends, and even if he did he couldn't ask them to buy him a thing like that. Pride, by God, pride. Only reason he even mentioned it to me is I'm practically the only guy he knows. Besides, look at him—he ain't got enough to buy a mirror like those. He might be savin' up, but where in hell in the world today can a dwarf work? Dime a dozen, drug on the market, outside of circuses."

"I feel awful. I feel sad." Aimee sat staring at the empty boardwalk. "Where does he live?"

"Flytrap down on the waterfront. The Ganghes Arms. Why?"

"I'm madly in love with him, if you must know."

He grinned around his cigar. "Aimee," he said. "You and your very funny jokes."

A warm night, a hot morning, and a blazing noon. The sea was a sheet of burning tinsel and glass.

Aimee came walking, in the locked-up carnival alleys out over the warm sea, keeping in the shade, half a dozen sun-bleached magazines under her arm. She opened a flaking door and called into hot darkness. "Ralph?" She picked her way through the black hall behind the mirrors, her heels tacking the wooden floor. "Ralph?"

Someone stirred sluggishly on the canvas cot. "Aimee?"

He sat up and screwed a dim light bulb into the dressing table socket. He squinted at her, half blinded. "Hey, you look like the cat that swallowed a canary."

"Ralph, I came about the midget!"

"Dwarf, Aimee honey, dwarf. A midget is in the cells, born that way. A dwarf is in the glands. . . ."

"Ralph! I just found out the most wonderful thing about him!"

"Honest to God," he said to his hands, holding them out as witnesses to his disbelief. "This woman! Who in hell gives two cents for some ugly little————"

"Ralph!" She held out the magazines, her eyes shining. "He's a writer! Think of that!"

"It's a pretty hot day for thinking." He lay back and examined her, smiling faintly.

"I just happened to pass the Ganghes Arms, and saw Mr. Greeley, the manager. He says the typewriter runs all night in Mr. Big's room!"

"Is *that* his name?" Ralph began to roar with laughter.

"Writes just enough pulp detective stories to live. I found one of his stories in the secondhand magazine place, and, Ralph, guess what?"

"I'm tired, Aimee."

"This little guy's got a soul as big as all outdoors; he's got *everything* in his head!"

"Why ain't he writin' for the big magazines, then, I ask you?"

"Because maybe he's afraid—maybe he doesn't know he can do it. That happens. People don't believe in themselves. But if he only tried, I bet he could sell stories anywhere in the world." *because*

"Why ain't he rich, I wonder?" *no one ever reviews*

"Maybe because ideas come slow because he's down in the dumps. Who wouldn't be? So small that way? I bet it's hard to think of anything except being so small and living in a one-room cheap apartment."

"Hell!" snorted Ralph. "You talk like Florence Nightingale's grandma."

She held up the magazine. "I'll read you part of his crime story. It's got all the guns and tough people, but it's told by a dwarf. I bet the editors never guessed the author knew what he was writing about. Oh, please don't sit there like that, Ralph! Listen."

And she began to read aloud.

"I am a dwarf and I am a murderer. The two things cannot be separated. One is the cause of the other.

"The man I murdered used to stop me on the street when I was twenty-one, pick me up in his arms, kiss my brow, croon wildly to me, sing Rock-a-bye Baby, haul me into meat markets, toss me on the scales and cry, 'Watch it. Don't weigh your thumb, there, butcher!'

"Do you *see* how our lives moved toward murder? This fool, this persecutor of my flesh and soul!

"As for my childhood: my parents were small people, not quite dwarfs, not quite. My father's inheritance kept us in a doll's house, an amazing thing like a white-scrolled wedding cake—little rooms, little chairs, miniature paintings, cameos, ambers with insects caught inside, everything tiny, tiny, tiny! The world of Giants far away, an ugly rumor beyond the garden wall. Poor mama, papa! They meant only the best for me. They kept me, like a porcelain vase, small and treasured, to themselves, in our ant world, our beehive rooms, our microscopic library, our land of beetle-sized doors and moth windows. Only now do I see the magnificent size of my parents' psychosis! They must have dreamed they would live forever, keeping me like a butterfly under glass. But first father died, and then fire ate up the little house, the wasp's nest, and every postage-stamp mirror and saltcellar closet within. Mama, too, gone!

And myself alone, watching the fallen embers, tossed out into a world of Monsters and Titans, caught in a landslide of reality, rushed, rolled, and smashed to the bottom of the cliff!

"It took me a year to adjust. A job with a sideshow was unthinkable. There seemed no place for me in the world. And then, a month ago, the Persecutor came into my life, clapped a bonnet on my unsuspecting head, and cried to friends, 'I want you to meet the little woman!'"

Aimee stopped reading. Her eyes were unsteady and the magazine shook as she handed it to Ralph. "You finish it. The rest is a murder story. It's all right. But don't you see? That little man. That little man."

Ralph tossed the magazine aside and lit a cigarette lazily. "I like Westerns better."

"Ralph, you got to read it. He needs someone to tell him how good he is and keep him writing."

Ralph looked at her, his head to one side. "And guess who's going to do it? Well, well, ain't we just the Saviour's right hand?"

"I won't listen!"

"Use your head, damn it! You go busting in on him he'll think you're handing him pity. He'll chase you screamin' outa his room."

She sat down, thinking about it slowly, trying to turn it over and see it from every side. "I don't know. Maybe you're right. Oh, it's not just pity, Ralph, honest. But maybe it'd look like it to him. I've got to be awful careful."

He shook her shoulder back and forth, pinching softly, with his fingers. "Hell, hell, lay off him, is all I ask; you'll get nothing but trouble for your dough. God, Aimee, I never *seen* you so hepped on anything. Look, you and me, let's make it a day, take a lunch, get us some gas, and just drive on down the coast as far as we can drive; swim, have supper, see a good show in some little town—to hell with the carnival, how about it? A damn nice day and no worries. I been savin' a coupla bucks."

"It's because I know he's different," she said, looking off into darkness. "It's because he's something we can never be—you and me and all the rest of us here on the pier. It's so funny, so funny. Life fixed him so he's good for nothing but carny shows, yet there he is on the land. And life made us so we wouldn't have to work in the carny shows, but here we are, anyway, way out here at sea on the pier. Sometimes it seems a million miles to shore. How come, Ralph, that we got the bodies, but he's got the brains and can think things we'll never even guess?"

"You haven't even been listening to me!" said Ralph.

She sat with him standing over her, his voice far away. Her eyes were half shut and her hands were in her lap, twitching.

"I don't like that shrewd look you're getting on," he said, finally.

She opened her purse slowly and took out a small roll of bills and started counting. "Thirty-five, forty dollars. There. I'm going to phone Billie Fine and have him send out one of those tall-type mirrors to Mr. Bigelow at the Ganghes Arms. Yes, I am!"

"What!"

"Think how wonderful for him, Ralph, having one in his own room any time he wants it. Can I use your phone?".

"Go ahead, *be* nutty."

Ralph turned quickly and walked off down the tunnel. A door slammed.

Aimee waited, then after a while put her hands to the phone and began to dial, with painful slowness. She paused between numbers, holding her breath, shutting her eyes, thinking how it might seem to be small in the world, and then one day someone sends a special mirror by. A mirror for your room where you can hide away with the big reflection of yourself, shining, and write stories and stories, never going out into the world unless you had to. How might it be then, alone, with the wonderful illusion all in one piece in the room. Would it make you happy or sad, would it help your writing or hurt it? She shook her head back and forth, back and forth. At least this way there would be no one to look down at you. Night after night, perhaps rising secretly at three in the cold morning, you could wink and dance around and smile and wave at yourself, so tall, so tall, so very fine and tall in the bright looking-glass.

A telephone voice said, "Billie Fine's."

"Oh, *Billie!*" she cried.

Night came in over the pier. The ocean lay dark and loud under the planks. Ralph sat cold and waxen in his glass coffin, laying out the cards, his eyes fixed, his mouth stiff. At his elbow, a growing pyramid of burnt cigarette butts grew larger. When Aimee walked along under the hot red and blue bulbs, smiling, waving, he did not stop setting the cards down slow and very slow. "Hi, Ralph!" she said.

"How's the love affair?" he asked, drinking from a dirty glass of iced water. "How's Charlie Boyer, or is it Cary Grant?"

"I just went and bought me a new hat," she said, smiling. "Gosh, I feel *good!* You know why? Billie Fine's sending a mirror out tomorrow! Can't you just see the nice little guy's face?"

"I'm not so hot at imagining."

"Oh, Lord, you'd think I was going to marry him or something."

"Why not? Carry him around in a suitcase. People say, Where's your husband? All you do is open your bag, yell, Here he is! Like a silver cornet. Take him outa his case any old hour, play a tune, stash him away. Keep a little sandbox for him on the back porch."

"I was feeling so good," she said.

"Benevolent is the word." Ralph did not look at her, his mouth tight. "Ben-ev-o-*lent.* I suppose this all comes from me watching him through that knothole, getting my kicks? That why you sent the mirror? People like you run around with tambourines, taking the joy out of my life."

"Remind me not to come to your place for drinks any more. I'd rather go with no people at all than mean people."

Ralph exhaled a deep breath. "Aimee, Aimee. Don't you know you can't help that guy? He's bats. And this crazy thing of yours is like saying, Go ahead, *be* batty, I'll help you, pal."

"Once in a lifetime anyway, it's nice to make a mistake if you think it'll do somebody some good," she said.

"God deliver me from do-gooders, Aimee."

"Shut up, shut up!" she cried, and then said nothing more.

He let the silence lie a while, and then got up, putting his fingerprinted glass aside. "Mind the booth for me?"

"Sure. Why?"

She saw ten thousand cold white images of him stalking down the glassy corridors, between mirrors, his mouth straight and his fingers working themselves.

She sat in the booth for a full minute and then suddenly shivered. A small clock ticked in the booth and she turned the deck of cards over, one by one, waiting. She heard a hammer pounding and knocking and pounding again, far away inside the Maze; a silence, more waiting, and then ten thousand images folding and refolding and dissolving, Ralph striding, looking out at ten thousand images of her in the booth. She heard his quiet laughter as he came down the ramp.

"Well, what's put you in such a good mood?" she asked, suspiciously.

"Aimee," he said, carelessly, "we shouldn't quarrel. You say tomorrow Billie's sending that mirror to Mr. Big's?"

"You're not going to try anything funny?"

"Me?" He moved her out of the booth and took over the cards, humming, his eyes bright. "Not me, oh no, not me." He did not look at her, but started quickly to slap out the cards. She stood behind him. Her right eye began to twitch a little. She folded and unfolded her arms. A minute ticked by. The only sound was the ocean under the night pier, Ralph breathing in the heat, the soft ruffle of the cards. The sky over the pier was hot and thick with clouds. Out at sea, faint glows of lightning were beginning to show.

"Ralph," she said at last.

"Relax, Aimee," he said.

"About that trip you wanted to take down the coast————"

"Tomorrow," he said. "Maybe next month. Maybe next year. Old Ralph Banghart's a patient guy. I'm not worried, Aimee. Look." He held up a hand. "I'm calm."

She waited for a roll of thunder at sea to fade away.

"I just don't want you mad, is all. I just don't want anything bad to happen, promise me."

The wind, now warm, now cool, blew along the pier. There was a smell of rain in the wind. The clock ticked. Aimee began to perspire heavily, watching the cards move and move. Distantly, you could hear targets being hit and the sound of the pistols at the shooting gallery.

And then, there he was.

Waddling along the lonely concourse, under the insect bulbs, his face twisted and dark, every movement an effort. From a long way down the pier he came, with Aimee watching. She wanted to say to him, This is your last night, the last time you'll have to embarrass yourself by coming here, the last time you'll have to put up with being watched by Ralph, even in secret. She wished she could cry out and laugh and say it right in front of Ralph. But she said nothing.

"Hello, hello!" shouted Ralph. "It's free, on the house, tonight! Special for old customers!"

The Dwarf looked up, startled, his little black eyes darting and swimming in confusion. His mouth formed the word thanks and he turned, one hand to his neck, pulling his tiny lapels tight up about his convulsing throat, the other hand clenching the silver dime secretly. Looking back, he gave a little nod, and then scores of dozens of compressed and tortured faces, burnt a strange dark color by the lights, wandered in the glass corridors.

"Ralph." Aimee took his elbow. "What's going on?"

He grinned. "I'm being benevolent, Aimee, benevolent."

"Ralph," she said.

"Sh," he said. *"Listen."*

They waited in the booth in the long warm silence.

Then, a long way off, muffled, there was a scream.

"Ralph!" said Aimee.

"Listen, listen!" he said.

There was another scream, and another and still another, and a threshing and a pounding and a breaking, a rushing around and through the maze. There, there, wildly colliding and ricocheting, from mirror to mirror, shrieking hysterically and sobbing, tears on his face, mouth gasped open, came Mr. Bigelow. He fell out in the blazing night air, glanced about wildly, wailed, and ran off down the pier.

"Ralph, what happened?"

Ralph sat laughing and slapping at his thighs.

She slapped his face. "What'd you *do?*"

He didn't quite stop laughing. "Come on. I'll show you!"

And then she was in the maze, rushed from white-hot mirror to mirror, seeing her lipstick all red fire a thousand times repeated on down a burning silver cavern where strange hysterical women much like herself followed a quick-moving, smiling man. "Come on!" he cried. And they broke free into a dust-smelling tiny room.

"Ralph!" she said.

They both stood on the threshold of the little room where the Dwarf had come every night for a year. They both stood where the Dwarf had stood each night, before opening his eyes to see the miraculous image in front of him.

Aimee shuffled slowly, one hand out, into the dim room.

The mirror had been changed.

This new mirror made even normal people small, small, small; it made even tall people little and dark and twisted smaller as you moved forward.

And Aimee stood before it thinking and thinking that if it made big people small, standing here, God, what would it do to a dwarf, a tiny dwarf, a dark dwarf, a startled and lonely dwarf?

She turned and almost fell. Ralph stood looking at her. "Ralph," she said. "God, why did you do it?"

"Aimee, come back!"

She ran out through the mirrors, crying. Staring with blurred eyes, it was hard to find the way, but she found it. She stood blinking at the empty pier, started to run one way, then another, then still another, then stopped. Ralph came up behind her, talking, but it was like a voice heard behind a wall late at night, remote and foreign.

"Don't talk to me," she said.

Someone came running up the pier. It was Mr. Kelly from the shooting gallery. "Hey, any you see a little guy just now? Little stiff swiped a pistol from my place, loaded, run off before I'd get a hand on him! You help me find him?"

And Kelly was gone, sprinting, turning his head to search between all the canvas sheds, on away under the hot blue and red and yellow strung bulbs.

Aimee rocked back and forth and took a step.

"Aimee, where you going?"

She looked at Ralph as if they had just turned a corner, strangers passing, and bumped into each other. "I guess," she said, "I'm going to help search."

"You won't be able to do nothing."

"I got to try, anyway. Oh God, Ralph, this is all my fault! I shouldn't have phoned Billie Fine! I shouldn't've ordered a mirror and got you so mad you did this! It's *me* should've gone to Mr. Big, not a crazy thing like I bought! I'm going to find him if it's the last thing I ever do in my life."

Swinging about slowly, her cheeks wet, she saw the quivery mirrors that stood in front of the Maze, Ralph's reflection was in one of them. She could not take her eyes away from the image; it held her in a cool and trembling fascination, with her mouth open.

"Aimee, what's wrong? What're you————"

He sensed where she was looking and twisted about to see what was going on. His eyes widened.

He scowled at the blazing mirror.

A horrid, ugly little man, two feet high, with a pale, squashed face under an ancient straw hat, scowled back at him. Ralph stood there glaring at himself, his hands at his sides.

Aimee walked slowly and then began to walk fast and then began to run. She ran down the empty pier and the wind blew warm and it blew large drops of hot rain out of the sky on her all the time she was running.

The President

DONALD BARTHELME

I AM NOT altogether sympathetic to the new President. He is, certainly, a strange fellow (only forty-eight inches high at the shoulder). But is strangeness alone enough? I spoke to Sylvia: "Is strangeness alone enough?" "I love you," Sylvia said. I regarded her with my warm kind eyes. "Your thumb?" I said. One thumb was a fiasco of tiny crusted slashes. "Pop-top beer cans," she said. "He is a *strange fellow,* all right. He has some magic charisma which makes people—" She stopped and began again. "When the band begins to launch into his campaign song, 'Struttin' with Some Barbecue,' I just . . . I can't . . ."

The darkness, strangeness, and complexity of the new President have touched everyone. There has been a great deal of fainting lately. Is the President at fault? I was sitting, I remember, in Row EE at City Center; the opera was *The Gypsy Baron.* Sylvia was singing in her green-and-blue gypsy costume in the gypsy encampment. I was thinking about the President. Is he, I wondered, right for this period? He is a *strange fellow,* I thought—not like the other Presidents we've had. Not like Garfield. Not like Taft. Not like Harding, Hoover, either of the Roosevelts, or Woodrow Wilson. Then I noticed a lady sitting in front of me, holding a baby. I tapped her on the shoulder. "Madam," I said, "your child has I believe fainted." "Giscard!" she cried, rotating the baby's head like a doll's. "Giscard, what has happened to you?" The President was smiling in his box.

"The President!" I said to Sylvia in the Italian restaurant. She raised her glass of warm red wine. "Do you think he liked me? My singing?" "He looked pleased," I said. "He was smiling." "A brilliant whirlwind campaign, I thought," Sylvia stated. "Winning was brilliant," I said. "He is the first President we've had from City College," Sylvia said. A waiter fainted behind us. "But is he right for the period?" I asked. "Our period is perhaps not so choice as the previous period, still—"

"He thinks a great deal about death, like all people from City," Sylvia said. "The death theme looms large in his consciousness. I've known a great many people from City, and these people, with no significant exceptions, are hung up on the death theme. It's an obsession, as it were." Other waiters carried the waiter who had fainted out into the kitchen.

"Our period will be characterized in future histories as a period of tentativeness and uncertainty, I feel," I said. "A kind of parenthesis. When he rides in his black limousine with the plastic top I see a little boy who has blown an enormous soap bubble which has trapped him. The look on his face—" "The other candidate was dazzled by his strangeness, newness, smallness, and philosophical grasp of the death theme," Sylvia said. "The other candidate didn't have a prayer," I said. Sylvia adjusted her green-and-blue veils in the Italian restaurant. "Not having gone to City College and sat around the cafeterias there discussing death," she said.

I am, as I say, not entirely sympathetic. Certain things about the new President are not clear. I can't make out what he is thinking. When he has finished speaking I can never remember what he has said. There remains only an impression of strangeness, darkness . . . On television, his face clouds when his name is mentioned. It is as if hearing his name frightens him. Then he stares directly into the camera (an actor's preempting gaze) and begins to speak. One hears only cadences. Newspaper accounts of his speeches always say only that he "touched on a number of matters in the realm of . . ." When he has finished speaking he appears nervous and unhappy. The camera credits fade in over an image of the President standing stiffly, with his arms rigid at his sides, looking to the right and to the left, as if awaiting instructions. On the other hand, the handsome meliorist who ran against him, all zest and programs, was defeated by a fantastic margin.

People are fainting. On Fifty-seventh Street, a young girl dropped in her tracks in front of Henri Bendel. I was shocked to discover that she wore only a garter belt under her dress. I picked her up and carried her into the store with the help of a Salvation Army major—a very tall man with an orange hairpiece. "She fainted," I said to the floorwalker. We talked about the new President, the Salvation Army major and I. "I'll tell you what *I* think," he said. "I think he's got something up his sleeve nobody knows about. I think he's keeping it under wraps. One of these days . . ." The Salvation Army major shook my hand. "I'm not saying that the problems he faces aren't tremendous, staggering. The awesome burden of the Presidency. But if anybody— any *one man* . . ."

What is going to happen? What is the President planning? No one knows. But everyone is convinced that he will bring it off. Our exhausted age wishes above everything to plunge into the heart of the problem, to be able to say,

Here is the difficulty. And the new President, that tiny, strange, and brilliant man, seems cankered and difficult enough to take us there. In the meantime, people are fainting. My secretary fell in the middle of a sentence. "Miss Kagle," I said. "Are you all right?" She was wearing an anklet of tiny silver circles. Each tiny silver circle held an initial: @@@@@@@@@@@@@@@@. Who is this person "A"? What is he in your life, Miss Kagle?

I gave her water with a little brandy in it. I speculated about the President's mother. Little is known about her. She presents herself in various guises:

A little lady, 5'2", with a cane.
A big lady, 7'1", with a dog.
A wonderful old lady, 4'3", with an indomitable spirit.
A noxious old sack, 6'8", excaudate, because of an operation.

Little is known about her. We are assured, however, that the same damnable involvements that obsess us obsess her too. Copulation. Strangeness. Applause. She must be pleased that her son is what he is—loved and looked up to, a mode of hope for millions. "Miss Kagle. Drink it down. It will put you on your feet again, Miss Kagle." I regarded her with my warm kind eyes.

At Town Hall I sat reading the program notes to *The Gypsy Baron*. Outside the building, eight mounted policemen collapsed en bloc. The well-trained horses planted their feet delicately among the bodies. Sylvia was singing. They said a small man could never be President (only forty-eight inches high at the shoulder). Our period is not the one I would have chosen, but it has chosen me. The new President must have certain intuitions. I am convinced that he has these intuitions (although I am certain of very little else about him; I have reservations, I am not sure). I could tell you about his mother's summer journey, in 1919, to western Tibet—about the dandymen and the red bear, and how she told off the Pathan headman, instructing him furiously to rub up his English or get out of her service—but what order of knowledge is this? Let me instead simply note his smallness, his strangeness, his brilliance, and say that we expect great things of him. "I love you," Sylvia said. The President stepped through the roaring curtain. We applauded until our arms hurt. We shouted until the ushers set off flares enforcing silence. The orchestra tuned itself. Sylvia sang the second lead. The President was smiling in his box. At the finale, the entire cast slipped into the orchestra pit in a great, swooning mass. We cheered until the ushers tore up our tickets.

Small Man

 EUGENE HIRSCH

I am a small man
in a tall room.

Women think
I cannot give them love.
They mock me.

Maria scrubs floors
on hands and knees.

I touched her neck
while she was working
and she smiles.

Perhaps one day
we can marry—
I, an attendant
in her royal household.

From The Dwarf

PÄR LAGERKVIST

I AM TWENTY-SIX inches tall, shapely and well proportioned, my head perhaps a trifle too large. My hair is not black like the others', but reddish, very stiff and thick, drawn back from the temples and the broad but not especially lofty brow. My face is beardless, but otherwise just like that of other men. My eyebrows meet. My bodily strength is considerable, particularly if I am annoyed. When the wrestling match was arranged between Jehoshaphat and myself I forced him onto his back after twenty minutes and strangled him. Since then I have been the only dwarf at this court.

Most dwarfs are buffoons. They have to make jokes and play tricks to make their masters and the guests laugh. I have never demeaned myself to anything like that. Nobody has even suggested that I should. My very appearance forbids such a use of me. My cast of countenance is unsuited to ridiculous pranks. And I never laugh. I am no buffoon. I am a dwarf and nothing but a dwarf.

On the other hand I have a sharp tongue which may occasionally give pleasure to some of those around me. That is not the same thing as being their buffoon.

I mentioned that my face was exactly like that of other men. That is not quite accurate, for it is very lined, covered with wrinkles. I do not look upon this as a blemish. I am made that way and I cannot help it if others are not. It shows me as I really am, unbeautified and undistorted. Maybe it was not meant to be like that, but that is exactly as I want to look.

The wrinkles make me look very old. I am not, but I have heard tell that we dwarfs are descended from a race older than that which now populates the world, and therefore we are old as soon as we are born. I do not know if this is true, but in that case we must be the original beings. I have nothing against belonging to a different race from the present one and showing it on my person.

I think that the others' faces are absolutely expressionless.

My masters are very gracious to me, particularly the Prince, who is a great and powerful man, a man of great schemes, and one who knows how to put them into execution. He is a man of action, but at the same time a scholar who finds time for everything and likes to discuss all manner of subjects under heaven and on earth. He conceals his true aims by talking about something else.

It may seem unnecessary to be so preoccupied by everything (always supposing he really is), but perhaps it has to be, perhaps as a prince he is obliged to comprehend everything. He gives the impression of being able to understand and master anything, or at least of wishing to do so. Undeniably he is an imposing personality, the only one I have ever known whom I do not despise.

He is very treacherous.

I am well acquainted with my lord, but I do not profess to know him inside and out. His is a complicated nature which it is not easy to understand. It would be wrong to say that he is full of hidden riddles—not at all—but somehow or other he is difficult to know. I do not quite understand him myself, and I do not really know why I follow him with such doglike devotion. On the other hand he does not understand me either.

He does not impress me as he does the others, but I like to be in the service of a master who is so impressive. I will not deny that he is a great man; but nobody is great to his dwarf.

I follow him constantly, like a shadow. . . .

There is a great difference between dwarfs and children. Because they are about the same size, people think that they are alike, and that they suit each other; but they do not. Dwarfs are set to play with children, forced to do so, without a thought being given to the fact that a dwarf is the opposite to a child and that he is born old. As far as I know, dwarf children never play—why should they? It would only look macabre, with their wizened old faces. It is nothing less than torture to use us dwarfs like that. But human beings know nothing about us.

My masters have never forced me to play with Angelica, but she herself has done so. I won't say that she did it out of spite, but when I look back on that time, especially when she was quite tiny, it seems as though I had been the victim of carefully thought-out malice. That infant, whom some people think so wonderful with her round blue eyes and her little pursed mouth, has tormented me almost more than anyone else at court. Every morning, from the time she could scarcely toddle, she would come staggering into the dwarf's apartment with her kitten under her arm. "Piccoline, will you play with us?" I answer: "I cannot, I have more important things to think about, my day is not meant for play." "Then what are you going to do?" she asks impertinently. "One cannot explain that to a child," I reply. "But at least you're going out, you aren't going to lie abed all day! I've been up such a long long time!" And I have to go out with her, I dare not refuse for fear of my masters, though inside I am raging with fury. She takes my hand as though I were her playmate; she is always wanting to hold my hand, though there is nothing I detest so much as sticky childish paws. I clench my fist in wrath, but she simply takes hold of my fist instead and drags me around everywhere, chattering all the time. We visit her dolls which have to be fed and dressed, the puppies sprawling half-blind outside the kennel, the rose garden where we have to play with the kitten. She takes a tiresome interest in all kinds of animals, not full-grown ones, but their young—in fact, in everything small. She can sit and play with her kitten for ages and expect me to join in. She believes that I too am a child with a child's delight in everything. I! I delight in nothing.

Sometimes it really seems as though a sensible idea were passing through her head when she notices how bored and bitter I am, for she looks surprisedly up at my furrowed old man's face. "Why don't you enjoy playing?"

And when she receives no answer from my compressed lips or from my cold dwarf's eyes with the centuries of experience in their depths, a shyness shadows her newborn baby eyes, and she is actually silent for a while.

What is play? A meaningless dabbling with nothing at all. A strange "let's pretend" way of dealing with things. They must not be treated as they really are, not seriously; one is only pretending. Astrologers play with the stars, the Prince plays with his building, his churches, the crucifixion scenes, and the campaniles, Angelica with her dolls—they all play, all pretend something. Only I despise this pretending. Only I *am*.

Once I crept into her room as she lay sleeping with her detestable kitten beside her in bed and cut off its head with my dagger. Then I threw it out onto the dungheap beneath the castle window. I was so furious that I hardly knew what I was doing. That is to say, I knew only too well. I was carrying out a plan which had long been germinating during those revolting playtimes in the rose garden. She was inconsolable when she saw that it was gone, and when everybody said that of course it must be dead, she sickened with an unknown fever and was ill for a long time, so that I, thank goodness, did not have to see her. When at last she got up again, I was obliged to listen all the more to her woeful narrative of her darling's fate, of the incredible thing which had happened. Nobody cared how the cat had disappeared, but the whole court had been upset because of some inexplicable drops of blood on the girl's neck, which could be interpreted as an evil omen. Anything which can possibly be taken as an omen is of tremendous interest to them.

In fact, throughout her childhood she never left me in peace although the games gradually changed. She was always hanging on to me and would have liked to confide in me, though I did not want her confidences. Sometimes I wonder if her importunate affection for me might not have had the same source as her weakness for kittens, puppies, ducklings, and so on; if, maybe, she were not happy in the grownup world, perhaps feared it, after some scare or other. It had nothing to do with me! It was no doing of mine if she wandered about in loneliness. But she always wanted to cling to me and this did not lessen after she had left her infancy behind her. Her mother ceased caring about her as soon as she stopped being doll-like. She was pretending too, everybody pretends. And her father, of course, had his own business to attend to. He may have had other reasons for not being interested in her, but that is a matter on which I will not give my opinion.

Not until she was ten or twelve did she begin to be silent and self-contained, and I was rid of her at last. Since then she has left me in peace, thank goodness, and keeps to herself. But I still fume when I think how much I have had to endure for her sake.

Now she is beginning to grow up, she is fifteen and will soon be reckoned a woman. But she is still very childish and does not conduct herself at all like a lady of quality. It is impossible to guess who is her father. It might be the Prince, but she may just as well be a bastard, and this treatment of her as though she were a princess may be quite superfluous. Some call her beautiful. I can see nothing beautiful in the childish face with its half-open mouth and big blue eyes which look as if they understand nothing at all. . . .

What is religion? I have given much thought to it, but in vain.

I pondered it especially that time a few years ago when I was compelled to officiate as a bishop in full canonicals at the carnival and give holy communion to the dwarfs of the Mantua court whom their Prince had brought here for the festival. We met at a miniature sanctuary which had been set up in one of the castle halls, and around us sat all the sniggering guests: knights and nobles and young coxcombs in their absurd apparel. I raised the crucifix and all the dwarfs fell on their knees. "Here is your savior," I declared in a sonorous voice, my eyes flaming with passion. "Here is the savior of all the dwarfs, himself a dwarf, who suffered under the great prince Pontius Pilate, and was nailed to his little toy cross for the joy and ease of all men." I took the chalice and held it up to them. "This is his dwarf's blood, in which all iniquities are cleansed and all dirty souls become as white as snow." Then I took the host and showed it to them and ate and drank of both in their sight, as is the custom, while I expounded the holy mysteries. "I eat his body which was deformed like yours. It tastes as bitter as gall, for it is full of hatred. May you all eat of it. I drink his blood, and it burns like a fire which cannot be quenched. It is as though I drink my own.

"Savior of all the dwarfs, may thy fire consume the whole world!"

And I threw the wine out over those who sat there, staring in gloom and amazement at our somber communion feast.

I am no blasphemer. It was they who blasphemed, not I, but the Prince had me clapped in irons for several days. The little jest had been intended to amuse, but I had spoiled it all and the guests had been very upset, almost scared. There were no chains small enough so they had to be specially made, and the smith thought that it was a great deal of trouble for such a short sentence. But the Prince said that it might be as well to have them for another time. He let me go sooner than had been planned, and I rather think he punished me merely for the sake of the guests, for as soon as they had left I was released. During the time that followed, however, he looked at me rather askance and did not seem to want to be alone with me; it was almost as though he were somewhat afraid of me.

Of course the dwarfs understood nothing. They cuttled around like frightened hens and squeaked with their miserable castrato voices. I don't know where they get those ridiculous voices; my own is rich and deep. But they are cowed and castrated to the depths of their souls, and most of them are buffoons who shame their race by their gross jests about their own bodies.

They are a contemptible clan. So that I need not see them, I have made the Prince sell all the dwarfs here, one after the other, until I am the only one at the court. I am glad they are gone and the dwarfs' apartment is empty and deserted when I sit there at night with my meditations. I am glad that Jehoshaphat is gone too, so that I am quit of his crumpled old woman's face and his piping voice. I am glad to be *alone.*

It is my fate that I hate my own people. My race is detestable to me.

But I hate myself too. I eat my own splenetic flesh. I drink my own poisoned blood. Every day I perform my solitary communion as the grim high priest of my people.

After this incident which caused so much offense, the Princess began to behave in a rather peculiar way. On the morning of my liberation she called me in to her, and when I entered the bedchamber she looked at me in silence with a thoughtful searching gaze. I had expected reproaches, perhaps more punishment, but when at last she spoke she admitted that my communion service had made a deep impression on her, that there had been something dark and terrible about it which had appealed to something within her. How had I been able to penetrate to her secret depths like that and speak to them?

I did not understand. I seized the opportunity to sneer as she lay there in the bed gazing vaguely past me.

She asked what I thought it felt like to hang on a cross. To be scourged, tortured, to die? And she said that she realized Christ must hate her, that He must be full of hatred while suffering for her sake.

I did not bother to reply, nor did she continue the conversation, but lay staring into space with dreaming eyes.

Then she dismissed me with a gesture of her beautiful hand and called to her tirewoman to fetch her crimson gown because she was going to get up.

I still don't understand what possessed her just then.

I have noticed that sometimes I frighten people; what they really fear is themselves. They think it is I who scare them, but it is the dwarf within them, the ape-faced manlike being who sticks up its head from the depths of their souls. They are afraid because they do not know that they have another being inside them. They are scared when anything rises to the surface, from their inside, out of some of the cesspools in their souls, something which they do not recognize and which is not a part of their real life. When nothing is visible above the surface, they are utterly fearless. They go about, tall and unconcerned, with their smooth faces which express nothing at all. But inside them is always something else which they ignore and, without knowing it, they are constantly living many kinds of lives. They are so strangely secretive and incoherent.

And they are deformed though it does not show on the outside. I live only my dwarf life. I never go around tall and smooth-featured. I am ever myself, always the same, I live *one* life alone. I have no other being inside me. And I recognize everything within me, nothing ever comes up from my inner depths, nothing there is shrouded in mystery. Therefore I do not fear the things which frighten them, the incoherent, the unknown, the mysterious. Such things do not exist for me. There is nothing "different" about me.

Fear? What is it? Is it what I feel when I lie alone in the dwarfs' apartment at night and see the ghost of Jehoshaphat nearing my bed, when he comes to me, deathly pale with blue marks around his neck and gaping mouth?

I feel no anguish and no regret, I am not unduly disturbed. When I see him I merely think that he is dead and that since his death I have been completely alone.

I want to be alone. I don't want there to be anyone else except me. And I can see that he is dead. It is only his ghost, and I am absolutely alone in the dark as I have been ever since I strangled him.

There is nothing frightening in that.

Hop-Frog

Edgar Allan Poe

I never knew any one so keenly alive to a joke as the king was. He seemed to live only for joking. To tell a good story of the joke kind, and to tell it well, was the surest road to his favor. Thus it happened that his seven ministers were all noted for their accomplishments as jokers. They all took after the king, too, in being large, corpulent, oily men, as well as inimitable jokers. Whether people grow fat by joking, or whether there is something in fat itself which predisposes to a joke, I have never been quite able to determine; but certain it is that a lean joker is a *rara avis in terris.*

About the refinements, or, as he called them, the "ghost" of wit, the king troubled himself very little. He had an especial admiration for *breadth* in a jest, and would often put up with *length,* for the sake of it. Over-niceties wearied him. He would have preferred Rabelais' "Gargantua" to the "Zadig" of Voltaire: and, upon the whole, practical jokes suited his taste far better than verbal ones.

At the date of my narrative, professing jesters had not altogether gone out of fashion at court. Several of the great continental "powers" still retained their "fools," who wore motley, with caps and bells, and who were expected to be always ready with sharp witticisms, at a moment's notice, in consideration of the crumbs that fell from the royal table.

Our king, as a matter of course, retained his "fool." The fact is, he *required* something in the way of folly—if only to counterbalance the heavy wisdom of the seven wise men who were his ministers—not to mention himself.

His fool, or professional jester, was not *only* a fool, however. His value was trebled in the eyes of the king by the fact of his being also a dwarf and a cripple. Dwarfs were as common at court, in those days, as fools; and many monarchs would have found it difficult to get through their days (days are rather longer at court than elsewhere) without both a jester to laugh *with,* and a dwarf to laugh *at.* But, as I have already observed, your jesters, in ninety-nine cases out of a hundred, are fat, round, and unwieldy—so that it was no small source of self-gratulation with our king that, in Hop-Frog (this was the fool's name), he possessed a triplicate treasure in one person.

I believe the name "Hop-Frog" was *not* that given to the dwarf by his sponsors at baptism, but it was conferred upon him, by general consent of the seven ministers, on account of his inability to walk as other men do. In fact, Hop-Frog could only get along by a sort of interjectional gait—something between a leap and a wriggle—a movement that afforded illimitable amusement, and of course consolation, to the king, for (notwithstanding the protuberance of his stomach and a constitutional swelling of the head) the king, by his whole court, was accounted a capital figure.

But although Hop-Frog, through the distortion of his legs, could move only with great pain and difficulty along a road or floor, the prodigious muscular power which nature seemed to have bestowed upon his arms, by way of compensation for deficiency in the lower limbs, enabled him to perform many feats of wonderful dexterity, where trees or ropes were in question, or anything else to climb. At such exercises he certainly much more resembled a squirrel, or a small monkey, than a frog.

I am not able to say, with precision, from what country Hop-Frog originally came. It was from some barbarous region, however, that no person ever heard of—a vast distance from the court of our king. Hop-Frog, and a young girl very little less dwarfish than himself (although of exquisite proportions, and a marvellous dancer), had been forcibly carried off from their respective homes in adjoining provinces, and sent as presents to the king, by one of his ever-victorious generals.

Under these circumstances, it is not to be wondered at that a close intimacy arose between the two little captives. Indeed, they soon became sworn friends. Hop-Frog, who, although he made a great deal of sport, was by no means popular, had it not in his power to render Trippetta many services; but *she*, on account of her grace and exquisite beauty (although a dwarf), was universally admired and petted; so she possessed much influence; and never failed to use it, whenever she could, for the benefit of Hop-Frog.

On some grand state occasion—I forgot what—the king determined to have a masquerade, and whenever a masquerade or anything of that kind occurred at our court, then the talents both of Hop-Frog and Trippetta were sure to be called into play. Hop-Frog, in especial, was so inventive in the way of getting up pageants, suggesting novel characters, and arranging costumes, for masked balls, that nothing could be done, it seems, without his assistance.

The night appointed for the *fête* had arrived. A gorgeous hall had been fitted up, under Trippetta's eye, with every kind of device which could possibly give *éclât* to a masquerade. The whole court was in a fever of expectation. As for costumes and characters, it might well be supposed that everybody had come to a decision on such points. Many had made up their minds (as to what *rôles* they should assume) a week, or even a month, in advance; and, in fact, there was not a particle of indecision anywhere—except in the case of the king and his seven ministers. Why *they* hesitated I never could tell, unless they did it by way of a joke. More probably, they found it difficult, on account of being so fat, to make up their minds. At all events, time flew; and, as a last resort, they sent for Trippetta and Hop-Frog.

When the two little friends obeyed the summons of the king, they found him sitting at his wine with the seven members of his cabinet council; but the monarch appeared to be in a very ill humor. He knew that Hop-Frog was not fond of wine; for it excited the poor cripple almost to madness; and madness is no comfortable feeling. But the king loved his practical jokes, and took pleasure in forcing Hop-Frog to drink and (as the king called it) "to be merry."

"Come here, Hop-Frog," said he, as the jester and his friend entered the room; "swallow this bumper to the health of your absent friends [here Hop-Frog sighed], and then let us have the benefit of your invention. We want characters—*characters*, man—something novel—out of the way. We are wearied with this everlasting sameness. Come, drink! the wine will brighten your wits."

Hop-Frog endeavored, as usual, to get up a jest in reply to these advances from the king; but the effort was too much. It happened to be the poor dwarf's birthday, and the command to drink to his "absent friends" forced the tears to his eyes. Many large, bitter drops fell into the goblet as he took it, humbly, from the hand of the tyrant.

"Ah! ha! ha! ha!" roared the latter, as the dwarf reluctantly drained the beaker. "See what a glass of good wine can do! Why, your eyes are shining already!"

Poor fellow! his large eyes *gleamed* rather than shone; for the effect of wine on his excitable brain was not more powerful than instantaneous. He placed the goblet nervously on the table, and looked round upon the company with a half-insane stare. They all seemed highly amused at the success of the king's "*joke.*"

"And now to business," said the prime minister, a *very* fat man.

"Yes," said the king. "Come, Hop-Frog, lend us your assistance. Characters, my fine fellow; we stand in need of characters—all of us—ha! ha! ha!" and as this was seriously meant for a joke, his laugh was chorused by the seven.

Hop-Frog also laughed, although feebly and somewhat vacantly.

"Come, come," said the king, impatiently, "have you nothing to suggest?"

"I am endeavoring to think of something *novel*," replied the dwarf, abstractedly, for he was quite bewildered by the wine.

"Endeavoring!" cried the tyrant, fiercely, "what do you mean by *that?* Ah, I perceive. You are sulky, and want more wine. Here, drink this!" and he poured out another goblet full and offered it to the cripple, who merely gazed at it, gasping for breath.

"Drink, I say!" shouted the monster, "or by the fiends—"

The dwarf hesitated. The king grew purple with rage. The courtiers smirked. Trippetta, pale as a corpse, advanced to the monarch's seat, and, falling on her knees before him, implored him to spare her friend.

The tyrant regarded her, for some moments, in evident wonder at her audacity. He seemed quite at a loss what to do or say—how most becomingly to express his indignation. At last, without uttering a syllable, he pushed her violently from him, and threw the contents of the brimming goblet in her face.

The poor girl got up the best she could, and, not daring even to sigh, resumed her position at the foot of the table.

There was a dead silence for about half a minute, during which the falling of a leaf, or of a feather, might have been heard. It was interrupted by a low, but harsh and protracted *grating* sound which seemed to come at once from every corner of the room.

"What—what—*what* are you making that noise for?" demanded the king, turning furiously to the dwarf.

The latter seemed to have recovered, in great measure, from his intoxication, and looking fixedly but quietly into the tyrant's face, merely ejaculated:

"I—I? How could it have been me?"

"The sound appeared to come from without," observed one of the courtiers. "I fancy it was the parrot at the window, whetting his bill upon his cage-wires."

"True," replied the monarch, as if much relieved by the suggestion; "but, on the honor of a knight, I could have sworn that it was the gritting of this vagabond's teeth."

Hereupon the dwarf laughed (the king was too confirmed a joker to object to any one's laughing), and displayed a set of large, powerful, and very repulsive teeth. Moreover, he avowed his perfect willingness to swallow as much wine as desired. The monarch was pacified; and having drained another bumper with no very perceptible ill effect, Hop-Frog entered at once, and with spirit, into the plans for the masquerade.

"I can not tell what was the association of idea," observed he, very tranquilly, and as if he had never tasted wine in his life, "but *just* after your majesty had struck the girl and thrown the wine in her face—*just after* your majesty had done this, and while the parrot was making that odd noise outside the window, there came into my mind a capital diversion—one of my own country frolics—often enacted among us, at our masquerades: but here it will be new altogether. Unfortunately, however, it requires a company of eight persons and—"

"Here we *are!*" cried the king, laughing at his acute discovery of the coincidence; "eight to a fraction—I and my seven ministers. Come! what is the diversion?"

"We call it," replied the cripple, "the Eight Chained Orang-Outangs, and it really is excellent sport if well enacted."

"*We* will enact it," remarked the king, drawing himself up, and lowering his eyelids.

"The beauty of the game," continued Hop-Frog, "lies in the fright it occasions among the women."

"Capital!" roared in chorus the monarch and his ministry.

"I will equip you as orang-outangs," proceeded the dwarf; "leave all that to me. The resemblance shall be so striking that the company of masqueraders will take you for real beasts—and of course they will be as much terrified as astonished."

"Oh, this is exquisite!" exclaimed the king. "Hop-Frog! I will make a man of you."

"The chains are for the purpose of increasing the confusion by their jangling. You are supposed to have escaped, *en masse,* from your keepers. Your majesty can not conceive the *effect* produced, at a masquerade, by eight chained orang-outangs, imagined to be real ones by most of the company; and rushing in with savage cries, among the crowd of delicately and gorgeously habited men and women. The *contrast* is inimitable."

"It *must* be," said the king: and the council arose hurriedly (as it was growing late), to put in execution the scheme of Hop-Frog.

His mode of equipping the party as orang-outangs was very simple, but effective enough for his purposes. The animals in question had, at the epoch of my story, very rarely been seen in any part of the civilized world; and as the imitations made by the dwarf were sufficiently beast-like and more than sufficiently hideous, their truthfulness to nature was thus thought to be secured.

The king and his ministers were first incased in tight-fitting stockinet shirts and drawers. They were then saturated with tar. At this stage of the process some one of the party suggested feathers; but the suggestion was at once overruled by the dwarf, who soon convinced the eight, by ocular demonstration, that the hair of such a brute as the orang-outang was much more efficiently represented by *flax*. A thick coating of the latter was accordingly plastered upon the coating of tar. A long chain was now procured. First, it was passed about the waist of the king, *and tied;* then about another of the party, and also tied; then about all successively, in the same manner. When this chaining arrangement was complete, and the party stood as far apart from each other as possible, they formed a circle; and to make all things appear natural, Hop-Frog passed the residue of the chain in two diameters, at right angles, across the circle, after the fashion adopted, at the present day, by those who capture chimpanzees, or other large apes, in Borneo.

The grand saloon in which the masquerade was to take place was a circular room, very lofty, and receiving the light of the sun only through a single window at top. At night (the season for which the apartment was especially designed) it was illuminated principally by a large chandelier, depending by a chain from the centre of the skylight, and lowered, or elevated, by means of a counterbalance as usual; but (in order not to look unsightly) this latter passed outside the cupola and over the roof.

The arrangements of the room had been left to Trippetta's superintendence; but, in some particulars, it seems she had been guided by the calmer judgment of her friend the dwarf. At his suggestion it was that, on this occasion, the chandelier was removed. Its waxen drippings (which, in weather so warm, it was quite impossible to prevent) would have been seriously detrimental to the rich dresses of the guests, who, on account of the crowded state of the saloon, could not *all* be expected to keep from out its centre—that is to say, from under the chandelier. Additional sconces were set in various parts of the hall, out of the way; and a flambeau, emitting sweet odor, was placed in the right hand of each of the Caryatides that stood against the wall—some fifty or sixty altogether.

The eight orang-outangs, taking Hop-Frog's advice, waited patiently until midnight (when the room was thoroughly filled with masqueraders) before making their appearance. No sooner had the clock ceased striking, however, than they rushed, or rather rolled in, all together—for the impediments of their chains caused most of the party to fall, and all to stumble as they entered.

The excitement among the masqueraders was prodigious, and filled the heart of the king with glee. As had been anticipated, there were not a few of the guests who supposed the ferocious-looking creatures to be beasts of *some* kind in reality, if not precisely orang-outangs. Many of the women swooned with affright; and had not the king taken the precaution to exclude all weapons from the saloon, his party might soon have expiated their frolic in their blood. As it was, a general rush was made for the doors; but the king had ordered them to be locked immediately upon his entrance; and, at the dwarf's suggestion, the keys had been deposited with *him*.

While the tumult was at its height, and each masquerader attentive only to his own safety (for, in fact, there was much *real* danger from the pressure of the excited crowd), the chain by which the chandelier ordinarily hung, and which had been drawn upon its removal, might have been seen very gradually to descend, until its hooked extremity came within three feet of the floor.

Soon after this, the king and his seven friends having reeled about the hall in all directions, found themselves, at length, in its centre, and, of course, in immediate contact with the chain. While they were thus situated, the dwarf, who had followed noiselessly at their heels, inciting them to keep up the commotion, took hold of their own chain at the intersection of the two portions which crossed the circle diametrically and at right angles. Here, with the rapidity of thought, he inserted the hook from which the chandelier had been wont to depend; and, in an instant, by some unseen agency, the chandelier-chain was drawn so far upward as to take the hook out of reach, and, as an inevitable consequence, to drag the orang-outangs together in close connection, and face to face.

The masqueraders, by this time, had recovered, in some measure, from their alarm; and, beginning to regard the whole matter as a well-contrived pleasantry, set up a loud shout of laughter at the predicament of the apes.

"Leave them to *me!*" now screamed Hop-Frog, his shrill voice making itself easily heard through all the din. "Leave them to *me*. I fancy *I* know them. If I can only get a good look at them *I* can soon tell who they are."

Here, scrambling over the heads of the crowd, he managed to get to the wall; when, seizing a flambeau from one of the Caryatides, he returned, as he went, to the centre of the room—leaped, with the agility of a monkey, upon the king's head—and thence clambered a few feet up the chain—holding down the torch to examine the group of orang-outangs, and still screaming: "*I* shall soon find out who they are!"

And now, while the whole assembly (the apes included) were convulsed with laughter, the jester suddenly uttered a shrill whistle; when the chain flew violently up for about thirty feet—dragging with it the dismayed and struggling orang-outangs, and leaving them suspended in mid-air between the skylight and the floor. Hop-Frog, clinging to the chain as it rose, still maintained his relative position in respect to the eight maskers, and still (as if nothing were the matter) continued to thrust his torch down toward them, as though endeavoring to discover who they were.

So thoroughly astonished was the whole company at this ascent that a dead silence of about a minute's duration ensued. It was broken by just such a low, harsh, *grating* sound as had before attracted the attention of the king and his councillors when the former threw the wine in the face of Trippetta. But, on the present occasion, there could be no question as to *whence* the sound issued. It came from the fang-like teeth of the dwarf, who ground them and gnashed them as he foamed at the mouth, and glared, with an expression of maniacal rage, into the upturned countenances of the king and his seven companions.

"Ah, ha!" said at length the infuriated jester. "Ah, ha! I begin to see who these people *are* now!" Here, pretending to scrutinize the king more closely, he held the flambeau to the flaxen coat which enveloped him, and which instantly burst into a sheet of vivid flame. In less than half a minute the whole eight orang-outangs were blazing fiercely, amid the shrieks of the multitude who gazed at them from below, horror-stricken, and without the power to render them the slightest assistance.

At length the flames, suddenly increasing in virulence, forced the jester to climb higher up the chain, to be out of their reach; and, as he made this movement, the crowd again sank, for a brief instant, into silence. The dwarf seized his opportunity, and once more spoke:

"I now see *distinctly*," he said, "what manner of people these maskers are. They are a great king and his seven privy-councillors—a king who does not scruple to strike a defenceless girl, and his seven councillors who abet him in the outrage. As for myself, I am simply Hop-Frog, the jester—and *this is my last jest.*"

Owing to the high combustibility of both the flax and the tar to which it adhered, the dwarf had scarcely made an end of his brief speech before the work of vengeance was complete. The eight corpses swung in their chains, a fetid, blackened, hideous, and indistinguishable mass. The cripple hurled his torch at them, clambered leisurely to the ceiling, and disappeared through the skylight.

It is supposed that Trippetta, stationed on the roof of the saloon, had been the accomplice of her friend in his fiery revenge, and that, together, they effected their escape to their own country; for neither was seen again.

Section C
Deformity & Disability

❧

Beauty

EUGENE HIRSCH

I see beauty in the window
of the downtown shop.
The mannequin's stilted shoes
trim the soles of her feet.
Her skirt suckles streams
of pin-sized hose.
She shows love
for the gaberdine guy
in the grey wearever smile
while he eyes the pose
of the diva, svelte blue,
who flows, annealed in grace,
for the fashionable ladies
of the district.

At home in the Elder Flats,
I disrobe. My sallow folds
of skin string vellum
on my splinty knobs of bone.
My lady love lies bare,
her laughing belly
waves of molten bread.
Her rolling
spreads across the selvage,
pleats the bedding
as we play.

Sometimes in the evening,
hand in hand, we wander down
to watch our frozen "friends,"
alive in strobes
which pierce the shop window
to the street,
swashing our coats
and those of passersby,
too hurried, now,
to sense the faint beauty
in the jealous night.

He

EUGENE HIRSCH

He was sitting, feet dangling
from the side of his bed,
faced by a tray of food on a stand.
He slowly took bits of beans,
each load, a basket of gravel,
each sip of juice, a pilgrimage
to the shrine for holy water, each taste
of bread, his very last. His black hands
were like prunes, the jagged purple marks
under his skin betraying the grape sludge
flowing through his veins. His head,
so recently plush, held only a few thin hairs.
His face and eyes were yellow-gaunt.
A gown hung over his shoulders
as over a hanger in a closet
with no clothes beneath. He looked up
when I came in with his daughter
and his new grandson. The sight
almost scared his cancer away,
as he smiled so wide, this warrior,
this young man whom we had sent to war
so few years ago, whom no one would now touch.

Neurology Rounds

WILLIAM D. HOSKIN

1

You balanced your way
to the teaching clinic
through corridors
that rolled and pitched under you
but not under us.
I wanted to take your arm.
We said "ataxia," hurried on.

2

Young and comely mother, you
offered a tremorous hand to me
and missed,
fought the random jerking of
your head, grimaced
a greeting. We turned away
to huddle over "palsy."

3

Desperately I watched
the ceaseless pursing of your lips,
grotesque but right
for mouths of fishes against aquarium glass,
heard the Greek label,
"choreiform dyskinesia."

4

Your face a frozen mask, you
tipped and tottered toward us
while your hands rolled
unseen pellets at your side.
I would not catch your
unblinking gaze of "paralysis agitans."

5

Pondering, staring, you knew
neither me nor you
but girlhood memories of
flags and warbonnets, the dust
of rodeos and stampedes
from your prairie past
put lights back in your eyes.
I wished this reverie could prove you well.
Our whispered word, "dementia."

You had your own proud names.
We dubbed you
Parkinson, Huntington, Alzheimer—
honored names and convenient
categories of anonymity.

I call you Courage
but it is not enough.

A Very Special Arts Festival

William D. Hoskin

Palsied ones make smooth
               strokes with computers
video sketches
               of us
instant replays
               when we ask

Black slashes red
               orange screams   yellow
green smiles as wide
               as the wall
speak for him
               he's seventeen

The deaf girl has
               her own quiet
spirit box
               ceramic and
free form to hold
               all the shapes
of her secrets inside.

The Anatomy of Desire

JOHN L'HEUREUX

BECAUSE HANLEY'S SKIN had been stripped off by the enemy, he could find no one who was willing to be with him for long. The nurses were obligated, of course, to see him now and then, and sometimes the doctor, but certainly not the other patients and certainly not his wife and children. He was raw, he was meat, and he would never be any better. He had a great and natural desire, therefore, to be possessed by someone.

He would walk around on his skinned feet, leaving bloody footprints up and down the corridors, looking for someone to love him.

"You're not supposed to be out here," the nurse said. And she added, somehow making it sound kind, "You untidy the floor, Hanley. "

"I want to be loved by someone," he said. "I'm human too. I'm like you."

But he knew he was not like her. Everybody called her the saint.

because of what he's told, he feels inferior

"Why couldn't it be you?" he said.

She was swabbing his legs with blood retardant, a new discovery that kept Hanley going. It was one of those miracle medications that just grew out of the war.

"I wasn't chosen," she said. "I have my skin."

"No," he said. "I mean why couldn't it be you who will love me, possess me? I have desires too," he said.

She considered this as she swabbed his shins and the soles of his feet.

"I have no desires," she said. "Or only one. It's the same thing."

He looked at her loving face. It was not a pretty face, but it was saintly.

"Then you will?" he said.

"If I come to know sometime that I must," she said.

The enemy had not chosen Hanley, they had just lucked upon him sleeping in his trench. They were a raid party of four, terrified and obedient, and they had been told to bring back an enemy to serve as an example of what is done to infiltrators.

They dragged Hanley back across the line and ran him, with his hands tied behind his back, the two kilometers to the general's tent.

The general dismissed the guards because he was very taken with Hanley. He untied the cords that bound his wrists and let his arms hang free. Then slowly, ritually, he tipped Hanley's face toward the light and examined it carefully. He kissed him on the brow and on the cheek and finally on the mouth. He gazed deep and long into Hanley's eyes until he saw his own reflection there looking back. He traced the lines of Hanley's eyebrows, gently, with the tip of his index finger. "Such a beautiful face," he said in his own language. He pressed his palms lightly against Hanley's forehead, against his cheekbones, his jaw. With his little finger he memorized the shape of Hanley's lips, the laugh lines at his eyes, the chin. The general did Hanley's face very thoroughly. Afterward he did some things down below, and so just before sunrise when the time came to lead Hanley out to the stripping post, he told the soldiers with the knives: "This young man could be my own son; so spare him here and here."

The stripping post stood dead-center in the line of barbed wire only a few meters beyond the range of gunfire. A loudspeaker was set up and began to blare the day's message. "This is what happens to infiltrators. No infiltrators will be spared." And then as troops from both sides watched through binoculars, the enemy cut the skin from Hanley's body, sparing—as the general had insisted—his face and his genitals. They were skilled men and the skin was stripped off expeditiously and they hung it, headless, on the barbed wire as an example. They lay Hanley himself on the ground where he could die.

He was rescued a little after noon when the enemy, for no good reason, went into sudden retreat.

Hanley was given emergency treatment at the field unit, and when they had done what they could for him, they sent him on to the vets' hospital. At least there, they told each other, he will be attended by the saint.

It was quite some time before the saint said yes, she would love him.

"Not just love me. Possess me."

"There are natural reluctancies," she said. "There are personal peculiarities," she said. "You will have to have patience with me."

"You're supposed to be a saint," he said.

So she lay down with him in his bloody bed and he found great satisfaction in holding this small woman in his arms. He kissed her and caressed her and felt young and whole again. He did not miss his wife and children. He did not miss his skin.

The saint did everything she must. She told him how handsome he was and what pleasure he gave her. She touched him in the way he liked best. She said he was her whole life, her fate. And at night when he woke her to staunch the blood, she whispered how she needed him, how she could not live without him.

This went on for some time.

The war was over and the occupying forces had made the general mayor of the capital city. He was about to run for senator and wanted his past to be beyond the reproach of any investigative committee. He wrote Hanley a letter which he sent through the International Red Cross.

"You could have been my own son," he said. "What we do in war is what we have to do. We do not choose cruelty or violence. I did only what was my duty."

"I am in love and I am loved," Hanley said. "Why isn't this enough?"

The saint was swabbing his chest and belly with blood retardant.

"Nothing is ever enough," she said.

"I love, but I am not possessed by love," he said, "I want to be surrounded by you. I want to be enclosed. I want to be enveloped. I don't have the words for it. But do you understand?"

"You want to be possessed," she said.

"I want to be inside you."

And so they made love, but afterward he said, "That was not enough. That is only a metaphor for what I want."

The general was elected senator and was made a trustee of three nuclear-arms conglomerates. But he was not well. And he was not sleeping well.

He wrote to Hanley, "I wake in the night and see your face before mine. I feel your forehead pressing against my palms. I taste your breath. I did only what I had to do. You could have been my son."

"I know what I want," Hanley said.

"If I can do it, I will," the saint said.

"I want your skin."

And so she lay down on the long white table, shuddering, while Hanley made his first incision. He cut along the shoulders and then down the arms and back up, then down the sides and the legs to the feet. It took him longer than he had expected. The saint shivered at the cold touch of the knife and she sobbed once at the sight of the blood, but by the time Hanley lifted the shroud of skin from her crimson body, she was resigned, satisfied even.

Hanley had spared her face and her genitals.

He spread the skin out to dry and, while he waited, he swabbed her raw body carefully with blood retardant. He whispered little words of love and thanks and desire to her. A smile played about her lips, but she said nothing.

It would be a week before he could put on her skin.

The general wrote to Hanley one last letter. "I can endure no more. I am possessed by you."

Hanley put on the skin of the saint. His genitals fitted nicely through the gap he had left and the skin at his neck matched hers exactly. He walked the corridors and for once left no bloody tracks behind. He stood before mirrors and admired himself. He touched his breasts and his belly and his thighs and there was no blood on his hands.

"Thank you," he said to her. "It is my heart's desire fulfilled. I am inside you. I am possessed by you."

And then, in the night, he kissed her on the brow and on the cheek and finally on the mouth. He gazed deep and long into her eyes. He traced the lines of her eyebrows gently, with the tip of his index finger. "Such a beautiful face," he said. He pressed his palms lightly against her forehead, her cheekbones, her jaw. With his little finger he memorized the shape of her lips.

And then it was that Hanley, loved, desperate to possess and be possessed, staring deep into the green and loving eyes of the saint, saw that there can be no possession, there is only desire. He plucked at his empty skin, and wept.

"1921"
From Sula

TONI MORRISON

SULA PEACE LIVED in a house of many rooms that had been built over a period of five years to the specifications of its owner, who kept on adding things: more stairways—there were three sets to the second floor—more rooms, doors and stoops. There were rooms that had three doors, others that opened out on the porch only and were inaccessible from any other part of the house; others that you could get to only by going through somebody's bedroom. The creator and sovereign of this enormous house with the four sickle-pear trees in the front yard and the single elm in the back yard was Eva Peace, who sat in a wagon on the third floor directing the lives of her children, friends, strays, and a constant stream of boarders. Fewer than nine people in the town remembered when Eva had two legs, and her oldest child, Hannah, was not one of them. Unless Eva herself introduced the subject, no one ever spoke of her disability; they pretended to ignore it, unless, in some mood of fancy, she began some fearful story about it—generally to entertain children. How the leg got up by itself one day and walked on off. How she hobbled after it but it ran too fast. Or how she had a corn on her toe and it just grew and grew and grew until her whole foot was a corn and then it traveled on up her leg and wouldn't stop growing until she put a red rag at the top but by that time it was already at her knee.

Somebody said Eva stuck it under a train and made them pay off. Another said she sold it to a hospital for $10,000—at which Mr. Reed opened his eyes and asked, "Nigger gal legs goin' for $10,000 a *piece?*" as though he could understand $10,000 a *pair*—but for *one?*

Whatever the fate of her lost leg, the remaining one was magnificent. It was stockinged and shod at all times and in all weather. Once in a while she got a felt slipper for Christmas or her birthday, but they soon disappeared, for Eva always wore a black laced-up shoe that came well above her ankle. Nor did she wear overlong dresses to disguise the empty place on her left side. Her dresses were mid-calf so that her one glamorous leg was always in view as well as the long fall of space below her left thigh. One of her men friends had fashioned a kind of wheelchair for her: a rocking-chair top fitted into a large child's wagon. In this contraption she wheeled around the room, from bedside to dresser to the balcony that opened out the north side of her room or to the window that looked out on the back yard. The wagon was so low that children who spoke to her standing up were eye level with her, and adults, standing or sitting, had to look down at her. But they didn't know it. They all had the impression that they were looking up at her, up into the open distances of her eyes, up into the soft black of her nostrils and up at the crest of her chin.

Eva had married a man named BoyBoy and had three children: Hannah, the eldest, and Eva, whom she named after herself but called Pearl, and a son named Ralph, whom she called Plum.

After five years of a sad and disgruntled marriage BoyBoy took off. During the time they were together he was very much preoccupied with other women and not home much. He did whatever he could that he liked, and he liked womanizing best, drinking second, and abusing Eva third. When he left in November, Eva had $1.65, five eggs, three beets and no idea of what or how to feel. The children needed her; she needed money, and needed to get on with her life. But the demands of feeding her three children were so acute she had to postpone her anger for two years until she had both the time and the energy for it. She was confused and desperately hungry. There were very few black families in those low hills then. The Suggs, who lived two hundred yards down the road, brought her a warm bowl of peas, as soon as they found out, and a plate of cold bread. She thanked them and asked if they had a little milk for the older ones. They said no, but Mrs. Jackson, they knew, had a cow still giving. Eva took a bucket over and Mrs. Jackson told her to come back and fill it up in the morning, because the evening milking had already been done. In this way, things went on until near December. People were very willing to help, but Eva felt she would soon run her welcome out; winters were hard and her neighbors were not that much better off. She would lie in bed with the baby boy, the two girls wrapped in quilts on the floor, thinking. The oldest child, Hannah, was five and too young to take care of the baby alone, and any housework Eva could find would keep her away from them from five thirty or earlier in the morning until dark—way past eight. The white people in the valley weren't rich enough then to want maids; they were small farmers and tradesmen and wanted hard-labor help if anything. She thought also of returning to some of her people in Virginia, but to come home dragging three young ones would have to be a step one rung before death for Eva. She would have to scrounge around and beg through the winter, until her baby was at least nine months old, then she could plant and maybe hire herself out to valley farms to weed or sow or feed stock until something steadier came along at harvest time. She thought she had probably been a fool to let BoyBoy haul her away from her people, but it had seemed so right at the time. He worked for a white carpenter and toolsmith who insisted on BoyBoy's accompanying him when he went West and set up in a squinchy little town called Medallion. BoyBoy brought his new wife and built them a one-room cabin sixty feet back from the road that wound up out of the valley, on up into the hills and was named for the man he worked for. They lived there a year before they had an outhouse.

Sometime before the middle of December, the baby, Plum, stopped having bowel movements. Eva massaged his stomach and gave him warm water. Something must be wrong with my milk, she thought. Mrs. Suggs gave her castor oil, but even that didn't work. He cried and fought so they couldn't get much down his throat anyway. He seemed in great pain and his shrieks were pitched high in outrage and suffering. At one point, maddened by his own crying, he gagged, choked and looked as though he was strangling to death. Eva rushed to him and kicked over the earthen slop jar, washing a small area of the floor with the child's urine. She managed to soothe him, but when he took up the cry again late that night, she resolved to end his misery once and for all. She wrapped him in blankets, ran her finger around the crevices and sides of the lard can and stumbled to the outhouse with him. Deep in its darkness and freezing stench she squatted down, turned the baby over on her knees, exposed his buttocks and shoved the last bit of food she had in the world (besides three beets) up his ass. Softening the insertion with the dab of lard, she probed with her middle finger to loosen his bowels. Her fingernail snagged what felt like a pebble; she pulled it out and others followed. Plum stopped crying as the black hard stools ricocheted onto the frozen ground. And now that it was over, Eva squatted there wondering why she had come all the way out there to free his stools, and what was she doing down on her haunches with her beloved baby boy warmed by her body in the almost total darkness, her shins and teeth freezing, her nostrils assailed. She shook her head as though to juggle her brains around, then said aloud, "Uh uh. Nooo." Thereupon she returned to the house and her bed. As the grateful Plum slept, the silence allowed her to think.

Two days later she left all of her children with Mrs. Suggs, saying she would be back the next day.

Eighteen months later she swept down from a wagon with two crutches, a new black pocketbook, and one leg. First she reclaimed her children, next she gave the surprised Mrs. Suggs a ten-dollar bill, later she started building a house on Carpenter's Road, sixty feet from BoyBoy's one-room cabin, which she rented out.

When Plum was three years old, BoyBoy came back to town and paid her a visit. When Eva got the word that he was on his way, she made some lemonade. She had no idea what she would do or feel during that encounter. Would she cry, cut his throat, beg him to make love to her? She couldn't imagine. So she just waited to see. She stirred lemonade in a green pitcher and waited.

BoyBoy danced up the steps and knocked on the door.

"Come on in," she hollered.

He opened the door and stood smiling, a picture of prosperity and good will. His shoes were a shiny orange, and he had on a citified straw hat, a light-blue suit, and a cat's-head stickpin in his tie. Eva smiled and told him to sit himself down. He smiled too.

"How you been, girl?"

"Pretty fair. What you know good?" When she heard those words come out of her own mouth she knew that their conversation would start off polite. Although it remained to be seen whether she would still run the ice pick through the cat's-head pin.

"Have some lemonade."

"Don't mind if I do." He swept his hat off with a satisfied gesture. His nails were long and shiny. "Sho is hot, and I been runnin' around all day."

Eva looked out of the screen door and saw a woman in a pea-green dress leaning on the smallest pear tree. Glancing back at him, she was reminded of Plum's face when he managed to get the meat out of a walnut all by himself. Eva smiled again, and poured the lemonade.

Their conversation was easy: she catching him up on all the gossip, he asking about this one and that one, and like everybody else avoiding any reference to her leg. It was like talking to somebody's cousin who just stopped by to say howdy before getting on back to wherever he came from. BoyBoy didn't ask to see the children, and Eva didn't bring them into the conversation.

After a while he rose to go. Talking about his appointments and exuding an odor of new money and idleness, he danced down the steps and strutted toward the pea-green dress. Eva watched. She looked at the back of his neck and the set of his shoulders. Underneath all of that shine she saw defeat in the stalk of his neck and the curious tight way he held his shoulders. But still she was not sure what she felt. Then he leaned forward and whispered into the ear of the woman in the green dress. She was still for a moment and then threw back her head and laughed. A high-pitched big-city laugh that reminded Eva of Chicago. It hit her like a sledge hammer, and it was then that she knew what to feel. A liquid trail of hate flooded her chest.

Knowing that she would hate him long and well filled her with pleasant anticipation, like when you know you are going to fall in love with someone and you wait for the happy signs. Hating BoyBoy, she could get on with it, and have the safety, the thrill, the consistency of that hatred as long as she wanted or needed it to define and strengthen her or protect her from routine vulnerabilities. (Once when Hannah accused her of hating colored people, Eva said she only hated one, Hannah's father BoyBoy, and it was hating him that kept her alive and happy.)

Happy or not, after BoyBoy's visit she began her retreat to her bedroom, leaving the bottom of the house more and more to those who lived there: cousins who were passing through, stray folks, and the many, many newly married couples she let rooms to with housekeeping privileges, and after 1910 she didn't willingly set foot on the stairs but once and that was to light a fire, the smoke of which was in her hair for years.

Among the tenants in that big old house were the children Eva took in. Operating on a private scheme of preference and prejudice, she sent off for children she had seen from the balcony of her bedroom or whose circumstances she had heard about from the gossipy old men who came to play checkers or read the *Courier*, or write her number. In 1921, when her granddaughter Sula was eleven, Eva had three such children. They came with woolen caps and names given to them by their mothers, or grandmothers, or somebody's best friend. Eva snatched the caps off their heads and ignored their names. She looked at the first child closely, his wrists, the shape of his head and the temperament that showed in his eyes and said, "Well. Look at Dewey. My my mymymy." When later that same year she sent for a child who kept falling down off the porch across the street, she said the same thing. Somebody said, "But, Miss Eva, you calls the other one Dewey."

"So? This here's another one."

When the third one was brought and Eva said "Dewey" again, everybody thought she had simply run out of names or that her faculties had finally softened.

"How is anybody going to tell them apart?" Hannah asked her.

"What you need to tell them apart for? They's all deweys."

When Hannah asked the question it didn't sound very bright, because each dewey was markedly different from the other two. Dewey one was a deeply black boy with a beautiful head and the golden eyes of chronic jaundice. Dewey two was light-skinned with freckles everywhere and a head of tight red hair. Dewey three was half Mexican with chocolate skin and black bangs. Besides, they were one and two years apart in age. It was Eva saying things like, "Send one of them deweys out to get me some Garret, if they don't have Garret, get Buttercup," or, "Tell them deweys to cut out that noise," or, "Come here, you dewey you," and, "Send me a dewey," that gave Hannah's question its weight.

Slowly each boy came out of whatever cocoon he was in at the time his mother or somebody gave him away, and accepted Eva's view, becoming in fact as well as in name a dewey—joining with the other two to become a trinity with a plural name . . . inseparable, loving nothing and no one but themselves. When the handle from the icebox fell off, all the deweys got whipped, and in dry-eyed silence watched their own feet as they turned their behinds high up into the air for the stroke. When the golden-eyed dewey was ready for school he would not go without the others. He was seven, freckled dewey was five, and Mexican dewey was only four. Eva solved the problem by having them all sent off together. Mr. Buckland Reed said, "But one of them's only four."

"How you know? They all come here the same year," Eva said.

"But that one there was one year old when he came, and that was three years ago."

"You don't know how old he was when he come here and neither do the teacher. Send 'em."

The teacher was startled but not unbelieving, for she had long ago given up trying to fathom the ways of the colored people in town. So when Mrs. Reed said that their names were Dewey King, that they were cousins, and all were six years old, the teacher gave only a tiny sigh and wrote them in the record book for the first grade. She too thought she would have no problem distinguishing among them, because they looked nothing alike, but like everyone else before her, she gradually found that she could not tell one from the other. The deweys would not allow it. They got all mixed up in her head, and finally she could not literally believe her eyes. They spoke with one voice, thought with one mind, and maintained an annoying privacy. Stouthearted, surly, and wholly unpredictable, the deweys remained a mystery not only during all of their lives in Medallion but after as well.

The deweys came in 1921, but the year before Eva had given a small room off the kitchen to Tar Baby, a beautiful, slight, quiet man who never spoke above a whisper. Most people said he was half white, but Eva said he was all white. That she knew blood when she saw it, and he didn't have none. When he first came to Medallion, the people called him Pretty Johnnie, but Eva looked at his milky skin and cornsilk hair and out of a mixture of fun and meanness called him Tar Baby. He was a mountain boy who stayed to himself, bothering no one, intent solely on drinking himself to death. At first he worked in a poultry market, and after wringing the necks of chickens all day, he came home and drank until he slept. Later he began to miss days at work and frequently did not have his rent money. When he lost his job altogether, he would go out in the morning, scrounge around for money doing odd jobs, bumming or whatever, and come home to drink. Because he was no bother, ate little, required nothing, and was a lover of cheap wine, no one found him a nuisance. Besides, he frequently went to Wednesday-night prayer meetings and sang with the sweetest hill voice imaginable "In the Sweet By-and-By." He sent the deweys out for his liquor and spent most of his time in a heap on the floor or sitting in a chair staring at the wall.

Hannah worried about him a little, but only a very little. For it soon became clear that he simply wanted a place to die privately but not quite alone. No one thought of suggesting to him that he pull himself together or see a doctor or anything. Even the women at prayer meeting who cried when he sang "In the Sweet By-and-By" never tried to get him to participate in the church activities. They just listened to him sing, wept and thought very graphically of their own imminent deaths. The people either accepted his own evaluation of his life, or were indifferent to it. There was, however, a measure of contempt in their indifference, for they had little patience with people who took themselves that seriously. Seriously enough to try to die. And it was natural that he, after all, became the first one to join Shadrack— Tar Baby and the deweys—on National Suicide Day.

Under Eva's distant eye, and prey to her idiosyncrasies, her own children grew up stealthily: Pearl married at fourteen and moved to Flint, Michigan, from where she posted frail letters to her mother with two dollars folded into the writing paper. Sad little nonsense letters about minor troubles, her husband's job and who the children favored. Hannah married a laughing man named Rekus who died when their daughter Sula was about three years old, at which time Hannah moved back into her mother's big house prepared to take care of it and her mother forever.

With the exception of BoyBoy, those Peace women loved all men. It was manlove that Eva bequeathed to her daughters. Probably, people said, because there were no men in the house, no men to run it. But actually that was not true. The Peace women simply loved maleness, for its own sake. Eva, old as she was, and with one leg, had a regular flock of gentleman callers, and although she did not participate in the act of love, there was a good deal of teasing and pecking and laughter. The men wanted to see her lovely calf, that neat shoe, and watch the focusing that sometimes swept down out of the distances in her eyes. They wanted to see the joy in her face as they settled down to play checkers, knowing that even when she beat them, as she almost always did, somehow, in her presence, it was they who had won something. They would read the newspaper aloud to her and make observations on its content, and Eva would listen feeling no obligation to agree and, in fact, would take them to task about their interpretation of events. But she argued with them with such an absence of bile, such a concentration of manlove, that they felt their convictions solidified by her disagreement.

With other people's affairs Eva was equally prejudiced about men. She fussed interminably with the brides of the newly wed couples for not getting their men's supper ready on time; about how to launder shirts, press them, etc. "Yo' man be here direc'lin. Ain't it 'bout time you got busy?"

"Aw, Miss Eva. It'll be ready. We just having spaghetti."

"Again?" Eva's eyebrows fluted up and the newlywed pressed her lips together in shame.

Hannah simply refused to live without the attentions of a man, and after Rekus' death had a steady sequence of lovers, mostly the husbands of her friends and neighbors. Her flirting was sweet, low and guileless. Without ever a pat of the hair, a rush to change clothes or a quick application of paint, with no gesture whatsoever, she rippled with sex. In her same old print wraparound, barefoot in the summer, in the winter her feet in a man's leather slippers with the backs flattened under her heels, she made men aware of her behind, her slim ankles, the dewsmooth skin and the incredible length of neck. Then the smile-eyes, the turn of the head—all so welcoming, light and playful. Her voice trailed, dipped and bowed; she gave a chord to the simplest words. Nobody, but nobody, could say "hey sugar" like Hannah. When he heard it, the man tipped his hat down a little over his eyes, hoisted his trousers and thought about the hollow place at the base of her neck. And all this without the slightest confusion about work and responsibilities. While Eva tested and argued with her men, leaving them feeling as though they had been in combat with a worthy, if amiable, foe, Hannah rubbed no edges, made no demands, made the man feel as though he were complete and wonderful just as he was—he didn't need fixing—and so he relaxed and swooned in the Hannah-light that shone on him simply because he was. If the man entered and Hannah was carrying a coal scuttle up from the basement, she handled it in such a way that it became a gesture of love. He made no move to help her with it simply because he wanted to see how her thighs looked when she bent to put it down, knowing that she wanted him to see them too.

But since in that crowded house there were no places for private and spontaneous lovemaking, Hannah would take the man down into the cellar in the summer where it was cool back behind the coal bin and the newspapers, or in the winter they would step into the pantry and stand up against the shelves she had filled with canned goods, or lie on the flour sack just under the rows of tiny green peppers. When those places were not available, she would slip into the seldom-used parlor, or even up to her bedroom. She liked the last place least, not because Sula slept in the room with her but because her love mate's tendency was always to fall asleep afterward and Hannah was fastidious about whom she slept with. She would fuck practically anything, but sleeping with someone implied for her a measure of trust and a definite commitment. So she ended up a daylight lover, and it was only once actually that Sula came home from school and found her mother in the bed, curled spoon in the arms of a man.

Seeing her step so easily into the pantry and emerge looking precisely as she did when she entered, only happier, taught Sula that sex was pleasant and frequent, but otherwise unremarkable. Outside the house, where children giggled about underwear, the message was different. So she watched her mother's face and the face of the men when they opened the pantry door and made up her own mind.

Hannah exasperated the women in the town—the "good" women, who said, "One thing I can't stand is a nasty woman"; the whores, who were hard put to find trade among black men anyway and who resented Hannah's generosity; the middling women, who had both husbands and affairs, because

Hannah seemed too unlike them, having no passion attached to her relationships and being wholly incapable of jealousy. Hannah's friendships with
women were, of course, seldom and short-lived, and the newly married
couples whom her mother took in soon learned what a hazard she was. She
could break up a marriage before it had even become one—she would make
love to the new groom and wash his wife's dishes all in an afternoon. What
she wanted, after Rekus died, and what she succeeded in having more often
than not, was some touching every day.

The men, surprisingly, never gossiped about her. She was unquestionably
a kind and generous woman and that, coupled with her extraordinary beauty
and funky elegance of manner, made them defend her and protect her from
any vitriol that newcomers or their wives might spill.

Eva's last child, Plum, to whom she hoped to bequeath everything, floated
in a constant swaddle of love and affection, until 1917 when he went to war.
He returned to the States in 1919 but did not get back to Medallion until 1920.
He wrote letters from New York, Washington, D.C., and Chicago full of promises of homecomings, but there was obviously something wrong. Finally some
two or three days after Christmas, he arrived with just the shadow of his old
dip-down walk. His hair had been neither cut nor combed in months, his
clothes were pointless and he had no socks. But he did have a black bag, a
paper sack, and a sweet, sweet smile. Everybody welcomed him and gave him
a warm room next to Tar Baby's and waited for him to tell them whatever it
was he wanted them to know. They waited in vain for his telling but not long
for the knowing. His habits were much like Tar Baby's but there were no
bottles, and Plum was sometimes cheerful and animated. Hannah watched
and Eva waited. Then he began to steal from them, take trips to Cincinnati
and sleep for days in his room with the record player going. He got even thinner, since he ate only snatches of things at beginnings or endings of meals. It
was Hannah who found the bent spoon black from steady cooking.

So late one night in 1921, Eva got up from her bed and put on her clothes.
Hoisting herself up on her crutches, she was amazed to find that she could
still manage them, although the pain in her armpits was severe. She practiced
a few steps around the room, and then opened the door. Slowly, she manipu-
lated herself down the long flights of stairs, two crutches under her left arm,
the right hand grasping the banister. The sound of her foot booming in comparison to the delicate pat of the crutch tip. On each landing she stopped for
breath. Annoyed at her physical condition, she closed her eyes and removed
the crutches from under her arms to relieve the unaccustomed pressure. At

the foot of the stairs she redistributed her weight between the crutches and swooped on through the front room, to the dining room, to the kitchen, swinging and swooping like a giant heron, so graceful sailing about in its own habitat but awkward and comical when it folded its wings and tried to walk. With a swing and a swoop she arrived at Plum's door and pushed it open with the tip of one crutch. He was lying in bed barely visible in the light coming from a single bulb. Eva swung over to the bed and propped her crutches at its foot. She sat down and gathered Plum into her arms. He woke, but only slightly.

"Hey, man. Hey. You holdin' me, Mamma?" His voice was drowsy and amused. He chuckled as though he had heard some private joke. Eva held him closer and began to rock. Back and forth she rocked him, her eyes wandering around his room. There in the corner was a half-eaten store-bought cherry pie. Balled up candy wrappers and empty pop bottles peeped from under the dresser. On the floor by her foot was a glass of strawberry crush and a *Liberty* magazine. Rocking, rocking, listening to Plum's occasional chuckles, Eva let her memory spin, loop and fall. Plum in the tub that time as she leaned over him. He reached up and dripped water into her bosom and laughed. She was angry, but not too, and laughed with him.

"Mamma, you so purty. You so purty, Mamma."

Eva lifted her tongue to the edge of her lip to stop the tears from running into her mouth. Rocking, rocking. Later she laid him down and looked at him a long time. Suddenly she was thirsty and reached for the glass of strawberry crush. She put it to her lips and discovered it was blood-tainted water and threw it to the floor. Plum woke up and said, "Hey, Mamma, whyn't you go on back to bed? I'm all right. Didn't I tell you? I'm all right. Go on, now."

"I'm going, Plum," she said. She shifted her weight and pulled her crutches toward her. Swinging and swooping, she left his room. She dragged herself to the kitchen and made grating noises.

Plum on the rim of a warm light sleep was still chuckling. Mamma. She sure was somethin'. He felt twilight. Now there seemed to be some kind of wet light traveling over his legs and stomach with a deeply attractive smell. It wound itself—this wet light—all about him, splashing and running into his skin. He opened his eyes and saw what he imagined was the great wing of an eagle pouring a wet lightness over him. Some kind of baptism, some kind of blessing, he thought. Everything is going to be all right, it said. Knowing that it was so he closed his eyes and sank back into the bright hole of sleep.

Eva stepped back from the bed and let the crutches rest under her arms. She rolled a bit of newspaper into a tight wick about six inches long, lit it and threw it onto the bed where the kerosene-soaked Plum lay in snug delight.

Quickly, as the *whoosh* of flames engulfed him, she shut the door and made her slow and painful journey back to the top of the house.

Just as she got to the third landing she could hear Hannah and some child's voice. She swung along, not even listening to the voices of alarm and the cries of the deweys. By the time she got to her bed someone was bounding up the stairs after her. Hannah opened the door. "Plum! Plum! He's burning, Mamma! We can't even open the door! Mamma!"

Eva looked into Hannah's eyes. "Is? My baby? Burning?" The two women did not speak, for the eyes of each were enough for the other. Then Hannah closed hers and ran toward the voices of neighbors calling for water.

From The Elephant Man

BERNARD POMERANCE

SCENE III: WHO HAS SEEN THE LIKE OF THIS?

TREVES *lectures.* MERRICK *contorts himself to approximate projected slides of the real Merrick.*

TREVES: The most striking feature about him was his enormous head. Its circumference was about that of a man's waist. From the brow there projected a huge bony mass like a loaf, while from the back of his head hung a bag of spongy fungous-looking skin, the surface of which was comparable to brown cauliflower. On the top of the skull were a few long lank hairs. The osseous growth on the forehead, at this stage about the size of a tangerine, almost occluded one eye. From the upper jaw there projected another mass of bone. It protruded from the mouth like a pink stump, turning the upper lip inside out, and making the mouth a wide slobbering aperture. The nose was merely a lump of flesh, only recognizable as a nose from its position. The deformities rendered the face utterly incapable of the expression of any emotion whatsoever. The back was horrible because from it hung, as far down as the middle of the thigh, huge sacklike masses of flesh covered by the same loathsome cauliflower stain. The right arm was of enormous size and shapeless. It suggested but was not elephantiasis, and was overgrown also with pendant masses of the same cauliflower-like skin. The right hand was large and clumsy—a fin or paddle rather than a hand. No distinction existed between the palm and back, the thumb was like a radish, the fingers like thick tuberous roots. As a limb it was useless. The other arm was remarkable by contrast. It was not only normal, but was moreover a delicately shaped limb covered with a fine skin and provided with a beautiful hand which any woman might have envied. From the chest hung a bag of the same repulsive flesh. It was like a dewlap suspended from the neck of a lizard. The lower limbs had the characters of the deformed arm. They were unwieldy, dropsical-looking, and grossly misshapen. There arose from the fungous skin growths a very sickening stench which was hard to tolerate. To add a further burden to his trouble, the wretched man when a boy developed hip disease which left him permanently lame, so that he could only walk with a stick. (*To* MERRICK) Please. (MERRICK *walks*.) He was thus denied all means of escape from his tormentors.

VOICE: Mr. Treves, you have shown a profound and unknown disorder to us. You have said when he leaves here it is for his exhibition again. I do not think it ought to be permitted. It is a disgrace. It is a pity and a disgrace. It is an indecency in fact. It may be a danger in ways we do not know. Something ought to be done about it.

TREVES: I am a doctor. What would you have me do?

VOICE: Well, I know what to do. *I* know.

Silence. A policeman enters as lights fade out.

SCENE XVIII: WE ARE DEALING WITH AN EPIDEMIC

TREVES *asleep.* MERRICK *at lectern.*

MERRICK: The most striking thing about him, note, is the terrifyingly normal head. This allowed him to lie down normally, and therefore to dream in the exclusive personal manner, without the weight of others' dreams accumulating to break his neck. From the brow projected a normal vision of benevolent enlightenment, what we believe to be a kind of self-mesmerized state. The mouth, deformed by satisfaction at being the hub of the best of existent worlds, was rendered therefore utterly incapable of self-critical speech, thus of the ability to change. The heart showed signs of worry at this unchanging yet untenable state. The back was horribly stiff from being kept against a wall to face the discontent of a world ordered for his convenience. The surgeon's hands were well-developed and strong, capable of the most delicate carvings-up, for others' own good. Due also to the normal head, the right arm was of enormous power; but, so incapable of the distinction between the assertion of authority and the charitable act of giving, that it was often to be found disgustingly beating others—for their own good. The left arm was slighter and fairer, and may be seen in typical position, hand covering the genitals which were treated as a sullen colony in constant need of restriction, governance, punishment. For their own good. To add a further burden to his trouble, the wretched man when a boy developed a disabling spiritual duality, therefore was unable to feel what others feel, nor reach harmony with them. Please. (TREVES *shrugs*.) He would thus be denied all means of escape from those he had tormented.

PINS *enter.*

FIRST PIN: Mr. Merrick. You have shown a profound and unknown disorder to us. You have said when he leaves here, it is for his prior life again. I do not think it ought to be permitted. It is a disgrace. It is a pity and a disgrace. It is an indecency in fact. It may be a danger in ways we do not know. Something ought to be done about it.

MERRICK: We hope in twenty years we will understand enough to put an end to this affliction.

FIRST PIN: Twenty years! Sir, that is unacceptable!

MERRICK: Had we caught it early, it might have been different. But his condition has already spread both East and West. The truth is, I am afraid, we are dealing with an epidemic.

MERRICK *puts another piece on St. Philip's.* PINS *exit.* TREVES *starts awake. Fadeout.*

The Leg

Karl Shapiro

Among the iodoform in twilight sleep,
What have I lost? he first enquires,
Peers in the middle distance where a pain,
Ghost of a nurse, hazily moves, and day,
Her blinding presence pressing in his eyes
And now his ears. They are handling him
With rubber hands. He wants to get up.

One day beside some flowers near his nose
He will be thinking, *When will I look at it?*
And pain, still in the middle distance, will reply,
At what? and he will know it's gone,
O where! and begin to tremble and cry.
He will begin to cry as a child cries
Whose puppy is mangled under a screaming wheel.

Later, as if deliberately, his fingers
Begin to explore the stump. He learns a shape
That is comfortable and tucked in like a sock.
This has a sense of humor, this can despise
The finest surgical limb, the dignity of limping,
The nonsense of wheel-chairs. Now he smiles to the wall:
The amputation becomes an acquisition.

For the leg is wondering where he is (all is not lost)
And surely he has a duty to the leg:
He is its injury, the leg is his orphan,
He must cultivate the mind of the leg,
Pray for the part that is missing, pray for peace
In the image of man, pray, pray for its safety,
And after a little while it will die quietly.

The body, what is it, Father, but a sign
To love the force that grows us, to give back
What in Thy palm is senselessness and mud?
Knead, knead the substance of our understanding
Which must be beautiful in flesh to walk,
That if Thou take me angrily in hand
And hurl me to the shark, I shall not die!

From The Journal of a Leper

John Updike

Oct. 31. I have long been a potter, a bachelor, and a leper. Leprosy is not exactly what I have, but what in the Bible is called leprosy (see Leviticus 13, Exodus 4:6, Luke 5:12–13) was probably this thing, which has a twisty Greek name it pains me to write. The form of the disease is as follows: spots, plaques, and avalanches of excess skin, manufactured by the dermis through some trifling but persistent error in its metabolic instructions, expand and slowly migrate across the body like lichen on a tombstone. I am silvery, scaly. Puddles of flakes form wherever I rest my flesh. Each morning, I vacuum my bed. My torture is skin deep: there is no pain, not even itching; we lepers live a long time, and are ironically healthy in other respects. Lusty, though we are loathsome to love. Keen-sighted, though we hate to look upon ourselves. The name of the disease, spiritually speaking, is Humiliation.

I have come back from Copley Square, to this basement where I pot. Himmelfahrer was here this morning, and praised my work, touching the glazes and rims in a bliss erotic and financial both. He is my retailer, my link with the world, my nurturing umbilicus. Thanks to him I can crouch unseen in clayey, kiln-lit dimness. His shop is on Newbury Street. Everything there is beautiful, expensive, blemishless; but nothing more so than my ceramics. If the merest pimple of captured dust mote reveal itself to my caress, I smash the bowl. The vaguest wobble in the banding, and damnation and destruction ensue. He calls me a genius. I call myself a leper. I should have been smashed at birth.

Tomorrow begins my cure. I ventured out for lunch to celebrate this, and to deposit Himmelfahrer's mammoth check. Boston was impeccable in the cold October sunlight, glazed and hardened by summer. The blue skin of the proud new Hancock folly rose sheer and unfractured into a sky of the same blue, mirrored. For a time, the building had shed windows as I shed scales, and with more legal reverberation, but it has been cured, they say. I look

toward it still, hoping to see some panes missing, its perfection still vulnerable. The strange yellow insect that cleans its windows is at work. In its lower
surfaces Trinity Church, a Venetian fantasy composed of two tones of tawny
stones, admires itself, undulating. The Square itself, a cruel slab laid upon
Back Bay's heart, is speckled with survivors—the season's last bongo drum-
mer, the last shell-necklace seller, the last saffron frond of Hare Krishna chant-
ers. They glance at me and glance away, pained. My hands and my face mark
me. In a month I can wear gloves, but even then my face will shout, *Enor-
mity:* the livid spots beside my nose, the crumbs in my eyelashes, the scurvy
patch skipping along my left cheek, the silver cupped in my ears. A bleary
rummy in a flapping overcoat comes up to me and halts his beggar's snarl,
gazing at my visage amazed. I give him a handful of coin nonetheless. Light
beats on my face mercilessly.

In the shadows of Ken's, I order matzo-ball soup and find it tepid. Still, it
is delicious to be out. The waitress is glorious, her arms pure kaolin, her
chiselled pout as she scribbles my order a masterpiece of Sèvres biscuit. When
she bends over, setting my pastrami sandwich before me, I want to hide forever between her cool, perfect, yet flexible breasts. She glances at me and
does not know I am a leper. If I bared my arms and chest she would run
screaming. A few integuments of wool and synthetic fibre save me from her
horror; my enrollment in humanity is so perilous. No wonder I despise and
adore my fellow-men—adore them for their normal human plainness, despise them for not detecting and destroying me. My hands would act as be-
trayers, but while eating I move them constantly, to blur them. Picking the
sandwich up, my right hand freezes; I had forgotten how hideous it was.
Usually, when I look down, it is covered with clay. It has two garish spots,
one large and one small, and in the same relation to one another as Australia
and Tasmania. The woman next to me at the counter, a hag in pancake makeup
and mink, glances down with me. Involuntarily she starts. Her fork clatters
to the floor. Deftly I pick it up and place it on the Formica between us, so she
does not have to touch me. Even so, she asks for another.

Nov. 1. The doctor whistles when I take off my clothes. "Quite a case." But he
is sure I will respond. "We have this type of light now." He is from Australia,
oddly, but does not linger over the spots on my hand. "First, a few photographs." The floor of his office, I notice, is sprinkled with flakes. There are
other lepers. At last, I am not alone. He squints and squats and clicks and
clucks. "Good. Seventy per cent I would say." He has me turn around, and

whistles again, more softly. "Then some blood tests, *pro forma.*" He explains the treatment. Internal medication will open me like a flower to lengthening doses of light. His own skin bears the dusty-rose ebb of a summer's tan. His scalp is flawlessly bald and dreamily smooth. I wonder what perversity drove him into dermatology. "When you clear," he says casually, toward the end. When I clear! The concept is staggering. I want to swoon, I want to embrace him, as one embraces, in primitive societies, a madman. On his desk there is a tawdry flesh-pink mug with a tea bag in it, and I vow to make him a perfect teacup if he makes good his promise. "Nasty turn in the weather today," he offers, buttoning up his camera; but it is a lame and somehow bestial business, polite conversation between two men of whom one is dressed and the other is naked. As I drag my clothes on, a shower of silver falls to the floor. He calls it, professionally, "scale." I call it, inwardly, filth.

I told Carlotta tonight of his casual promise to make me "clear." She says she loves me the way I am. "How *can* you!" I blurt. She shrugs. She was late this evening, having been hours at devotions. It is All Saints' Day. We make love. Stroking her buttocks, I think of the doctor's skull.

Nov. 8. First treatment. The "light box" has six sides lined with vertical tubes. A hexagonal prism, as the Hancock Tower is a rhomboidal prism and a Toblerone chocolate bar is a triangular one. A roaring when it switches on, so one has astronautical sensations; also sensations of absurdity, standing nude as in a "daring" play where the stage lights have consumed the audience. The attendant, a tremulous young man with a diabolically pointed beard, gave me goggles to protect my retinas; I look down. I am on fire! In this kiln my feet, my legs, my arms, wherever there are scales, glow with a violet-white intensity like nothing but certain moments of developing prints in a darkroom pan. To make sure the legs are mine, I do a little dance. The Dance of Shiva, his body smeared with ashes, his hair matted and foul. My legs, chalky as logs about to fall into embers, vibrate and swing in the cleansing fire. The dance is short-lived; the first dose is but a minute. The box has a nasty, rebuking snort when it shuts off.

Dressed, stepping out from behind the curtain, I make future arrangements with the attendant and wonder what has led him into work of this sort. Dealing with people like me is a foul business, I am certain.

Nov. 12. No perceptible change. Carlotta tells me to relax. Dr. Aus (his real name keeps escaping me) says two weeks pass before the first noticeable effects. Himmelfahrer tells me Christmas is coming. I work past midnight on an epic course of vases, rimmed and banded with a very thin slip tinctured with cobalt oxide. The decoration should not strike the appraiser at first glance; he should think first "vase," and then "blue," and then "blue and not-blue." The Chinese knew how to imbue this mystery, this blush in the glaze, this plenitude of nothingness. I scorn incision, sgraffito, wax resist, relief. Smoothness is the essence, the fingers must not be perturbed. The wheel turns. My hand vanishes up past the wrist into the orifice of whistling, whispering clay, confiding the slither of its womb-wall to me, while the previous vase dries.

My dose was two minutes today.

The disease is frightened. Its surface feigns indifference, but deeper it itches with subtle rage, so that I cannot sleep. It has spread across my shoulders, to the insides of my arms, to my fingernails, whitening and warping them with ridges that grow out from beneath the cuticle like buried terrors coming to light.

Nov. 13. I have been taken off the treatment!

A leper among lepers, doubly untouchable.

Aus says my antibody count is sinisterly high. "A few more tests, to be on the safe side." Tells me stories of other lepers—cardiac patients, claustrophobes, arthritics—who had to be excluded. "Don't want to cure the disease and kill the patient." Please do, I beg him. He tut-tuts, his Commonwealth sanity recoiling from our dark American streak. Tells me that like all lepers I have very naturally "fallen in love with the lights."

I cannot work, I cannot smile.

I know now the box *exists,* that is the torture. It is there, out there, a magical prism in this city of dungeons and coffins and telephone booths. Boston, that honeycomb of hospitals, has a single hexagon of divine nectar, a decompression chamber admitting me to Paradise, and it is locked. I marvel at, in the long history of trapped mankind, the inability of our thoughts to transport bodies, to remove them cell by cell from the burning attic, the sunk submarine. Mine is the ancient prayer, *Deliver me.* Carlotta says that all her prayers are that I be granted the strength and grace to bear my disappointments. A vapid petition, I narrowly refrain from telling her. Confessionals, lavatories, one-room apartments, tellers' booths—they rattle through my mind like dud machine-gun cartridges. I want to be in my light box.

Nov. 15. Blood tests all morning. The nurse drawing the samples from my veins looms comely as the dawn, solid-muscled as a young puma. She handles my horrible arm without comment. I glance down and imagine that the leprosy on its underside shines less brightly. She chatters over my head to a sister nurse of childish things, of downtown movies and horny internes and TV talk shows, her slender jaw ruminating on a wad of chewing gum. In her forgetfulness of me, as I fill vial after vial, her breasts drift in their starched carapace inches from my nose. I want to nurse, to counteract the outward flow of my blood. Yin and yang, mutually feeding.

Carlotta, coming tonight to console me, finds me almost excessively manly.

Nov. 18. Dreams. I am skiing on a white slope, beneath a white sky. I look down at my feet and they are also white, and my skis are engulfed by the powder. I am exhilarated. Then the dream transfers me to an interior, a ski hut where the white walls merge into the domed ceiling indistinguishably. There is an Eskimo maiden, muscular, brown, naked. I am dressed like a doctor, but more stiffly, in large white cards. I awaken, immensely ashamed.

In the negative print of this dream, I am sitting on a white bowl and my excrement overflows, unstoppably, unwipably, engulfing my feet, my thighs in patches I try to scrape. I awaken and am relieved to be in bed, between clean sheets. Then I look at my arms in the half-light of dawn and a nightmarish horror sweeps over me. This is real. This skin is me, I can't get out.

Himmelfahrer adores my new vases. He fairly danced with anticipation of his profit, stroked their surface—mat white and finely crackled à la early T'ang ware—as if touching something holy. I feel his visits indignantly, as invasions of my cave of dimness. I wear gloves at all times now, save when molding the clay. If I could only wear a mask—ski, African, Halloween—my costume would be impregnable.

3 A.M. I was in a dark room. A narrow crack of light marked a doorway. I tiptoed near, seeking escape, and there is no door to open; the light is a long fluorescent tube. I grip it and it is my own phallus.

Nov. 22. Miracle!

Aus called before nine and said the tests appear normal; the first must have been a lab error. It showed, he confessed, that I was fatally ill with lupus, and ultraviolet light was pure poison to me. I am reinstated. Come Thursday and resume.

Carlotta brings champagne this evening to celebrate, and I am secretly offended. She does *not* love me the way I am, apparently. She shyly asks if I want to give thanks and I coldly reply, "To whom?"

Nov. 25. The attendant welcomed me back without enthusiasm or acknowledgment of my hiatus. His face pale as candle tallow above the wispy inverted flame of his beard. I scan the remnant of his face left beardless and detect no trace of leprosy. Also, my fellow lepers, piled like so many over-coats in the tiny anteroom, waiting for their minutes of light, have perfect skin to my eyes. Most are men: squat, swarthy, ostentatiously dapper type—rug or insurance salesmen, their out-of-season tans bespeaking connections in Florida. There is a youngish woman, too. Her skin is so deeply brown her lips look pale by contrast. She sits primly, as before confession. Her plump throat, her tapered fingers and round wrists betray a sumptuous body—the brown vision of my Eskimo maiden, adipose to withstand the embrace of ice. I follow her in with my eyes, see her feet step out of their shoes beneath the white curtain, and then be disengaged by a naked hand from the silken tangle of fallen tights. Desire fills me. I take my own turn, in an adjacent box, with some impatience, as something my due, like breathing, like walking on unbroken legs. My time is two minutes—where I left off. It seems longer. I fall to counting the tubes, and notice that one is burnt out. I discover, touch-ing it to effect a repair, that all the tubes are touchable, they are not the skin of the sun. I tell the attendant of the malfunctioning tube, and he nods bleakly.

And walking home, through the twilight that comes earlier and earlier, I look up and see that a pane has fallen from my beloved, vexed Hancock Tower. It wasn't in the newspapers.   *even perfection has flaws*

And Himmelfahrer, his rather abrasive voice close to tears, calls to cry that two of the vases have turned up cracked in his storeroom. In the mood of benevolence that the renewal of my treatment has imbued me with, I vol-unteer that the flaw may have been in my firing, and we agree to share the loss. He is grateful.

Dec. 7. I am up to eight minutes. Carlotta says that my skin feels different. She confesses that my bumps had become a pattern in her mind, that my shoulders had felt as dry and ragged to her fingers as unplaned lumber, that she had had to steel herself to touch me ardently, fearful that I would hurt. It had startled her, she says, to wake up in the morning and find herself dusted with my flakes. She confides all this lightly, uncomplainingly, but her tone of relaxation implies that a trial for her is past. I had dared to dream that I was beautiful, if not in her eyes and to her touch, then in her heart, in the glow-ing heart of her love. But even there, I see now, I was a leper, loved in one of those acts of inner surmounting that are the pride and the insufferable vanity of the female race. Drunk on wine, I had an urge to pollute her, and I glazed her breasts with an *englobe* of honey, peanut butter, and California Chablis.

In the mirror I see little visible change—just a grudging sort of darkening in the isthmuses of normal skin between the continental daubs of silver and scarlet. The cure is quackery. I am a slave of quackery and crockery. And lechery. I long to see again the lovely female leper, whose ankles, as I remember my glimpse beneath the curtain, bore a feathery hint of scaliness. Papagena. We are all dreadful, but how worse to be a woman, when men have so little capacity for inner surmounting. Yet how correspondingly grateful and ardent to be touched. Yet she is never there. If there is any pattern in their appointments, it is that no leper sees another more than once.

In the corridors, though, we see cripples and comatose post-operatics being wheeled from the elevator, the dwarfed and the maimed, the drugged and the baffled, the sick and the relatives of the sick, bearing flowers and complaints. The visitors bring into the halls chill whiffs of the city, and a snuffly air of having been wronged; they merge indistinguishably with the sick, and altogether these crowds, lifted by the random hand of misfortune from the streets, make in these overburdened halls a metropolis of their own. A strange, medieval effect of *thronging*. Of Judgment Day and of humanity posing for the panoramic camera disaster carries. Monstrous moving clumps of faces, granular, asymmetrical, earthen.

Dec. 12. Small bowls on the little wheel all week, and some commissioned eggshell cups and saucers. The handles no thicker than a grape tendril. Stacking the kiln a tricky, teetery business. The bisque firing on Tuesday, and then the glaze: feldspar and kaolin for body, frits and colemanite for flux, seven-per-cent zircopax for semi-opacity, a touch of nickel oxide for the aloof, timeless gray I visualize. Kiln up to 2250 ; Cone No. 6 doffed its tip in the peephole, Cone 5 melted on its side, Cone 7 upright, an impervious soldier at attention in Hell. Turned kiln off at midnight. Eyes smarting, dots dancing. Nicest time to sleep, while kiln cools, the stoneware tucked safe into its fixed extremity of hardness.

In the morning, the gray a touch more urgent, less aloof than I had hoped. Two rims crystallized. Smashed these, then five more of the twenty, favoring the palest. Held the eighth in my hand, remembering my impulse to give a teacup to Dr. Aus. He has kept his promise. The mirror notices a difference, so does Carlotta. I find something crass lately in her needs, her bestowals, her observations. She says my tan is exciting, on my bottom as well, like a man in a blue movie. We used to go to blue movies, the darkest theatres, to hide me; I would marvel at all the skin. A strange recurring fantasy: when we spend the night together her skin and mine will melt together, like the glazes of two pots set too close together in the kiln.

Dec. 13. St. Lucy's Day. The saint of dim-sightedness, of the winter dark, Carlotta tells me. My stomach feels queasy—perhaps the pills that compel my skin to interact with the light. Couldn't get going all day. My brain feels soft.

Dec. 16. Aus whistles when I take off my clothes. "Quite an improvement." Yet he scarcely examines me, smiles dismissively when I try to show him the recalcitrant spots, the uneven topography of the healing. "You've forgotten the shape you were in, my friend." It is true. My life up to now has been unreal, a nightmare. He offers to show me the "snaps" he took. I say no. He takes new photographs. I elaborate my sensation that the leprosy, chased from my skin, is fleeing to deeper tissue, and will wait there to be reborn, in more loathsome and devilish form. He scorns this notion. "All you lepers get greedy." A clinical stage, evidently, like anger in the dying. I am *good enough,* his manner states. He accepts the teacup indifferently, with a grazing glance. "My wife'll adore it." My stomach turns. I should have saved out two. It never occurred to me he was married. Did he choose her, I wonder, for her pelt? One of the wonders of our world: the love life of gynecologists, etc.

Dec. 17. When I ask Himmelfahrer how our Beacon Hill patroness liked the cups, he replies she was rapturous. But his manner of relating this is not rapturous. He seems dull, I feel dull. Instead of working the afternoon through, I leave a few pieces to airdry and walk in the city, parading my passable face, my fair hands. I tend to underdress these days. I have caught cold. I never catch colds.

Dec. 21. The nadir of the year. The faces in Copley Square are winter-thinned and opaque. I miss the thronging, gaudy effect of the hospital halls. Here, on the pavements, the faces drift like newspapers of two days ago, printed in a language we will never take the trouble to learn. Their death masks settle upon their features, the curve toward disintegration implicit in the present fit. I used to love people; they seemed lordly, in permitting me to walk among them, a spy from the scabrous surface of another planet. Now I am aware of loving only the Hancock Tower, which has had its missing pane restored and is again perfect, unoccupied, changeably blue, taking upon itself the insubstantial shapes of clouds, their porcelain gauze, their adamant dreaming. I reflect that all art, all beauty, is reflection. The faces on Boylston Street appear to me sodden, spongy, drenched with time, self-absorbed. The waitress at Ken's, whom I once thought exquisite, seems sullen and doughy. Her chest is pale blubber. The matzo-ball soup is so tepid I push it away, into the arm of the man next to me at the counter. I wait for him to apologize, and he does. Afterward, picking the pastrami from between my teeth, I cross Copley Square and look at myself in the Hancock panes. There I am, distorted so that parts of me seem a yard broad and others narrow as the waist of an hourglass. I look up and the foreshortened height of the structure, along its acute angle, looms like the lifted prow of a ship. I wait for it to topple, and it doesn't.

Carlotta tells me I am less passionate. It is morning. She has just left, leaving behind her a musky afterscent of dissatisfaction.

Dec. 25. I am beautiful. I keep unwrapping myself to be sure. Even on my shins leprosy has vanished, leaving a fine crackle of dry skin, à la T'ang ware, that bath oil will ease. On my thighs, a faint pink shadow such as a whiff of copper oxide produces in a reduction atmosphere. The skin looks babyish, startled, disarmed: the well-known blankness of health. I feel between my self and my epiderm a gap, a thin space where a wedge of spiritual dissociation could be set. I have a thin headache, from last eve's boozy spat with Carlotta. And a tooth that is shrinking away from its porcelain filling seems to be dying; at least there is a neuralgic soft spot under my cheekbone. Perhaps, too, it hurts me to be alone. The light box is closed for the holiday. Carlotta is spending Christmas in religious retreat with an order of Episcopalian nuns on Louisburg Square.

Notes for a new line of stoneware: bigger, rougher, rude, with granulations and leonine stains of iron oxide.

Dec. 29. Caressing Carlotta, my fingertips discovered a pimple at the nape of her neck. Taking her to the window, I saw that the skin of her upper chest, stretched taut across the clavicles, was marred by a hundred imperfections—

freckles, inflamed follicles, a mole with a hair like a clot of earth supporting the stem of a single dead flower, the red indentations left by the chain of her crucifix, the whitish trace of an old wound or boil, indescribably fine curdlings and mottlings. My hand in contrast bore nothing of the kind; even the ghostly shadow of my Australia-shaped lesion had been smoothed away. We discovered, Carlotta and I, that while examining her shoulders I had lost my readiness for love; nothing we did could will it back. An incident unprecedented in our relationship. She seized the opportunity to exercise her womanly capacity for forgiveness, but I was not gulled, knowing who, at bottom, was to blame. Her spots danced on the insides of my lids.

Jan. 6. Dr. Aus has pronounced me "clear." He, by the way, is going home for a month, during which time I am to be given, like a new car, "maintenance checks." He takes my photographs for his collection, and looks forward to being away. It will be high summer Down Under. "We live on the beaches." I picture him suspended upside down in a parallelepiped of intense white sun, and feel abandoned.

Jan. 11. Carlotta says we should cool it. She has been seeing another man, a lay priest. I have been impotent with her twice since the initial fiasco, but she says that is not it. She will always love me, it is just that a woman needs to be needed, if I can understand. I pretend that I do. A worse blow falls when Himmelfahrer visits. He surveys my new work, pyramids of it, some of it still warm from the kiln, which I have enlarged. He appears disconsolate. He agrees to take only half, and that on consignment. He says it is the slow season. He touches a gargoylish pitcher (the spout a snout, the handle a tail) and observes there has been a change. I say the design is a joke, a fancy. He says he is speaking not of intent but of texture. He says these are good pots but not fanatic, that in today's highly competitive world you got to be fanatic to be even good. He is a heavy gray man, who moves with many leaden sighs. I feel a pang of guilt, knowing that I spend fewer hours than formerly in my studio, preferring to walk out into the city, clad as lightly as the cold allows, immersing myself in mankind and in the snow, which has been falling abundantly. A contagion of bliss in a city, in its air of digested disaster— the sirens wailing from the rooftops, the unexplained volume of smoke down the block, the blotchy-faced drunk shrieking at phantoms and hawking into the war-memorial urn.

Himmelfahrer apologizes for his own disappointment, and relents. He offers to take this new batch on our former terms if I will revert to my former small scale and muted tone and exquisite finish. I spurn him, of course. I see the plot. He and Carlotta are trying to make me again their own, their toy within the gilded cage of my disease. No more. I am free, as other men. I am whole.

Everyday Use

Alice Walker

for your grandmama

I WILL WAIT for her in the yard that Maggie and I made so clean and wavy yesterday afternoon. A yard like this is more comfortable than most people know. It is not just a yard. It is like an extended living room. When the hard clay is swept clean as a floor and the fine sand around the edges lined with tiny, irregular grooves, anyone can come and sit and look up into the elm tree and wait for the breezes that never come inside the house.

Maggie will be nervous until after her sister goes: she will stand hopelessly in corners, homely and ashamed of the burn scars down her arms and legs, eying her sister with a mixture of envy and awe. She thinks her sister has held life always in the palm of one hand, that "no" is a word the world never learned to say to her.

You've no doubt seen those TV shows where the child who has "made it" is confronted, as a surprise, by her own mother and father, tottering in weakly from backstage. (A pleasant surprise, of course: What would they do if parent and child came on the show only to curse out and insult each other?) On TV mother and child embrace and smile into each other's faces. Sometimes the mother and father weep, the child wraps them in her arms and leans across the table to tell how she would not have made it without their help. I have seen these programs.

Sometimes I dream a dream in which Dee and I are suddenly brought together on a TV program of this sort. Out of a dark and soft-seated limousine I am ushered into a bright room filled with many people. There I meet a smiling, gray, sporty man like Johnny Carson who shakes my hand and tells me what a fine girl I have. Then we are on the stage and Dee is embracing me with tears in her eyes. She pins on my dress a large orchid, even though she has told me once that she thinks orchids are tacky flowers.

In real life I am a large, big-boned woman with rough, man-working hands. In the winter I wear flannel nightgowns to bed and overalls during the day. I can kill and clean a hog as mercilessly as a man. My fat keeps me hot in zero weather. I can work outside all day, breaking ice to get water for washing; I can eat pork liver cooked over the open fire minutes after it comes steaming from the hog. One winter I knocked a bull calf straight in the brain between the eyes with a sledge hammer and had the meat hung up to chill before nightfall. But of course all this does not show on television. I am the way my daughter would want me to be: a hundred pounds lighter, my skin like an uncooked barley pancake. My hair glistens in the hot bright lights. Johnny Carson has much to do to keep up with my quick and witty tongue.

But that is a mistake. I know even before I wake up. Who ever knew a Johnson with a quick tongue? Who can even imagine me looking a strange white man in the eye? It seems to me I have talked to them always with one foot raised in flight, with my head turned in whichever way is farthest from them. Dee, though. She would always look anyone in the eye. Hesitation was no part of her nature.

"How do I look, Mama?" Maggie says, showing just enough of her thin body enveloped in pink skirt and red blouse for me to know she's there, almost hidden by the door.

"Come out into the yard," I say.

Have you ever seen a lame animal, perhaps a dog run over by some care- less person rich enough to own a car, sidle up to someone who is ignorant enough to be kind to him? That is the way my Maggie walks. She has been like this, chin on chest, eyes on ground, feet in shuffle, ever since the fire that burned the other house to the ground.

Dee is lighter than Maggie, with nicer hair and a fuller figure. She's a woman now, though sometimes I forget. How long ago was it that the other house burned? Ten, twelve years? Sometimes I can still hear the flames and feel Maggie's arms sticking to me, her hair smoking and her dress falling off her in little black papery flakes. Her eyes seemed stretched open, blazed open by the flames reflected in them. And Dee. I see her standing off under the sweet gum tree she used to dig gum out of; a look of concentration on her face as she watched the last dingy gray board of the house fall in toward the red-hot brick chimney. Why don't you do a dance around the ashes? I'd wanted to ask her. She had hated the house that much.

I used to think she hated Maggie, too. But that was before we raised the money, the church and me, to send her to Augusta to school. She used to read to us without pity; forcing words, lies, other folks' habits, whole lives upon us two, sitting trapped and ignorant underneath her voice. She washed us in a river of make-believe, burned us with a lot of knowledge we didn't necessarily need to know. Pressed us to her with the serious way she read, to shove us away at just the moment, like dimwits, we seemed about to understand.

Dee wanted nice things. A yellow organdy dress to wear to her graduation from high school; black pumps to match a green suit she'd made from an old suit somebody gave me. She was determined to stare down any disaster in her efforts. Her eyelids would not flicker for minutes at a time. Often I fought off the temptation to shake her. At sixteen she had a style of her own: and knew what style was.

I never had an education myself. After second grade the school was closed down. Don't ask me why: in 1927 colored asked fewer questions than they do now. Sometimes Maggie reads to me. She stumbles along good-naturedly but can't see well. She knows she is not bright. Like good looks and money, quickness passed her by. She will marry John Thomas (who has mossy teeth in an earnest face) and then I'll be free to sit here and I guess just sing church songs to myself. Although I never was a good singer. Never could carry a tune. I was always better at a man's job. I used to love to milk till I was hooked in the side in '49. Cows are soothing and slow and don't bother you, unless you try to milk them the wrong way.

I have deliberately turned my back on the house. It is three rooms, just like the one that burned, except the roof is tin; they don't make shingle roofs any more. There are no real windows, just some holes cut in the sides, like the portholes in a ship, but not round and not square, with rawhide holding the shutters up on the outside. This house is in a pasture, too, like the other one. No doubt when Dee sees it she will want to tear it down. She wrote me once that no matter where we "choose" to live, she will manage to come see us. But she will never bring her friends. Maggie and I thought about this and Maggie asked me, "Mama, when did Dee ever *have* any friends?"

She had a few. Furtive boys in pink shirts hanging about on washday after school. Nervous girls who never laughed. Impressed with her they worshiped the well-turned phrase, the cute shape, the scalding humor that erupted like bubbles in lye. She read to them.

When she was courting Jimmy T she didn't have much time to pay to us, but turned all her faultfinding power on him. He *flew* to marry a cheap city girl from a family of ignorant flashy people. She hardly had time to recompose herself.

When she comes I will meet—but there they are!

Maggie attempts to make a dash for the house, in her shuffling way, but I stay her with my hand. "Come back here," I say. And she stops and tries to dig a well in the sand with her toe.

It is hard to see them clearly through the strong sun. But even the first glimpse of leg out of the car tells me it is Dee. Her feet were always neat-looking, as if God himself had shaped them with a certain style. From the other side of the car comes a short, stocky man. Hair is all over his head a foot long and hanging from his chin like a kinky mule tail. I hear Maggie suck in her breath. "Uhnnnh," is what it sounds like. Like when you see the wriggling end of a snake just in front of your foot on the road. "Uhnnnh."

Dee next. A dress down to the ground, in this hot weather. A dress so loud it hurts my eyes. There are yellows and oranges enough to throw back the light of the sun. I feel my whole face warming from the heat waves it throws out. Earrings gold, too, and hanging down to her shoulders. Bracelets dangling and making noises when she moves her arm up to shake the folds of the dress out of her armpits. The dress is loose and flows, and as she walks closer, I like it. I hear Maggie go "Uhnnnh" again. It is her sister's hair. It stands straight up like the wool on a sheep. It is black as night and around the edges are two long pigtails that rope about like small lizards disappearing behind her ears.

"Wa-su-zo-Tean-o!" she says, coming on in that gliding way the dress makes her move. The short stocky fellow with the hair to his navel is all grinning and he follows up with "Asalamalakim, my mother and sister!" He moves to hug Maggie but she falls back, right up against the back of my chair. I feel her trembling there and when I look up I see the perspiration falling off her chin.

"Don't get up," says Dee. Since I am stout it takes something of a push. You can see me trying to move a second or two before I make it. She turns, showing white heels through her sandals, and goes back to the car. Out she peeks next with a Polaroid. She stoops down quickly and lines up picture after picture of me sitting there in front of the house with Maggie cowering behind me. She never takes a shot without making sure the house is included. When a cow comes nibbling around the edge of the yard she snaps it and me and Maggie *and* the house. Then she puts the Polaroid in the back seat of the car, and comes up and kisses me on the forehead.

Meanwhile Asalamalakim is going through motions with Maggie's hand. Maggie's hand is as limp as a fish, and probably as cold, despite the sweat, and she keeps trying to pull it back. It looks like Asalamalakim wants to shake hands but wants to do it fancy. Or maybe he don't know how people shake hands. Anyhow, he soon gives up on Maggie.

"Well," I say. "Dee."

"No, Mama," she says. "Not 'Dee', Wangero Leewanika Kemanjo!"

"What happened to 'Dee'?" I wanted to know.

"She's dead," Wangero said. "I couldn't bear it any longer, being named after the people who oppress me."

"You know as well as me you was named after your aunt Dicie," I said. Dicie is my sister. She named Dee. We called her "Big Dee" after Dee was born.

"But who was *she* named after?" asked Wangero.

"I guess after Grandma Dee," I said.

"And who was she named after?" asked Wangero.

"Her mother," I said, and saw Wangero was getting tired. "That's about as far back as I can trace it," I said. Though, in fact, I probably could have carried it back beyond the Civil War through the branches.

"Well," said Asalamalakim, "there you are."

"Uhnnnh," I heard Maggie say.

"There I was not," I said, "before 'Dicie' cropped up in our family, so why should I try to trace it that far back?"

He just stood there grinning, looking down on me like somebody inspecting a Model A car. Every once in a while he and Wangero sent eye signals over my head.

"How do you pronounce this name?" I asked.

"You don't have to call me by it if you don't want to," said Wangero.

"Why shouldn't I?" I asked. "If that's what you want us to call you, we'll call you."

"I know it might sound awkward at first," said Wangero.

"I'll get used to it," I said. "Ream it out again."

Well, soon we got the name out of the way. Asalamalakim had a name twice as long and three times as hard. After I tripped over it two or three times he told me to just call him Hakim-a-barber. I wanted to ask him was he a barber, but I didn't really think he was, so I didn't ask.

"You must belong to those beef-cattle peoples down the road," I said. They said "Asalamalakim" when they met you, too, but they didn't shake hands. Always too busy: feeding the cattle, fixing the fences, putting up salt-lick shelters, throwing down hay. When the white folks poisoned some of the herd the men stayed up all night with rifles in their hands. I walked a mile and a half just to see the sight.

Hakim-a-barber said, "I accept some of their doctrines, but farming and raising cattle is not my style." (They didn't tell me, and I didn't ask, whether Wangero (Dee) had really gone and married him.)

We sat down to eat and right away he said he didn't eat collards and pork was unclean. Wangero, though, went on through the chitlins and corn bread, the greens and everything else. She talked a blue streak over the sweet potatoes. Everything delighted her. Even the fact that we still used the benches her daddy made for the table when we couldn't afford to buy chairs.

"Oh, Mama!" she cried. Then turned to Hakim-a-barber. "I never knew how lovely these benches are. You can feel the rump prints," she said, running her hands underneath her and along the bench. Then she gave a sigh and her hand closed over Grandma Dee's butter dish. "That's it!" she said. "I knew there was something I wanted to ask you if I could have." She jumped up from the table and went over in the corner where the churn stood, the milk in it clabber by now. She looked at the churn and looked at it.

"This churn top is what I need," she said. "Didn't Uncle Buddy whittle it out of a tree you all used to have?"

"Yes," I said.

"Uh huh," she said happily. "And I want the dasher, too."

"Uncle Buddy whittle that, too?" asked the barber.

Dee (Wangero) looked up at me.

"Aunt Dee's first husband whittled the dash," said Maggie so low you almost couldn't hear her. "His name was Henry, but they called him Stash."

"Maggie's brain is like an elephant's," Wangero said, laughing. "I can use the churn top as a centerpiece for the alcove table," she said, sliding a plate over the churn, "and I'll think of something artistic to do with the dasher."

When she finished wrapping the dasher the handle stuck out. I took it for a moment in my hands. You didn't even have to look close to see where hands pushing the dasher up and down to make butter had left a kind of sink in the wood. In fact, there were a lot of small sinks; you could see where thumbs and fingers had sunk into the wood. It was beautiful light yellow wood, from a tree that grew in the yard where Big Dee and Stash had lived.

After dinner Dee (Wangero) went to the trunk at the foot of my bed and started rifling through it. Maggie hung back in the kitchen over the dishpan. Out came Wangero with two quilts. They had been pieced by Grandma Dee and then Big Dee and me had hung them on the quilt frames on the front porch and quilted them. One was in the Lone Star pattern. The other was Walk Around the Mountain. In both of them were scraps of dresses Grandma Dee had worn fifty and more years ago. Bits and pieces of Grandpa Jarrell's Paisley shirts. And one teeny faded blue piece, about the size of a penny matchbox, that was from Great Grandpa Ezra's uniform that he wore in the Civil War.

"Mama," Wangero said sweet as a bird. "Can I have these old quilts?"

I heard something fall in the kitchen, and a minute later the kitchen door slammed.

"Why don't you take one or two of the others?" I asked. "These old things was just done by me and Big Dee from some tops your grandma pieced before she died."

"No," said Wangero. "I don't want those. They are stitched around the borders by machine."

"That'll make them last better," I said.

"That's not the point," said Wangero. "These are all pieces of dresses Grandma used to wear. She did all this stitching by hand. Imagine!" She held the quilts securely in her arms, stroking them.

"Some of the pieces, like those lavender ones, come from old clothes her mother handed down to her," I said, moving up to touch the quilts. Dee (Wangero) moved back just enough so that I couldn't reach the quilts. They already belonged to her.

"Imagine!" she breathed again, clutching them closely to her bosom.

"The truth is," I said, "I promised to give them quilts to Maggie, for when she marries John Thomas."

She gasped like a bee had stung her.

"Maggie can't appreciate these quilts!" she said. "She'd probably be backward enough to put them to everyday use."

"I reckon she would," I said. "God knows I been saving 'em for long enough with nobody using 'em. I hope she will!" I didn't want to bring up how I had offered Dee (Wangero) a quilt when she went away to college. Then she had told me they were old-fashioned, out of style.

"But they're *priceless!*" she was saying now, furiously; for she has a temper. "Maggie would put them on the bed and in five years they'd be in rags. Less than that!"

"She can always make some more," I said. "Maggie knows how to quilt."

Dee (Wangero) looked at me with hatred. "You just will not understand. The point is these quilts, *these* quilts!"

"Well," I said, stumped. "What would you do with them?"

"Hang them," she said. As if that was the only thing you *could* do with quilts.

Maggie by now was standing in the door. I could almost hear the sound her feet made as they scraped over each other.

"She can have them, Mama," she said, like somebody used to never winning anything, or having anything reserved for her. "I can' member Grandma Dee without the quilts."

I looked at her hard. She had filled her bottom lip with checkerberry snuff and it gave her face a kind of dopey, hangdog look. It was Grandma Dee and Big Dee who taught her how to quilt herself. She stood there with her scarred hands hidden in the folds of her skirt. She looked at her sister with something like fear but she wasn't mad at her. This was Maggie's portion. This was the way she knew God to work.

When I looked at her like that something hit me in the top of my head and ran down to the soles of my feet. Just like when I'm in church and the spirit of God touches me and I get happy and shout. I did something I never had done before: hugged Maggie to me, then dragged her on into the room, snatched the quilts out of Miss Wangero's hands and dumped them into Maggie's lap. Maggie just sat there on my bed with her mouth open.

"Take one or two of the others," I said to Dee.

But she turned without a word and went out to Hakim-a-barber.

"You just don't understand," she said, as Maggie and I came out to the car.

"What don't I understand?" I wanted to know.

"Your heritage," she said. And then she turned to Maggie, kissed her, and said, "You ought to try to make something of yourself, too, Maggie. It's really a new day for us. But from the way you and Mama still live you'd never know it."

She put on some sunglasses that hid everything above the tip of her nose and her chin.

Maggie smiled; maybe at the sunglasses. But a real smile, not scared. After we watched the car dust settle I asked Maggie to bring me a dip of snuff. And then the two of us sat there just enjoying, until it was time to go in the house and go to bed.

Song For My Son

MARILYN DAVIS

a wooden puppet with tangled
strings   he bobs and bounces
in mid-air   head flopping
arms waving   my hands
under his arms sustain
his spastic stiffness
the Blue Fairy cradling
sweet Pinocchio

He loves to rock and roll
feet prancing   a crazy
puppet dance   his face glows
with the light   of the wishing
star   and borrowing his
brilliance   we too dance
heads bobbing   arms waving
faster and faster until
cast off puppets all
we fall to the floor   laughing
while the fading light
of the wishing star
caresses his face

The Ones that are Thrown Out

Miller Williams

One has flippers. This one is like a seal.
One has gills. This one is like a fish.
One has webbed hands, is like a duck.
One has a little tail, is like a pig.
One is like a frog
with no dome at all above the eyes.

They call them bad babies.

They didn't mean to be bad
but who does.

Good Country People

FLANNERY O'CONNOR

BESIDES THE NEUTRAL expression that she wore when she was alone, Mrs. Freeman had two others, forward and reverse, that she used for all her human dealings. Her forward expression was steady and driving like the advance of a heavy truck. Her eyes never swerved to left or right but turned as the story turned as if they followed a yellow line down the center of it. She seldom used the other expression because it was not often necessary for her to retract a statement, but when she did, her face came to a complete stop, there was an almost imperceptible movement of her black eyes, during which they seemed to be receding, and then the observer would see that Mrs. Freeman, though she might stand there as real as several grain sacks thrown on top of each other, was no longer there in spirit. As for getting anything across to her when this was the case, Mrs. Hopewell had given it up. She might talk her head off. Mrs. Freeman could never be brought to admit herself wrong on any point. She would stand there and if she could be brought to say anything, it was something like, "Well, I wouldn't of said it was and I wouldn't of said it wasn't," or letting her gaze range over the top kitchen shelf where there was an assortment of dusty bottles, she might remark, "I see you ain't ate many of them figs you put up last summer."

They carried on their most important business in the kitchen at breakfast. Every morning Mrs. Hopewell got up at seven o'clock and lit her gas heater and Joy's. Joy was her daughter, a large blonde girl who had an artificial leg. Mrs. Hopewell thought of her as a child though she was thirty-two years old and highly educated. Joy would get up while her mother was eating and lumber into the bathroom and slam the door, and before long, Mrs. Freeman would arrive at the back door. Joy would hear her mother call, "Come on in," and then they would talk for a while in low voices that were indistinguishable in the bathroom. By the time Joy came in, they had usually finished the weather report and were on one or the other of Mrs. Freeman's daughters, Glynese or Carramae. Joy called them Glycerin and Caramel. Glynese, a redhead, was eighteen and had many admirers; Carramae, a blonde, was only fifteen but already married and pregnant. She could not keep anything on her stomach. Every morning Mrs. Freeman told Mrs. Hopewell how many times she had vomited since the last report.

Mrs. Hopewell liked to tell people that Glynese and Carramae were two of the finest girls she knew and that Mrs. Freeman was a *lady* and that she was never ashamed to take her anywhere or introduce her to anybody they might meet. Then she would tell how she had happened to hire the Freemans in the first place and how they were a godsend to her and how she had had them four years. The reason for her keeping them so long was that they were not trash. They were good country people. She had telephoned the man whose name they had given as a reference and he had told her that Mr. Freeman was a good farmer but that his wife was the nosiest woman ever to walk the earth. "She's got to be into everything," the man said. "If she don't get there before the dust settles, you can bet she's dead, that's all. She'll want to know all your business. I can stand him real good," he had said, "but me nor my wife neither could have stood that woman one more minute on this place." That had put Mrs. Hopewell off for a few days.

She had hired them in the end because there were no other applicants but she had made up her mind beforehand exactly how she would handle the woman. Since she was the type who had to be into everything, then, Mrs. Hopewell had decided, she would not only let her be into everything, she would *see to it* that she was into everything—she would give her the responsibility of everything, she would put her in charge. Mrs. Hopewell had no bad qualities of her own but she was able to use other people's in such a constructive way that she never felt the lack. She had hired the Freemans and she had kept them four years.

Nothing is perfect. This was one of Mrs. Hopewell's favorite sayings. Another was: that is life! And still another, the most important, was: well, other people have their opinions too. She would make these statements, usually at the table, in a tone of gentle insistence as if no one held them but her, and the large hulking Joy, whose constant outrage had obliterated every expression from her face, would stare just a little to the side of her, her eyes icy blue, with the look of someone who has achieved blindness by an act of will and means to keep it.

When Mrs. Hopewell said to Mrs. Freeman that life was like that, Mrs. Freeman would say, "I always said so myself." Nothing had been arrived at by anyone that had not first been arrived at by her. She was quicker than Mr. Freeman. When Mrs. Hopewell said to her after they had been on the place a while, "You know, you're the wheel behind the wheel," and winked, Mrs. Freeman had said, "I know it. I've always been quick. It's some that are quicker than others."

"Everybody is different," Mrs. Hopewell said.

"Yes, most people is," Mrs. Freeman said.

"It takes all kinds to make the world."

"I always said it did myself."

The girl was used to this kind of dialogue for breakfast and more of it for dinner; sometimes they had it for supper too. When they had no guest they ate in the kitchen because that was easier. Mrs. Freeman always managed to arrive at some point during the meal and to watch them finish it. She would stand in the doorway if it were summer but in the winter she would stand with one elbow on top of the refrigerator and look down on them, or she would stand by the gas heater, lifting the back of her skirt slightly. Occasionally she would stand against the wall and roll her head from side to side. At no time was she in any hurry to leave. All this was very trying on Mrs. Hopewell but she was a woman of great patience. She realized that nothing is perfect and that in the Freemans she had good country people and that if, in this day and age, you get good country people you had better hang onto them.

She had had plenty of experience with trash. Before the Freemans she had averaged one tenant family a year. The wives of these farmers were not the kind you would want to be around you for very long. Mrs. Hopewell, who had divorced her husband long ago, needed someone to walk over the fields with her; and when Joy had to be impressed for these services, her remarks were usually so ugly and her face so glum that Mrs. Hopewell would say, "If you can't come pleasantly, I don't want you at all," to which the girl, standing square and rigid-shouldered with her neck thrust slightly forward, would reply, "If you want me, here I am—LIKE I AM."

Mrs. Hopewell excused this attitude because of the leg (which had been shot off in a hunting accident when Joy was ten). It was hard for Mrs. Hopewell to realize that her child was thirty-two now and that for more than twenty years she had had only one leg. She thought of her still as a child because it tore her heart to think instead of the poor stout girl in her thirties who had never danced a step or had any normal good times. Her name was really Joy but as soon as she was twenty-one and away from home, she had had it legally changed. Mrs. Hopewell was certain that she had thought and thought until she had hit upon the ugliest name in any language. Then she had gone and had the beautiful name, Joy, changed without telling her mother until after she had done it. Her legal name was Hulga.

When Mrs. Hopewell thought the name, Hulga, she thought of the broad blank hull of a battleship. She would not use it. She continued to call her Joy to which the girl responded but in a purely mechanical way.

Hulga had learned to tolerate Mrs. Freeman who saved her from taking walks with her mother. Even Glynese and Carramae were useful when they occupied attention that might otherwise have been directed at her. At first she had thought she could not stand Mrs. Freeman for she had found that it was not possible to be rude to her. Mrs. Freeman would take on strange resentments and for days together she would be sullen but the source of her displeasure was always obscure; a direct attack, a positive leer, blatant ugliness to her face—these never touched her. And without warning one day, she began calling her Hulga.

She did not call her that in front of Mrs. Hopewell who would have been incensed but when she and the girl happened to be out of the house together, she would say something and add the name Hulga to the end of it, and the big spectacled Joy-Hulga would scowl and redden as if her privacy had been intruded upon. She considered the name her personal affair. She had arrived at it first purely on the basis of its ugly sound and then the full genius of its fitness had struck her. She had a vision of the name working like the ugly sweating Vulcan who stayed in the furnace and to whom, presumably, the goddess had to come when called. She saw it as the name of her highest creative act. One of her major triumphs was that her mother had not been able to turn her dust into Joy, but the greater one was that she had been able to turn it herself into Hulga. However, Mrs. Freeman's relish for using the name only irritated her. It was as if Mrs. Freeman's beady steel-pointed eyes had penetrated far enough behind her face to reach some secret fact. Something about her seemed to fascinate Mrs. Freeman and then one day Hulga realized that it was the artificial leg. Mrs. Freeman had a special fondness for the details of secret infections, hidden deformities, assaults upon children. Of diseases, she preferred the lingering or incurable. Hulga had heard Mrs. Hopewell give her the details of the hunting accident, how the leg had been literally blasted off, how she had never lost consciousness. Mrs. Freeman could listen to it any time as if it had happened an hour ago.

When Hulga stumped into the kitchen in the morning (she could walk without making the awful noise but she made it—Mrs. Hopewell was certain—because it was ugly-sounding), she glanced at them and did not speak. Mrs. Hopewell would be in her red kimono with her hair tied around her head in rags. She would be sitting at the table, finishing her breakfast and Mrs. Freeman would be hanging by her elbow outward from the refrigerator, looking down at the table. Hulga always put her eggs on the stove to boil and then stood over them with her arms folded, and Mrs. Hopewell would look at her—a kind of indirect gaze divided between her and Mrs. Freeman— and would think that if she would only keep herself up a little, she wouldn't be so bad looking. There was nothing wrong with her face that a pleasant expression wouldn't help. Mrs. Hopewell said that people who looked on the bright side of things would be beautiful even if they were not.

Whenever she looked at Joy this way, she could not help but feel that it would have been better if the child had not taken the Ph.D. It had certainly not brought her out any and now that she had it, there was no more excuse for her to go to school again. Mrs. Hopewell thought it was nice for girls to go to school to have a good time but Joy had "gone through." Anyhow, she would not have been strong enough to go again. The doctors had told Mrs. Hopewell that with the best of care, Joy might see forty-five. She had a weak heart. Joy had made it plain that if it had not been for this condition, she would be far from these red hills and good country people. She would be in a university lecturing to people who knew what she was talking about. And Mrs. Hopewell could very well picture her there, looking like a scarecrow and lecturing to more of the same. Here she went about all day in a six-year-old skirt and a yellow sweat shirt with a faded cowboy on a horse embossed on it. She thought this was funny; Mrs. Hopewell thought it was idiotic and showed simply that she was still a child. She was brilliant but she didn't have a grain of sense. It seemed to Mrs. Hopewell that every year she grew less like other people and more like herself—bloated, rude, and squint-eyed. And she said such strange things! To her own mother she had said—without warning, without excuse, standing up in the middle of a meal with her face purple and her mouth half full—"Woman! do you ever look inside? Do you ever look inside and see what you are *not*? God!" she had cried sinking down again and staring at her plate, "Malebranche was right: we are not our own light. We are not our own light!" Mrs. Hopewell had no idea to this day what brought that on. She had only made the remark, hoping Joy would take it in, that a smile never hurt anyone.

The girl had taken the Ph.D. in philosophy and this left Mrs. Hopewell at a complete loss. You could say, "My daughter is a nurse," or "My daughter is a school teacher," or even, "My daughter is a chemical engineer." You could not say, "My daughter is a philosopher." That was something that had ended with the Greeks and Romans. All day Joy sat on her neck in a deep chair, reading. Sometimes she went for walks but she didn't like dogs or cats or birds or flowers or nature or nice young men. She looked at nice young men as if she could smell their stupidity.

One day Mrs. Hopewell had picked up one of the books the girl had just put down and opening it at random, she read, "Science, on the other hand, has to assert its soberness and seriousness afresh and declare that it is concerned solely with what-is. Nothing—how can it be for science anything but a horror and a phantasm? If science is right, then one thing stands firm: science wishes to know nothing of nothing. Such is after all the strictly scientific approach to Nothing. We know it by wishing to know nothing of Nothing." These words had been underlined with a blue pencil and they worked on Mrs. Hopewell like some evil incantation in gibberish. She shut the book quickly and went out of the room as if she were having a chill.

This morning when the girl came in, Mrs. Freeman was on Carramae. "She thrown up four times after supper," she said, "and was up twice in the night after three o'clock. Yesterday she didn't do nothing but ramble in the bureau drawer. All she did. Stand up there and see what she could run up on."

"She's got to eat," Mrs. Hopewell muttered, sipping her coffee, while she watched Joy's back at the stove. She was wondering what the child had said to the Bible salesman. She could not imagine what kind of a conversation she could possibly have had with him.

He was a tall gaunt hatless youth who had called yesterday to sell them a Bible. He had appeared at the door, carrying a large black suitcase that weighted him so heavily on one side that he had to brace himself against the door facing. He seemed on the point of collapse but he said in a cheerful voice, "Good morning, Mrs. Cedars!" and set the suitcase down on the mat. He was not a bad-looking young man though he had on a bright blue suit and yellow socks that were not pulled up far enough. He had prominent face bones and a streak of sticky-looking brown hair falling across his forehead.

"I'm Mrs. Hopewell," she said.

"Oh!" he said, pretending to look puzzled but with his eyes sparkling, "I saw it said 'The Cedars,' on the mailbox so I thought you was Mrs. Cedars!" and he burst out in a pleasant laugh. He picked up the satchel and under cover of a pant, he fell forward into her hall. It was rather as if the suitcase had moved first, jerking him after it. "Mrs. Hopewell!" he said and grabbed her hand. "I hope you are well!" and he laughed again and then all at once his face sobered completely. He paused and gave her a straight earnest look and said, "Lady, I've come to speak of serious things."

"Well, come in," she muttered, none too pleased because her dinner was almost ready. He came into the parlor and sat down on the edge of a straight chair and put the suitcase between his feet and glanced around the room as if he were sizing her up by it. Her silver gleamed on the two sideboards; she decided he had never been in a room as elegant as this.

"Mrs. Hopewell," he began, using her name in a way that sounded almost intimate, "I know you believe in Chrustian service."

"Well yes," she murmured.

"I know," he said and paused, looking very wise with his head cocked on one side, "that you're a good woman. Friends have told me."

Mrs. Hopewell never liked to be taken for a fool. "What are you selling?" she asked.

"Bibles," the young man said and his eye raced around the room before he added, "I see you have no family Bible in your parlor, I see that is the one lack you got!"

Mrs. Hopewell could not say, "My daughter is an atheist and won't let me keep the Bible in the parlor." She said, stiffening slightly, "I keep my Bible by my bedside." This was not the truth. It was in the attic somewhere.

"Lady," he said, "the word of God ought to be in the parlor."

"Well, I think that's a matter of taste," she began. "I think . . ."

"Lady," he said, "for a Chrustian, the word of God ought to be in every room in the house besides in his heart. I know you're a Chrustian because I can see it in every line of your face."

She stood up and said, "Well, young man, I don't want to buy a Bible and I smell my dinner burning."

He didn't get up. He began to twist his hands and looking down at them, he said softly, "Well lady, I'll tell you the truth—not many people want to buy one nowadays and besides, I know I'm real simple. I don't know how to say a thing but to say it. I'm just a country boy." He glanced up into her unfriendly face. "People like you don't like to fool with country people like me!"

"Why!" she cried, "good country people are the salt of the earth! Besides, we all have different ways of doing, it takes all kinds to make the world go 'round. That's life!"

"You said a mouthful," he said.

"Why, I think there aren't enough good country people in the world!" she said, stirred. "I think that's what's wrong with it!"

His face had brightened. "I didn't introduce myself," he said. "I'm Manley Pointer from out in the country around Willohobie, not even from a place, just from near a place."

"You wait a minute," she said. "I have to see about my dinner." She went out to the kitchen and found Joy standing near the door where she had been listening.

"Get rid of the salt of the earth," she said, "and let's eat."

Mrs. Hopewell gave her a pained look and turned the heat down under the vegetables. "*I* can't be rude to anybody," she murmured and went back into the parlor.

He had opened the suitcase and was sitting with a Bible on each knee.

"You might as well put those up," she told him. "I don't want one."

"I appreciate your honesty," he said. "You don't see any more real honest people unless you go way out in the country."

"I know," she said, "real genuine folks!" Through the crack in the door she heard a groan.

"I guess a lot of boys come telling you they're working their way through college," he said, "but I'm not going to tell you that. Somehow," he said, "I don't want to go to college. I want to devote my life to Chrustian service. See," he said, lowering his voice, "I got this heart condition. I may not live long. When you know it's something wrong with you and you may not live long, well then, lady . . ." He paused, with his mouth open, and stared at her.

He and Joy had the same condition! She knew that her eyes were filling with tears but she collected herself quickly and murmured, "Won't you stay for dinner? We'd love to have you!" and was sorry the instant she heard herself say it.

"Yes mam," he said in an abashed voice, "I would sher love to do that!"

Joy had given him one look on being introduced to him and then throughout the meal had not glanced at him again. He had addressed several remarks to her, which she had pretended not to hear. Mrs. Hopewell could not understand deliberate rudeness, although she lived with it, and she felt she had always to overflow with hospitality to make up for Joy's lack of courtesy. She urged him to talk about himself and he did. He said he was the seventh child of twelve and that his father had been crushed under a tree when he himself was eight year old. He had been crushed very badly, in fact, almost cut in two and was practically not recognizable. His mother had got along the best she could by hard working and she had always seen that her children went to Sunday School and that they read the Bible every evening. He was now nineteen year old and he had been selling Bibles for four months. In that time he had sold seventy-seven Bibles and had the promise of two more sales. He wanted to become a missionary because he thought that was the way you could do most for people. "He who losest his life shall find it," he said simply and he was so sincere, so genuine and earnest that Mrs. Hopewell would not for the world have smiled. He prevented his peas from sliding onto the table by blocking them with a piece of bread which he later cleaned his plate with. She could see Joy observing sidewise how he handled his knife and fork and she saw too that every few minutes, the boy would dart a keen appraising glance at the girl as if he were trying to attract her attention.

After dinner Joy cleared the dishes off the table and disappeared and Mrs. Hopewell was left to talk with him. He told her again about his childhood and his father's accident and about various things that had happened to him. Every five minutes or so she would stifle a yawn. He sat for two hours until finally she told him she must go because she had an appointment in town. He packed his Bibles and thanked her and prepared to leave, but in the doorway he stopped and wrung her hand and said that not on any of his trips had he met a lady as nice as her and he asked if he could come again. She had said she would always be happy to see him.

Joy had been standing in the road, apparently looking at something in the distance, when he came down the steps toward her, bent to the side with his heavy valise. He stopped where she was standing and confronted her directly. Mrs. Hopewell could not hear what he said but she trembled to think what Joy would say to him. She could see that after a minute Joy said something and that then the boy began to speak again, making an excited gesture with his free hand. After a minute Joy said something else at which the boy began to speak once more. Then to her amazement, Mrs. Hopewell saw the two of them walk off together, toward the gate. Joy had walked all the way to the gate with him and Mrs. Hopewell could not imagine what they had said to each other, and she had not yet dared to ask.

Mrs. Freeman was insisting upon her attention. She had moved from the refrigerator to the heater so that Mrs. Hopewell had to turn and face her in order to seem to be listening. "Glynese gone out with Harvey Hill again last night," she said. "She had this sty."

"Hill," Mrs. Hopewell said absently, "is that the one who works in the garage?"

"Nome, he's the one that goes to chiropractor school," Mrs. Freeman said. "She had this sty. Been had it two days. So she says when he brought her in the other night he says, 'Lemme get rid of that sty for you,' and she says, 'How?' and he says, 'You just lay yourself down acrost the seat of that car and I'll show you.' So she done it and he popped her neck. Kept on a-popping it several times until she made him quit. This morning," Mrs. Freeman said, "she ain't got no sty. She ain't got no traces of a sty."

"I never heard of that before," Mrs. Hopewell said.

"He ast her to marry him before the Ordinary," Mrs. Freeman went on, "and she told him she wasn't going to be married in no *office*."

"Well, Glynese is a fine girl," Mrs. Hopewell said. "Glynese and Carramae are both fine girls."

"Carramae said when her and Lyman was married Lyman said it sure felt sacred to him. She said he said he wouldn't take five hundred dollars for being married by a preacher."

"How much would he take?" the girl asked from the stove.

"He said he wouldn't take five hundred dollars," Mrs. Freeman repeated.

"Well we all have work to do," Mrs. Hopewell said.

"Lyman said it just felt more sacred to him," Mrs. Freeman said. "The doctor wants Carramae to eat prunes. Says instead of medicine. Says them cramps is coming from pressure. You know where I think it is?"

"She'll be better in a few weeks," Mrs. Hopewell said.

"In the tube," Mrs. Freeman said. "Else she wouldn't be as sick as she is."

Hulga had cracked her two eggs into a saucer and was bringing them to the table along with a cup of coffee that she had filled too full. She sat down carefully and began to eat, meaning to keep Mrs. Freeman there by questions if for any reason she showed an inclination to leave. She could perceive her mother's eye on her. The first round-about question would be about the Bible salesman and she did not wish to bring it on. "How did he pop her neck?" she asked.

Mrs. Freeman went into a description of how he had popped her neck. She said he owned a '55 Mercury but that Glynese said she would rather marry a man with only a '36 Plymouth who would be married by a preacher. The girl asked what if he had a '32 Plymouth and Mrs. Freeman said what Glynese had said was a '36 Plymouth.

Mrs. Hopewell said there were not many girls with Glynese's common sense. She said what she admired in those girls was their common sense. She said that reminded her that they had had a nice visitor yesterday, a young man selling Bibles. "Lord," she said, "he bored me to death but he was so sincere and genuine I couldn't be rude to him. He was just good country people, you know," she said, "—just the salt of the earth."

"I seen him walk up," Mrs. Freeman said, "and then later—I seen him walk off," and Hulga could feel the slight shift in her voice, the slight insinuation, that he had not walked off alone, had he? Her face remained expressionless but the color rose into her neck and she seemed to swallow it down with the next spoonful of egg. Mrs. Freeman was looking at her as if they had a secret together.

"Well, it takes all kinds of people to make the world go 'round," Mrs. Hopewell said. "It's very good we aren't all alike."

"Some people are more alike than others," Mrs. Freeman said.

Hulga got up and stumped, with about twice the noise that was necessary, into her room and locked the door. She was to meet the Bible salesman at ten o'clock at the gate. She had thought about it half the night. She had started thinking of it as a great joke and then she had begun to see profound implications in it. She had lain in bed imagining dialogues for them that were insane on the surface but that reached below to depths that no Bible salesman would be aware of. Their conversation yesterday had been of this kind.

He had stopped in front of her and had simply stood there. His face was bony and sweaty and bright, with a little pointed nose in the center of it, and his look was different from what it had been at the dinner table. He was gazing at her with open curiosity, with fascination, like a child watching a new fantastic animal at the zoo, and he was breathing as if he had run a great distance to reach her. His gaze seemed somehow familiar but she could not think where she had been regarded with it before. For almost a minute he didn't say anything. Then on what seemed an insuck of breath, he whispered, "You ever ate a chicken that was two days old?"

The girl looked at him stonily. He might have just put this question up for consideration at the meeting of a philosophical association. "Yes," she presently replied as if she had considered it from all angles.

"It must have been mighty small!" he said triumphantly and shook all over with little nervous giggles, getting very red in the face, and subsiding finally into his gaze of complete admiration, while the girl's expression remained exactly the same.

"How old are you?" he asked softly.

She waited some time before she answered. Then in a flat voice she said, "Seventeen."

His smiles came in succession like waves breaking on the surface of a little lake. "I see you got a wooden leg," he said. "I think you're real brave. I think you're real sweet."

The girl stood blank and solid and silent.

"Walk to the gate with me," he said. "You're a brave sweet little thing and I liked you the minute I seen you walk in the door."

Hulga began to move forward.

"What's your name?" he asked, smiling down on the top of her head.

"Hulga," she said.

"Hulga," he murmured, "Hulga. Hulga. I never heard of anybody name Hulga before. You're shy, aren't you, Hulga?" he asked.

She nodded, watching his large red hand on the handle of the giant valise.

"I like girls that wear glasses," he said. "I think a lot. I'm not like these people that a serious thought don't ever enter their heads. It's because I may die."

"I may die too," she said suddenly and looked up at him. His eyes were very small and brown, glittering feverishly.

"Listen," he said, "don't you think some people was meant to meet on account of what all they got in common and all? Like they both think serious thoughts and all?" He shifted the valise to his other hand so that the hand nearest her was free. He caught hold of her elbow and shook it a little. "I don't work on Saturday," he said. "I like to walk in the woods and see what Mother Nature is wearing. O'er the hills and far away. Pic-nics and things. Couldn't we go on a pic-nic tomorrow? Say yes, Hulga," he said and gave her a dying look as if he felt his insides about to drop out of him. He had even seemed to sway slightly toward her.

During the night she had imagined that she seduced him. She imagined that the two of them walked on the place until they came to the storage barn beyond the two back fields and there, she imagined, that things came to such a pass that she very easily seduced him and that then, of course, she had to reckon with his remorse. True genius can get an idea across even to an inferior mind. She imagined that she took his remorse in hand and changed it into a deeper understanding of life. She took all his shame away and turned it into something useful.

She set off for the gate at exactly ten o'clock, escaping without drawing Mrs. Hopewell's attention. She didn't take anything to eat, forgetting that food is usually taken on a picnic. She wore a pair of slacks and a dirty white shirt, and as an afterthought, she had put some Vapex on the collar of it since she did not own any perfume. When she reached the gate no one was there.

She looked up and down the empty highway and had the furious feeling that she had been tricked, that he had only meant to make her walk to the gate after the idea of him. Then suddenly he stood up, very tall, from behind a bush on the opposite embankment. Smiling, he lifted his hat which was new and wide-brimmed. He had not worn it yesterday and she wondered if he had bought it for the occasion. It was toast-colored with a red and white band around it and was slightly too large for him. He stepped from behind the bush still carrying the black valise. He had on the same suit and the same yellow socks sucked down in his shoes from walking. He crossed the highway and said, "I knew you'd come!"

The girl wondered acidly how he had known this. She pointed to the valise and asked, "Why did you bring your Bibles?"

He took her elbow, smiling down on her as if he could not stop. "You can never tell when you'll need the word of God, Hulga," he said. She had a moment in which she doubted that this was actually happening and then they began to climb the embankment. They went down into the pasture toward the woods. The boy walked lightly by her side, bouncing on his toes. The valise did not seem to be heavy today; he even swung it. They crossed half the pasture without saying anything and then, putting his hand easily on the small of her back, he asked softly, "Where does your wooden leg join on?"

She turned an ugly red and glared at him and for an instant the boy looked abashed. "I didn't mean you no harm," he said. "I only meant you're so brave and all. I guess God takes care of you."

"No," she said, looking forward and walking fast, "I don't even believe in God."

At this he stopped and whistled. "No!" he exclaimed as if he were too astonished to say anything else.

She walked on and in a second he was bouncing at her side, fanning with his hat. "That's very unusual for a girl," he remarked, watching her out of the corner of his eye. When they reached the edge of the wood, he put his hand on her back again and drew her against him without a word and kissed her heavily.

The kiss, which had more pressure than feeling behind it, produced that extra surge of adrenalin in the girl that enables one to carry a packed trunk out of a burning house, but in her, the power went at once to the brain. Even before he released her, her mind, clear and detached and ironic anyway, was regarding him from a great distance, with amusement but with pity. She had never been kissed before and she was pleased to discover that it was an unexceptional experience and all a matter of the mind's control. Some people might enjoy drain water if they were told it was vodka. When the boy, looking expectant but uncertain, pushed her gently away, she turned and walked on, saying nothing as if such business, for her, were common enough.

He came along panting at her side, trying to help her when he saw a root that she might trip over. He caught and held back the long swaying blades of thorn vine until she had passed beyond them. She led the way and he came breathing heavily behind her. Then they came out on a sunlit hillside, sloping softly into another one a little smaller. Beyond, they could see the rusted top of the old barn where the extra hay was stored.

The hill was sprinkled with small pink weeds. "Then you ain't saved?" he asked suddenly, stopping.

The girl smiled. It was the first time she had smiled at him at all. "In my economy," she said, "I'm saved and you are damned but I told you I didn't believe in God."

Nothing seemed to destroy the boy's look of admiration. He gazed at her now as if the fantastic animal at the zoo had put its paw through the bars and given him a loving poke. She thought he looked as if he wanted to kiss her again and she walked on before he had the chance.

"Ain't there somewheres we can sit down sometime?" he murmured, his voice softening toward the end of the sentence.

"In that barn," she said.

They made for it rapidly as if it might slide away like a train. It was a large two-story barn, cool and dark inside. The boy pointed up the ladder that led into the loft and said, "It's too bad we can't go up there."

"Why can't we?" she asked.

"Yer leg," he said reverently.

The girl gave him a contemptuous look and putting both hands on the ladder, she climbed it while he stood below, apparently awestruck. She pulled herself expertly through the opening and then looked down at him and said,

"Well, come on if you're coming," and he began to climb the ladder, awkwardly bringing the suitcase with him.

"We won't need the Bible," she observed.

"You never can tell," he said, panting. After he had got into the loft, he was a few seconds catching his breath. She had sat down in a pile of straw. A wide sheath of sunlight, filled with dust particles, slanted over her. She lay back against a bale, her face turned away, looking out the front opening of the barn where hay was thrown from a wagon into the loft. The two pink-speckled hillsides lay back against a dark ridge of woods. The sky was cloudless and cold blue. The boy dropped down by her side and put one arm under her and the other over her and began methodically kissing her face, making little noises like a fish. He did not remove his hat but it was pushed far enough back not to interfere. When her glasses got in his way, he took them off of her and slipped them into his pocket.

The girl at first did not return any of the kisses but presently she began to and after she had put several on his cheek, she reached his lips and remained there, kissing him again and again as if she were trying to draw all the breath out of him. His breath was clear and sweet like a child's and the kisses were sticky like a child's. He mumbled about loving her and about knowing when he first seen her that he loved her, but the mumbling was like the sleepy fretting of a child being put to sleep by his mother. Her mind, throughout this, never stopped or lost itself for a second to her feelings. "You ain't said you loved me none," he whispered finally, pulling back from her. "You got to say that."

She looked away from him off into the hollow sky and then down at a black ridge and then down farther into what appeared to be two green swelling lakes. She didn't realize he had taken her glasses but this landscape could not seem exceptional to her for she seldom paid any close attention to her surroundings.

"You got to say it," he repeated. "You got to say you love me."

She was always careful how she committed herself. "In a sense," she began, "if you use the word loosely, you might say that. But it's not a word I use. I don't have illusions. I'm one of those people who see *through* to nothing."

The boy was frowning. "You got to say it. I said it and you got to say it," he said.

The girl looked at him almost tenderly. "You poor baby," she murmured. "It's just as well you don't understand," and she pulled him by the neck, facedown, against her. "We are all damned," she said, "but some of us have taken off our blindfolds and see that there's nothing to see. It's a kind of salvation."

The boy's astonished eyes looked blankly through the ends of her hair. "Okay," he almost whined, "but do you love me or don'tcher?"

"Yes," she said and added, "in a sense. But I must tell you something. There mustn't be anything dishonest between us." She lifted his head and looked him in the eye. "I am thirty years old," she said. "I have a number of degrees."

The boy's look was irritated but dogged. "I don't care," he said. "I don't care a thing about what all you done. I just want to know if you love me or don'tcher?" and he caught her to him and wildly planted her face with kisses until she said, "Yes, yes."

"Okay then," he said, letting her go. "Prove it."

She smiled, looking dreamily out on the shifty landscape. She had seduced him without even making up her mind to try. "How?" she asked, feeling that he should be delayed a little.

He leaned over and put his lips to her ear. "Show me where your wooden leg joins on," he whispered.

The girl uttered a sharp little cry and her face instantly drained of color. The obscenity of the suggestion was not what shocked her. As a child she had sometimes been subject to feelings of shame but education had removed the last traces of that as a good surgeon scrapes for cancer; she would no more have felt it over what he was asking than she would have believed in his Bible. But she was as sensitive about the artificial leg as a peacock about his tail. No one ever touched it but her. She took care of it as someone else would his soul, in private and almost with her own eyes turned away. "No," she said.

"I known it," he muttered, sitting up. "You're just playing me for a sucker."

"Oh no no!" she cried. "It joins on at the knee. Only at the knee. Why do you want to see it?"

The boy gave her a long penetrating look. "Because," he said, "it's what makes you different. You ain't like anybody else."

She sat staring at him. There was nothing about her face or her round freezing blue eyes to indicate that this had moved her; but she felt as if her heart had stopped and left her mind to pump her blood. She decided that for the first time in her life she was face to face with real innocence. This boy, with an instinct that came from beyond wisdom, had touched the truth about her. When after a minute, she said in a hoarse high voice, "All right," it was like surrendering to him completely. It was like losing her own life and finding it again, miraculously, in his.

Very gently he began to roll the slack leg up. The artificial limb, in a white sock and brown flat shoe, was bound in a heavy material like canvas and ended in an ugly jointure where it was attached to the stump. The boy's face and his voice were entirely reverent as he uncovered it and said, "Now show me how to take it off and on."

She took it off for him and put it back on again and then he took it off himself, handling it as tenderly as if it were a real one. "See!" he said with a delighted child's face. "Now I can do it myself!"

"Put it back on," she said. She was thinking that she would run away with him and that every night he would take the leg off and every morning put it back on again. "Put it back on," she said.

"Not yet," he murmured, setting it on its foot out of her reach. "Leave it off for a while. You got me instead."

She gave a little cry of alarm but he pushed her down and began to kiss her again. Without the leg she felt entirely dependent on him. Her brain seemed to have stopped thinking altogether and to be about some other function that it was not very good at. Different expressions raced back and forth over her face. Every now and then the boy, his eyes like two steel spikes, would glance behind him where the leg stood. Finally she pushed him off and said, "Put it back on me now."

"Wait," he said. He leaned the other way and pulled the valise toward him and opened it. It had a pale blue spotted lining and there were only two Bibles in it. He took one of these out and opened the cover of it. It was hollow and contained a pocket flask of whiskey, a pack of cards, and a small blue box with printing on it. He laid these out in front of her one at a time in an evenly-spaced row, like one presenting offerings at the shrine of a goddess. He put the blue box in her hand. THIS PRODUCT TO BE USED ONLY FOR THE PREVENTION OF DISEASE, she read, and dropped it. The boy was unscrewing the top of the flask. He stopped and pointed, with a smile, to the deck of cards. It was not an ordinary deck but one with an obscene picture on the back of each card. "Take a swig," he said, offering her the bottle first. He held it in front of her, but like one mesmerized, she did not move.

Her voice when she spoke had an almost pleading sound. "Aren't you," she murmured, "aren't you just good country people?"

The boy cocked his head. He looked as if he were just beginning to understand that she might be trying to insult him. "Yeah," he said, curling his lip slightly, "but it ain't held me back none. I'm as good as you any day in the week."

"Give me my leg," she said.

He pushed it farther away with his foot. "Come on now, let's begin to have us a good time," he said coaxingly. "We ain't got to know one another good yet."

"Give me my leg!" she screamed and tried to lunge for it but he pushed her down easily.

"What's the matter with you all of a sudden?" he asked, frowning as he screwed the top on the flask and put it quickly back inside the Bible. "You just a while ago said you didn't believe in nothing. I thought you was some girl!"

Her face was almost purple. "You're a Christian!" she hissed. "You're a fine Christian! You're just like them all—say one thing and do another. You're a perfect Christian, you're . . ."

The boy's mouth was set angrily. "I hope you don't think," he said in a lofty indignant tone, "that I believe in that crap! I may sell Bibles but I know which end is up and I wasn't born yesterday and I know where I'm going!"

"Give me my leg!" she screeched. He jumped up so quickly that she barely saw him sweep the cards and the blue box back into the Bible and throw the Bible into the valise. She saw him grab the leg and then she saw it for an instant slanted forlornly across the inside of the suitcase with a Bible at either side of its opposite ends. He slammed the lid shut and snatched up the valise and swung it down the hole and then stepped through himself.

When all of him had passed but his head, he turned and regarded her with a look that no longer had any admiration in it. "I've gotten a lot of interesting things," he said. "One time I got a woman's glass eye this way. And you needn't to think you'll catch me because Pointer ain't really my name. I use a different name at every house I call at and don't stay nowhere long. And I'll tell you another thing, Hulga," he said, using the name as if he didn't think much of it, "you ain't so smart. I been believing in nothing ever since I was born!" and then the toast-colored hat disappeared down the hole and the girl was left, sitting on the straw in the dusty sunlight. When she turned her churning face toward the opening, she saw his blue figure struggling successfully over the green speckled lake.

Mrs. Hopewell and Mrs. Freeman, who were in the back pasture, digging up onions, saw him emerge a little later from the woods and head across the meadow toward the highway. "Why, that looks like that nice dull young man that tried to sell me a Bible yesterday," Mrs. Hopewell said, squinting. "He must have been selling them to the Negroes back in there. He was so simple," she said, "but I guess the world would be better off if we were all that simple."

Mrs. Freeman's gaze drove forward and just touched him before he disappeared under the hill. Then she returned her attention to the evil-smelling onion shoot she was lifting from the ground. "Some can't be that simple," she said. "I know I never could."

To: The Access Committee

H. N. BECKERMAN

To:
  The Access Committee
Attention:
  Handicapped Romeo.
    There is now a suitable ramp
  installed at my balcony.
    Impatiently,
    Miss Juliet

Just Another Year in Chronic IA

DALLAS DENNY

WE'RE ON THE big damned yellow and black school bus, on our way to a "picnic," which means that we will stop at a roadside park with three trees and two concrete picnic tables and eat extra crispy recipe Kentucky Fried Chicken, bones and all, and maybe even the plastic sporks, the hungrier of us. Then we will be put back on the bus and ride back to the hospital, where we will disembark and be rolled back to the musty, dusty, and always gloomy buildings, back to the chronic wards. The hydraulic wheelchair lift of the bus is broken, which means that the technicians have to load and unload us through the fire door at the back of the bus, sweating and cursing, and occasionally letting one of us bang on the asphalt, warping our rubber-rimmed wheels.

Once, on such an outing, I was unloaded first, and rolled away down a hill as the technicians struggled with Mordred Holmes, who was fighting to stay on the bus. They didn't notice as my wheelchair gathered momentum, passing surprised picnickers and campers, whizzing past tents and oak trees until the wheels hit a root and the wheelchair stopped. I didn't stop. I was thrown forward and plowed into a yellow-and-green umbrella tent, collapsing it and scaring hell out of the young couple inside. I got a nasty cut out of that one, just over my eye, from a tentpeg. I remember staring at the sun through the treetops, feeling bodies under me, under the canvas, wriggling into clothes, and then a circle of people around me, staring, questioning, until two of the white-suited technicians came running down the hill, and then everybody understood, and looked away, or looked at me in that pitying way, and the young couple whose tent I had wrecked looked at each other and then down at the ground.

I have a bruise on that same eye today, because the techs sat me beside Jack Oliver, whom I dislike. When they wheeled me up beside Oliver, he said,

"Why did you go and put him there for? You know he's going to spit on me and then I'll pop him one." The technicians just shrugged and left, and I spit at Oliver, and he plugged me one, and then there was a fight as the technicians wrestled him to the floor in the aisle of the bus and gave him an injection of Valium in his buttocks. Now Oliver is just sitting there, enjoying the high from the drug.

O'Rourke is driving the bus today, his whites yellowed to the exact shade of his teeth. O'Rourke has figured out exactly how much gasoline his car uses, and measures it by the drop. He tells Stoner, who usually works with him, that it takes him exactly three-eighths of a gallon to get to work from his house, and seven-sixteenths of a gallon to get home, because there are more hills on the way home than there are on the way to work. At break time every evening, O'Rourke goes down to his car, a 1968 Oldsmobile, and pours in gasoline from milk jugs he keeps in the trunk. I try to look out the window every afternoon about 3 PM, when O'Rourke comes in. He never varies by more than one minute, and usually his car is choking and gasping, running out of gas, as he pulls into the parking lot. It's fun to watch him run out, which he does on occasion, a couple of hundred yards short of the parking lot. It ruins his whole day.

O'Rourke drives the bus like he drives his car, as if there were an egg between his foot and the gas pedal. He accelerates very slowly, but if a car in front of him happens to be moving too slowly to suit him, he becomes absolutely apoplectic. Stoner tells me in confidence that O'Rourke is crazy. But Stoner is crazy, too. For one thing, he is insanely jealous of his wife. He spends his suppertime parked in his car, across campus at the building where she works, peering at her through cheap binoculars. Stoner is the kind of guy who has everything, but none of it is very good. You know what I mean. Formica dining set, imitation crushed velvet sofa and chair, velvet painting of Christ on the wall of the living room, K-Mart stereo, a console color television set that spends about six months a year in the shop, an eight-year-old Buick with a broken air conditioner. That kind of stuff. Every month he gets a "great classic" book in the mail and carries it about on the ward for two or three days, showing off the imitation leather binding, but of course not reading it. Stoner has not read some of the best—Tolstoy, Joyce, Melville, Conrad, Dickens. What he does read are magazines from the top racks of mini-marts. I never liked pornography myself. But Stoner is always waving a picture of some nude in front of my face, knowing I can do little about it. He shows the stuff to Margaret, who he has figured is a lesbian, and to Stelson, who has Gilles de la Tourette Syndrome, and who curses uncontrollably when he sees the pictures.

Stelson's disease has not been diagnosed (except by me, and I do not count). He has a neurological condition which causes his facial tics, his barks, his cursing. The psychiatrists think he is crazy. He sees the shrink every week for an hour of taxpayers' time, so the good doctor can find out what repressed childhood event causes his continual cursing. Stelson has been seeing the shrink for about four years now.

I have spastic quadriplegia (severe). That's what I read in my chart. Doritos (like the tortilla chips) showed it to me. It is caused by spinal cord and brain damage I got when I wiped my car out on the night of my senior prom. I've been here, in the hospital, on the chronic wards, ever since the insurance money ran out. I can't care for myself, except for feeding myself with a special spoon on my better days. I can't even turn the pages of books or magazines without tearing them, due to the tremors. Most of the staff figure that my brain was fried in the wreck, but Doritos and Johnny Walker knew better. They used to call me Spaz, and the name has stuck (unofficially, of course). Spaz. Spaz-I-Am. Do you like green eggs and ham? Do you like them, Spaz-I-Am?

Doritos and Johnny Walker were a welcome change from the dour-faced, middle-aged, middle-class pinheads like O'Rourke and Stoner who usually work the ward. Doritos and Walker used to let me sit in the nursing station while they dug drugs out of the medicine cabinet and looked them up in the PDR and maybe took a couple. They would eat Quaaludes like candy, long before anyone else figured out that they had potential for being abused. They would get twisted and bent, looking progressively more like the patients on Chronic III A as the night wore on. Doritos would bring me books like *Fear and Loathing in Las Vegas* and *One Flew Over the Cuckoo's Nest,* tearing the pages out and handing them to me one at a time, or reading aloud his favorite parts. "As your attorney," he would screech to Johnny Walker, "I advise you to take six Phenergan." I wanted to yell, "Get out! Get out while you still can! Just look what the bastards have done to me!" But of course, I couldn't. And now Doritos is doing five-to-ten in the slammer, and Johnny Walker is in a pharmacy program at Duke. I saw Doritos on the 6:00 news the day he was busted. Seems he went into the bathroom of an Exxon station, he and a buddy, and the attendant, who noticed them lurching around the lot, went into the john and dug their works out of the trash can and called the cops, who picked them up with a pocketful of ampules stolen from the hospital.

When Stoner and O'Rourke and Kelly work, they sit around with their keys on little chains on their belts and tell bad jokes and say disparaging things about various minorities. They never do any work. One day, while Doritos and Johnny Walker were still around, old Jim Peach hobbled up to the nursing station and in his backroom voice asked for a cigarette. Kelly gave him a ready-rolled, but Peach just looked at it with his lip curled up in a kind of half-sneer and said, as he put the cigarette in his pocket, "No, I want one like those long-haired boys gave me." Kelly didn't catch it, just like he didn't understand why Frank Lee, the screamer, kept talking about "the lights" the day Johnny Walker fed him some mescaline.

Doritos and Walker were replaced by two young guys. One, J. Michaels (that's what his nametag says), is OK, but the other is being broken in "right" by the old men, and is already learning to turn a cold and calloused eye on everything that happens on the ward.

I can see Stoner flirting with the clerk at the KFC as she stacks red-and-white boxes three feet deep on the counter. If I were her, I would just keep on piling up boxes until I had built a red-and-white wall between me and Stoner and this busload of freaks! I can picture her frantically slapping box on top of box, using the Colonel's mashed potatoes for mortar, spreading it with deft strokes with the plastic top of a cole slaw cup, or maybe with a spork. What would the archaeologists make of that wall when they unearthed it in 5000 years? Would they see us as a culture of chicken worshippers, entombing the bones of our revered sacred fowl after a sacramental dip in holy hot oils, in caskets emblazoned with the smiling face of our benevolent white-haired leader? Perhaps . . .

I am shaken from my musings by a lurch of the bus as O'Rourke leaves the parking lot. He has slammed on the brakes to miss a Corvette. My wheelchair, which is not fastened securely, tips me into Jack Oliver's lap. Jack, despite the Valium, is only too happy to pound the side of my face with his meaty fists. Stoner can't see me because of the pile of chicken boxes, and O'Rourke is too busy cursing the driver of the Corvette and worrying about wasted gas to bother looking in the rear-view mirror. Nobody else is going to stop Jack; that's for sure. The other patients are all too spaced out to care. It looks like it's going to be a long trip.

Letter from the Rehabilitation Institute

LUCIA CORDELL GETSI

Mostly bandaged, Joe looks like the Elephant Man
or the Creature from the Black Lagoon, in white.
Without blinking, he says he wished he'd died
in the fire his twelve year strength failed
to pull his mother from. He still smells her flesh,
like a cinder in his nose, or what is left
of nose. *It's too hard,* he says, *alone, and like this.*

LaToya is quiet in her bed or rolling cart,
seems to be observant. Her small body, amoeba-like,
responds to voice probes: *Sit up, LaToya, raise
your arm.* No one can tell if she understands
her mother was killed by the train that smacked
the speech out of her mouth. One drooped eye
tracks my arms that pivot Manon* to the chair.

Danny tried to beat the express lane traffic
on foot. He wears seamed legs and crushed hips,
a patchwork body pieced by surgeons who speak of him
as a masterwork. He pops wheelies in his motorized
chair, bothers the girls as though he'll have one.
When he goes home, Frankenstein with cane, his mother
clicks her high heels quickly away, as far ahead
of him as she can get. He jerks along behind.

"G." got shot in the back like the other Black
and Chicago boys here, wears his colon in a pouch.
He walks. The only one who can. These boys call
each other Mutha, slap hands in greeting, manage

a tired strut in their wheelchairs. In art therapy
G. paints a light like a jack-o'-lantern grinning
in a shadow, a richochet of motherlessness
that writhes like an orange ghost trapped in paper.

Arnold "fell" from three storeys, lay on concrete
one whole morning. His mother never visits.
Little cuddler, the nurses vie to tuck him
in. Earphones on his ears, he snaps his fingers and
jives, baby hips rocking to music that sings
him finally to sleep. At 3 A.M. he howls
and whimpers like a puppy lost from the litter.

Jimmy dived and struck the bottom he thought was
deeper. He'll never pull water over his head
again, or a blanket when he's cold, or feel
below his broken neck. Bone thin, his body
is flat, enormous eyes grab like hands.
His trache gurgles when he whispers he is scared.

I could tell about Lily, the university student
who woke in a tremor of electric shock up one side
of her body and down the other. After months
of paralysis she can sit well enough to withstand
the long flight home to Japan, strapped
in her seat. Or Aileen, the six-year-old
ballerina who struggles to speak again
after her fourth stroke.

In this place of broken children
I don't know who *you* are—*you* are different
in the way I was different before
I arrived and thought I would be the same,
in the way Manon tries to find an adolescence, falling
in love with a snazzy wheelchair, a funny
story, someone else's need. No,
there is nothing to be done about difference.
It leaves a mark.

*Manon is the poet's daughter

The Birthmark

NATHANIEL HAWTHORNE

IN THE LATTER part of the last century there lived a man of science, an eminent proficient in every branch of natural philosophy, who not long before our story opens had made experience of a spiritual affinity more attractive than any chemical one. He had left his laboratory to the care of an assistant, cleared his fine countenance from the furnace smoke, washed the stain of acids from his fingers, and persuaded a beautiful woman to become his wife. In those days when the comparatively recent discovery of electricity and other kindred mysteries of Nature seemed to open paths into the region of miracle, it was not unusual for the love of science to rival the love of woman in its depth and absorbing energy. The higher intellect, the imagination, the spirit, and even the heart might all find their congenial ailment in pursuits which, as some of their ardent votaries believed, would ascend from one step of powerful intelligence to another, until the philosopher should lay his hand on the secret of creative force and perhaps make new worlds for himself. We know not whether Aylmer possessed this degree of faith in man's ultimate control over Nature. He had devoted himself, however, too unreservedly to scientific studies ever to be weaned from them by any second passion. His love for his young wife might prove the stronger of the two; but it could only be by intertwining itself with his love of science and uniting the strength of the latter to his own.

Such a union accordingly took place, and was attended with truly remarkable consequences and a deeply impressive moral. One day, very soon after their marriage, Aylmer sat gazing at his wife with a trouble in his countenance that grew stronger until he spoke.

"Georgiana," said he, "has it never occurred to you that the mark upon your cheek might be removed?"

"No, indeed," said she, smiling; but perceiving the seriousness of his manner, she blushed deeply. "To tell you the truth it has been so often called a charm that I was simple enough to imagine it might be so."

"Ah, upon another face perhaps it might," replied her husband; "but never on yours. No, dearest Georgiana, you came so nearly perfect from the hand of Nature that this slightest possible defect, which we hesitate whether to term a defect or a beauty, shocks me, as being the visible mark of earthly imperfection."

"Shocks you, my husband!" cried Georgiana, deeply hurt, at first reddening with momentary anger, but then bursting into tears. "Then why did you take me from my mother's side? You cannot love what shocks you!"

To explain this conversation it must be mentioned that in the center of Georgiana's left cheek there was a singular mark, deeply interwoven, as it were, with the texture and substance of her face. In the usual state of her complexion—a healthy though delicate bloom—the mark wore a tint of deeper crimson, which imperfectly defined its shape amid the surrounding rosiness. When she blushed it gradually became more indistinct, and finally vanished amid the triumphant rush of blood that bathed the whole cheek with its brilliant glow. But if any shifting emotion caused her to turn pale there was the mark again, a crimson stain upon the snow, in what Aylmer sometimes deemed an almost fearful distinctness. Its shape bore not a little similarity to the human hand, though of the smallest pygmy size. Georgiana's lovers were wont to say that some fairy at her birth hour had laid her tiny hand upon the infant's cheek, and left this impress there in token of the magic endowments that were to give her such sway over all hearts. Many a desperate swain would have risked life for the privilege of pressing his lips to the mysterious hand. It must not be concealed, however, that the impression wrought by this fairy sign-manual varied exceedingly according to the difference of temperament in the beholders. Some fastidious persons—but they were exclusively of her own sex—affirmed that the bloody hand, as they chose to call it, quite destroyed the effect of Georgiana's beauty, and rendered her countenance even hideous. But it would be as reasonable to say that one of those small blue stains which sometimes occur in the purest statuary marble would convert the Eve of Powers to a monster. Masculine observers, if the birthmark did not heighten their admiration, contented themselves with wishing it away, that the world might possess one living specimen of ideal loveliness without the semblance of a flaw.

After his marriage—for he thought little or nothing of the matter before— Aylmer discovered that this was the case with himself. Had she been less beautiful—if Envy's self could have found aught else to sneer at—he might have felt his affection heightened by the prettiness of this mimic hand, now vaguely portrayed, now lost, now stealing forth again and glimmering to and fro with every pulse of emotion that throbbed within her heart; but seeing her otherwise so perfect, he found this one defect grow more and more intolerable with every moment of their united lives. It was the fatal flaw of humanity which Nature, in one shape or another, stamps ineffaceably on all her productions, either to imply that they are temporary and finite, or that their perfection must be wrought by toil and pain. The crimson hand expressed the ineludible grip in which mortality clutches the highest and purest of earthly mold, degrading them into kindred with the lowest, and even with the very brutes, like whom their visible frames return to dust. In this manner, selecting it as the symbol of his wife's liability to sin, sorrow, decay, and death, Aylmer's sombre imagination was not long in rendering the birthmark a frightful object, causing him more trouble and horror than ever Georgiana's beauty, whether of soul or sense, had given him delight.

At all the seasons which should have been their happiest, he invariably and without intending it—nay, in spite of a purpose to the contrary—reverted to this one disastrous topic. Trifling as it at first appeared, it so connected itself with innumerable trains of thought and modes of feeling that it became the central point of all. With the morning twilight Aylmer opened his eyes upon his wife's face and recognized the symbol of imperfection; and when they sat together at the evening hearth his eyes wandered stealthily to her cheek, and beheld, flickering with the blaze of the wood fire, the spectral hand that wrote mortality where he would fain have worshipped. Georgiana soon learned to shudder at his gaze. It needed but a glance with the peculiar expression that his face often wore to change the roses of her cheek into a deathlike paleness, amid which the crimson hand was brought strongly out, like a bas-relief of ruby on the whitest marble.

Late one night when the lights were growing dim, so as hardly to betray the stain on the poor wife's cheek, she herself, for the first time, voluntarily took up the subject.

"Do you remember, my dear Aylmer," said she, with a feeble attempt at a smile, "have you any recollection of a dream last night about this odious hand?"

"None! none whatever!" replied Aylmer, starting; but then he added, in a dry, cold tone, affected for the sake of concealing the real depth of his emotion, "I might well dream of it; for before I fell asleep it had taken a pretty firm hold of my fancy."

"And you did dream of it?" continued Georgiana, hastily; for she dreaded lest a gush of tears should interrupt what she had to say. "A terrible dream! I

wonder that you can forget it. Is it possible to forget this one expression?—
'It is in her heart now; we must have it out!' Reflect, my husband; for by all
means I would have you recall that dream."

The mind is in a sad state when Sleep, the all-involving, cannot confine
her specters within the dim region of her sway, but suffers them to break
forth, affrighting this actual life with secrets that perchance belong to a deeper
one. Aylmer now remembered his dream. He had fancied himself with his
servant Aminadab, attempting an operation for the removal of the birthmark. But the deeper went the knife, the deeper sank the hand, until at length
its tiny grasp appeared to have caught hold of Georgiana's heart, whence,
however, her husband was inexorably resolved to cut or wrench it away.

When the dream had shaped itself perfectly in his memory, Aylmer sat in
his wife's presence with a guilty feeling. Truth often finds its way to the mind
close muffled in robes of sleep, and then speaks with uncompromising di-
rectness of matters in regard to which we practise an unconscious self-
deception during our waking moments. Until now he had not been aware of
the tyrannizing influence acquired by one idea over his mind, and of the
lengths which he might find in his heart to go for the sake of giving himself
peace.

"Aylmer," resumed Georgiana, solemnly, "I know not what may be the
cost to both of us to rid me of this fatal birthmark. Perhaps its removal may
cause cureless deformity; or it may be the stain goes as deep as life itself.
Again: do we know that there is a possibility, on any terms, of unclasping the
firm grip of this little hand which was laid upon me before I came into the
world?"

"Dearest Georgiana, I have spent much thought upon the subject," hastily
interrupted Aylmer. "I am convinced of the perfect practicability of its removal."

"If there be the remotest possibility of it," continued Georgiana, "let the
attempt be made at whatever risk. Danger is nothing to me, for life, while this
hateful mark makes me the object of your horror and disgust—life is a burden which I would fling down with joy. Either remove this dreadful hand, or
take my wretched life! You have deep science. All the world bears witness of it.
You have achieved great wonders. Cannot you remove this little, little mark,
which I cover with the tips of two small fingers? Is this beyond your power,
for the sake of your own peace, and to save your poor wife from madness?"

"Noblest, dearest, tenderest wife," cried Aylmer, rapturously, "doubt not
my power. I have already given this matter the deepest thought—thought

which might almost have enlightened me to create a being less perfect than yourself. Georgiana, you have led me deeper than ever into the heart of science. I feel myself fully competent to render this dear cheek as faultless as its fellow; and then, most beloved, what will be my triumph when I shall have corrected what Nature left imperfect in her fairest work! Even Pygmalion, when his sculptured woman assumed life, felt not greater ecstasy than mine will be."

"It is resolved, then," said Georgiana, faintly smiling. "And, Aylmer, spare me not, though you should find the birthmark take refuge in my heart at last."

Her husband tenderly kissed her cheek—her right cheek—not that which bore the impress of the crimson hand.

The next day Aylmer apprised his wife of a plan that he had formed whereby he might have opportunity for the intense thought and constant watchfulness which the proposed operation would require; while Georgiana, likewise, would enjoy the perfect repose essential to its success. They were to seclude themselves in the extensive apartments occupied by Aylmer as a laboratory, and where, during his toilsome youth, he had made discoveries in the elemental powers of Nature that had roused the admiration of all the learned societies in Europe. Seated calmly in this laboratory, the pale philosopher had investigated the secrets of the highest cloud region and of the profoundest mines; he had satisfied himself of the causes that kindled and kept alive the fires of the volcano; and had explained the mystery of fountains, and how it is that they gush forth, some so bright and pure, and others with such rich medicinal virtues, from the dark bosom of the earth. Here, too, at an earlier period, he had studied the wonders of the human frame, and attempted to fathom the very process by which Nature assimilates all her precious influences from earth and air, and from the spiritual world, to create and foster man, her masterpiece. The latter pursuit, however, Aylmer had long laid aside in unwilling recognition of the truth—against which all seekers sooner or later stumble—that our great creative Mother, while she amuses us with apparently working in the broadest sunshine, is yet severely careful to keep her own secrets, and, in spite of her pretended openness, shows us nothing but results. She permits us, indeed, to mar, but seldom to mend, and, like a jealous patentee, on no account to make. Now, however, Aylmer resumed these half-forgotten investigations; not, of course, with such hopes or wishes as first suggested them; but because they involved much physiological truth and lay in the path of his proposed scheme for the treatment of Georgiana.

As he led her over the threshold of the laboratory, Georgiana was cold and tremulous. Aylmer looked cheerfully into her face, with intent to reassure her, but was so startled with the intense glow of the birthmark upon the whiteness of her cheek that he could not restrain a strong convulsive shudder. His wife fainted.

"Aminadab! Aminadab!" shouted Aylmer, stamping violently on the floor.

Forthwith there issued from an inner apartment a man of low stature, but bulky frame, with shaggy hair hanging about his visage, which was grimed with the vapors of the furnace. This personage had been Aylmer's underworker during his whole scientific career, and was admirably fitted for that office by his great mechanical readiness, and the skill with which, while incapable of comprehending a single principle, he executed all the details of his master's experiments. With his vast strength, his shaggy hair, his smoky aspect, and the indescribable earthiness that incrusted him, he seemed to represent man's physical nature; while Aylmer's slender figure, and pale, intellectual face, were no less apt a type of the spiritual element.

"Throw open the door of the boudoir, Aminadab," said Aylmer, "and burn a pastil."

"Yes, master," answered Aminadab, looking intently at the lifeless form of Georgiana; and then he muttered to himself, "If she were my wife, I'd never part with that birthmark."

When Georgiana recovered consciousness she found herself breathing an atmosphere of penetrating fragrance, the gentle potency of which had recalled her from her deathlike faintness. The scene around her looked like enchantment. Aylmer had converted those smoky, dingy, sombre rooms, where he had spent his brightest years in recondite pursuits, into a series of beautiful apartments not unfit to be the secluded abode of a lovely woman. The walls were hung with gorgeous curtains, which imparted the combination of grandeur and grace that no other species of adornment can achieve; and as they fell from the ceiling to the floor, their rich and ponderous folds, concealing all angles and straight lines, appeared to shut in the scene from infinite space. For aught Georgiana knew, it might be a pavilion among the clouds. And Aylmer, excluding the sunshine, which would have interfered with his chemical processes, had supplied its place with perfumed lamps, emitting flames of various hue, but all uniting in a soft, impurpled radiance. He now knelt by his wife's side, watching her earnestly, but without alarm; for he was confident in his science, and felt that he could draw a magic circle round her within which no evil might intrude.

"Where am I? Ah, I remember," said Georgiana, faintly; and she placed her hand over her cheek to hide the terrible mark from her husband's eyes.

"Fear not, dearest!" exclaimed he. "Do not shrink from me! Believe me, Georgiana, I even rejoice in this single imperfection, since it will be such a rapture to remove it."

"Oh, spare me!" sadly replied his wife. "Pray do not look at it again. I never can forget that convulsive shudder."

In order to soothe Georgiana, and, as it were, to release her mind from the burden of actual things, Aylmer now put in practice some of the light and playful secrets which science had taught him among its profounder lore. Airy figures, absolutely bodiless ideas, and forms of unsubstantial beauty came and danced before her, imprinting their momentary footsteps on beams of light. Though she had some indistinct idea of the method of these optical phenomena, still the illusion was almost perfect enough to warrant the belief that her husband possessed sway over the spiritual world. Then again, when she felt a wish to look forth from her seclusion, immediately, as if her thoughts were answered, the procession of external existence flitted across a screen. The scenery and the figures of actual life were perfectly represented, but with that bewitching, yet indescribable difference which always makes a picture, an image, or a shadow so much more attractive than the original. When wearied of this, Aylmer bade her cast her eyes upon a vessel containing a quantity of earth. She did so, with little interest at first; but was soon startled to perceive the germ of a plant shooting upward from the soil. Then came the slender stalk; the leaves gradually unfolded themselves, and amid them was a perfect and lovely flower.

"It is magical!" cried Georgiana. "I dare not touch it."

"Nay, pluck it," answered Aylmer—"pluck it, and inhale its brief perfume while you may. The flower will wither in a few moments and leave nothing save its brown seed vessels; but thence may be perpetuated a race as ephemeral as itself."

But Georgiana had no sooner touched the flower than the whole plant suffered a blight, its leaves turning coal-black as if by the agency of fire.

"There was too powerful a stimulus," said Aylmer, thoughtfully.

To make up for this abortive experiment, he proposed to take her portrait by a scientific process of his own invention. It was to be effected by rays of light striking upon a polished plate of metal. Georgiana assented; but, on looking at the result, was affrighted to find the features of the portrait blurred and indefinable; while the minute figure of a hand appeared where the cheek should have been. Aylmer snatched the metallic plate and threw it into a jar of corrosive acid.

Soon, however, he forgot these mortifying failures. In the intervals of study and chemical experiment he came to her flushed and exhausted, but seemed invigorated by her presence, and spoke in glowing language of the resources of his art. He gave a history of the long dynasty of the alchemists, who spent so many ages in quest of the universal solvent by which the golden principle might be elicited from all things vile and base. Aylmer appeared to believe that, by the plainest scientific logic, it was altogether within the limits of possibility to discover this long-sought medium; "but," he added, "a philosopher who should go deep enough to acquire the power would attain too lofty a wisdom to stoop to the exercise of it." Not less singular were his opinions in regard to the elixir vita. He more than intimated that it was at his option to concoct a liquid that should prolong life for years, perhaps interminably; but that it would produce a discord in Nature which all the world, and chiefly the quaffer of the immortal nostrum, would find cause to curse.

"Aylmer, are you in earnest?" asked Georgiana, looking at him with amazement and fear. "It is terrible to possess such power, or even to dream of possessing it."

"Oh, do not tremble, my love," said her husband. "I would not wrong either you or myself by working such inharmonious effects upon our lives; but I would have you consider how trifling, in comparison, is the skill requisite to remove this little hand."

At the mention of the birthmark, Georgiana, as usual, shrank as if a redhot iron had touched her cheek.

Again Aylmer applied himself to his labors. She could hear his voice in the distant furnace room giving directions to Aminadab, whose harsh, uncouth, misshapen tones were audible in response, more like the grunt or growl of a brute than human speech. After hours of absence, Aylmer reappeared and proposed that she should now examine his cabinet of chemical products and natural treasures of the earth. Among the former he showed her a small vial, in which, he remarked, was contained a gentle yet most powerful fragrance, capable of impregnating all the breezes that blow across a kingdom. They were of inestimable value, the contents of that little vial; and, as he said so, he threw some of the perfume into the air and filled the room with piercing and invigorating delight.

"And what is this?" asked Georgiana, pointing to a small crystal globe containing a gold-colored liquid. "It is so beautiful to the eye that I could imagine it the elixir of life."

"In one sense it is," replied Aylmer; "or, rather, the elixir of immortality. It is the most precious poison that ever was concocted in this world. By its aid I could apportion the lifetime of any mortal at whom you might point your finger. The strength of the dose would determine whether he were to linger out years, or drop dead in the midst of a breath. No king on his guarded throne could keep his life if I, in my private station, should deem that the welfare of millions justified me in depriving him of it."

"Why do you keep such a terrific drug?" inquired Georgiana in horror.

"Do not mistrust me, dearest," said her husband, smiling; "its virtuous potency is yet greater than its harmful one. But see! here is a powerful cosmetic. With a few drops of this in a vase of water, freckles may be washed away as easily as the hands are cleansed. A stronger infusion would take the blood out of the cheek, and leave the rosiest beauty a pale ghost."

"Is it with this lotion that you intend to bathe my cheek?" asked Georgiana, anxiously.

"Oh, no," hastily replied her husband; "this is merely superficial. Your case demands a remedy that shall go deeper."

In his interviews with Georgiana, Aylmer generally made minute inquiries as to her sensations and whether the confinement of the rooms and the temperature of the atmosphere agreed with her. These questions had such a particular drift that Georgiana began to conjecture that she was already subjected to certain physical influences, either breathed in with the fragrant air or taken with her food. She fancied likewise, but it might be altogether fancy, that there was a stirring up of her system—a strange, indefinite sensation creeping through her veins, and tingling, half painfully, half pleasurably, at her heart. Still, whenever she dared to look into the mirror, there she beheld herself pale as a white rose and with the crimson birthmark stamped upon her cheek. Not even Aylmer now hated it so much as she.

To dispel the tedium of the hours which her husband found it necessary to devote to the processes of combination and analysis, Georgiana turned over the volumes of his scientific library. In many dark old tomes she met with chapters full of romance and poetry. They were the works of the philosophers of the middle ages, such as Albertus Magnus, Cornelius Agrippa, Paracelsus, and the famous friar who created the prophetic Brazen Head. All these antique naturalists stood in advance of their centuries, yet were imbued with some of their credulity, and therefore were believed, and perhaps imagined themselves to have acquired from the investigation of Nature a power above Nature, and from physics a sway over the spiritual world. Hardly less curious and imaginative were the early volumes of the "Transactions of the Royal Society," in which the members, knowing little of the limits of natural possibility, were continually recording wonders or proposing methods whereby wonders might be wrought.

But to Georgiana the most engrossing volume was a large folio from her husband's own hand, in which he had recorded every experiment of his scientific career, its original aim, the methods adopted for its development, and its final success or failure, with the circumstances to which either event was attributable. The book, in truth, was both the history and emblem of his ardent, ambitious, imaginative, yet practical and laborious life. He handled physical details as if there were nothing beyond them; yet spiritualized them all, and redeemed himself from materialism by his strong and eager aspiration towards the infinite. In his grasp the veriest clod of earth assumed a soul. Georgiana, as she read, reverenced Aylmer and loved him more profoundly than ever, but with a less entire dependence on his judgment than heretofore. Much as he had accomplished, she could not but observe that his most splendid successes were almost invariably failures, if compared with the ideal at which he aimed. His brightest diamonds were the merest pebbles, and felt to be so by himself, in comparison with the inestimable gems which lay hidden beyond his reach. The volume, rich with achievements that had won renown for its author, was yet as melancholy a record as ever mortal hand had penned. It was the sad confession and continual exemplification of the shortcomings of the composite man, the spirit burdened with clay and working in matter, and of the despair that assails the higher nature at finding itself so miserably thwarted by the earthly part. Perhaps every man of genius in whatever sphere might recognize the image of his own experience in Aylmer's journal.

So deeply did these reflections affect Georgiana that she laid her face upon the open volume and burst into tears. In this situation she was found by her husband.

"It is dangerous to read in a sorcerer's books," said he, with a smile, though his countenance was uneasy and displeased. "Georgiana, there are pages in that volume which I can scarcely glance over and keep my senses. Take heed lest it prove as detrimental to you."

"It has made me worship you more than ever," said she.

"Ah, wait for this one success," rejoined he, "then worship me if you will.

I shall deem myself hardly unworthy of it. But come, I have sought you for the luxury of your voice. Sing to me, dearest."

So she poured out the liquid music of her voice to quench the thirst of his spirit. He then took his leave with a boyish exuberance of gayety, assuring her that her seclusion would endure but a little longer, and that the result was already certain. Scarcely had he departed when Georgiana felt irresistibly impelled to follow him. She had forgotten to inform Aylmer of a symptom which for two or three hours past had begun to excite her attention. It was a sensation in the fatal birthmark, not painful, but which induced a restlessness throughout her system. Hastening after her husband, she intruded for the first time into the laboratory.

The first thing that struck her eye was the furnace, that hot and feverish worker, with the intense glow of its fire, which by the quantities of soot clustered above it seemed to have been burning for ages. There was a distilling apparatus in full operation. Around the room were retorts, tubes, cylinders, crucibles, and other apparatus of chemical research. An electrical machine stood ready for immediate use. The atmosphere felt oppressively close, and was tainted with gaseous odors which had been tormented forth by the processes of science. The severe and homely simplicity of the apartment, with its naked walls and brick pavement, looked strange, accustomed as Georgiana had become to the fantastic elegance of her boudoir. But what chiefly, indeed almost solely, drew her attention, was the aspect of Aylmer himself.

He was pale as death, anxious and absorbed, and hung over the furnace as if it depended upon his utmost watchfulness whether the liquid which it was distilling should be the draught of immortal happiness or misery. How different from the sanguine and joyous mien that he had assumed for Georgiana's encouragement!

"Carefully now, Aminadab; carefully, thou human machine; carefully, thou man of clay!" muttered Aylmer, more to himself than his assistant. "Now, if there be a thought too much or too little, it is all over."

"Ho! ho!" mumbled Aminadab. "Look, master! look!"

Aylmer raised his eyes hastily and at first reddened, then grew paler than ever, on beholding Georgiana. He rushed towards her and seized her arm with a grip that left the print of his fingers upon it.

"Why do you come hither? Have you no trust in your husband?" cried he, impetuously. "Would you throw the blight of that fatal birthmark over my labors? It is not well done. Go, prying woman, go!"

"Nay, Aylmer," said Georgiana with the firmness of which she possessed no stinted endowment, "it is not you that have a right to complain. You mistrust your wife; you have concealed the anxiety with which you watch the development of this experiment. Think not so unworthily of me, my husband. Tell me all the risk we run and fear not that I shall shrink; for my share in it is far less than your own."

"No, no, Georgiana!" said Aylmer, impatiently; "it must not be."

"I submit," replied she calmly. "And Aylmer, I shall quaff whatever draught you bring me; but it will be on the same principle that would induce me to take a dose of poison if offered by your hand."

"My noble wife," said Aylmer, deeply moved, "I knew not the height and depth of your nature until now. Nothing shall be concealed. Know, then, that this crimson hand, superficial as it seems, has clutched its grasp into your being with a strength of which I had no previous conception. I have already administered agents powerful enough to do aught except to change your entire physical system. Only one thing remains to be tried. If that fails us we are ruined."

"Why did you hesitate to tell me this?" asked she.

"Because, Georgiana," said Aylmer, in a low voice, "there is danger."

"Danger? There is but one danger—that this horrible stigma shall be left upon my cheek!" cried Georgiana. "Remove it, remove it, whatever be the cost, or we shall both go mad!"

"Heaven knows your words are too true," said Aylmer, sadly. "And now, dearest, return to your boudoir. In a little while all will be tested."

He conducted her back and took leave of her with a solemn tenderness which spoke far more than his words how much was now at stake.

After his departure Georgiana became rapt in musings. She considered the character of Aylmer, and did it completer justice than at any previous moment. Her heart exulted, while it trembled, at his honorable love—so pure and lofty that it would accept nothing less than perfection nor miserably make itself contented with an earthlier nature than he had dreamed of. She felt how much more precious was such a sentiment than that meaner kind which would have borne with the imperfection for her sake, and have been guilty of treason to holy love by degrading its perfect idea to the level of the actual; and with her whole spirit she prayed that, for a single moment, she might satisfy his highest and deepest conception. Longer than one moment she well knew it could not be; for his spirit was ever on the march, ever ascending, and each instant required something that was beyond the scope of the instant before.

The sound of her husband's footsteps aroused her. He bore a crystal goblet containing a liquor colorless as water, but bright enough to be the draught of immortality. Aylmer was pale; but it seemed rather the consequence of a highly wrought state of mind and tension of spirit than of fear or doubt.

"The concoction of the draught has been perfect," said he, in answer to Georgiana's look. "Unless all my science have deceived me, it cannot fail."

"Save on your account, my dearest Aylmer," observed his wife, "I might wish to put off this birthmark of mortality by relinquishing mortality itself in preference to any other mode. Life is but a sad possession to those who have attained precisely the degree of moral advancement at which I stand. Were I weaker and blinder it might be happiness. Were I stronger, it might be endured hopefully. But, being what I find myself, methinks I am of all mortals the most fit to die."

"You are fit for heaven without tasting death!" replied her husband. "But why do we speak of dying? The draught cannot fail. Behold its effect upon this plant."

On the window seat there stood a geranium diseased with yellow blotches, which had overspread all its leaves. Aylmer poured a small quantity of the liquid upon the soil in which it grew. In a little time, when the roots of the plant had taken up the moisture, the unsightly blotches began to be extinguished in a living verdure.

"There needed no proof," said Georgiana, quietly. "Give me the goblet. I joyfully stake all upon your word."

"Drink, then, thou lofty creature!" exclaimed Aylmer, with fervid admiration. "There is no taint of imperfection on thy spirit. Thy sensible frame, too, shall soon be all perfect."

She quaffed the liquid and returned the goblet to his hand.

"It is grateful," said she with a placid smile. "Methinks it is like water from a heavenly fountain; for it contains I know not what of unobtrusive fragrance and deliciousness. It allays a feverish thirst that had parched me for many days. Now, dearest, let me sleep. My earthly senses are closing over my spirit like the leaves around the heart of a rose at sunset."

She spoke the last words with a gentle reluctance, as if it required almost more energy than she could command to pronounce the faint and lingering syllables. Scarcely had they loitered through her lips ere she was lost in slumber. Aylmer sat by her side, watching her aspect with the emotions proper to a man the whole value of whose existence was involved in the process now to be tested. Mingled with this mood, however, was the philosophic investigation characteristic of the man of science. Not the minutest symptom escaped him. A heightened flush of the cheeks, a slight irregularity of breath, a quiver of the eyelids, a hardly perceptible tremor through the frame—such were the details which, as the moments passed, he wrote down in his folio volume. Intense thought had set its stamp upon every previous page of that volume, but the thoughts of years were all concentrated upon the last.

While thus employed, he failed not to gaze often at the fatal hand, and not without a shudder. Yet once, by a strange and unaccountable impulse, he pressed it with his lips. His spirit recoiled, however, in the very act; and Georgiana, out of the midst of her deep sleep, moved uneasily and murmured as if in remonstrance. Again Aylmer resumed his watch. Nor was it without avail. The crimson hand, which at first had been strongly visible upon the marble paleness of Georgiana's cheek, now grew more faintly outlined. She remained not less pale than ever; but the birthmark, with every breath that came and went, lost somewhat of its former distinctness. Its presence had been awful; its departure was more awful still. Watch the stain of the rainbow fading out of the sky, and you will know how that mysterious symbol passed away.

"By Heaven! it is well-nigh gone!" said Aylmer to himself, in almost irrepressible ecstasy. "I can scarcely trace it now. Success! success! And now it is like the faintest rose color. The lightest flush of blood across her cheek would overcome it. But she is so pale!"

He drew aside the window curtain and suffered the light of natural day to fall into the room and rest upon her cheek. At the same time he heard a gross, hoarse chuckle, which he had long known as his servant Aminadab's expression of delight.

"Ah, clod! ah, earthly mass!" cried Aylmer, laughing in a sort of frenzy, "you have served me well! Matter and spirit—earth and heaven—have both done their part in this! Laugh, thing of the senses! You have earned the right to laugh."

These exclamations broke Georgiana's sleep. She slowly unclosed her eyes and gazed into the mirror which her husband had arranged for that purpose. A faint smile flitted over her lips when she recognized how barely perceptible was now that crimson hand which had once blazed forth with such disastrous brilliancy as to scare away all their happiness. But then her eyes sought Aylmer's face with a trouble and anxiety that he could by no means account for.

"My poor Aylmer!" murmured she.

"Poor? Nay, richest, happiest, most favored!" exclaimed he. "My peerless bride, it is successful! You are perfect!"

"My poor Aylmer," she repeated, with a more than human tenderness, "you have aimed loftily; you have done nobly. Do not repent that with so high and pure a feeling, you have rejected the best the earth could offer. Aylmer, dearest Aylmer, I am dying!"

Alas! it was too true! The fatal hand had grappled with the mystery of life, and was the bond by which an angelic spirit kept itself in union with a mortal frame. As the last crimson tint of the birthmark—that sole token of human imperfection—faded from her cheek, the parting breath of the now perfect woman passed into the atmosphere, and her soul, lingering a moment near her husband, took its heavenward flight. Then a hoarse, chuckling laugh was heard again! Thus ever does the gross fatality of earth exult in its invariable triumph over the immortal essence which, in this dim sphere of half development, demands the completeness of a higher state. Yet, had Aylmer reached a profounder wisdom, he need not thus have flung away the happiness which would have woven his mortal life of the selfsame texture with the celestial. The momentary circumstance was too strong for him; he failed to look beyond the shadowy scope of time, and, living once for all in eternity, to find the perfect future in the present.

From The Hunchback of Notre Dame

VICTOR HUGO

BOOK VIII

Chapter III: A Human Heart in a Form Scarcely Human

NEXT MORNING SHE perceived on awakening that she had slept. This singular circumstance surprised her—it was so long that she had been unaccustomed to sleep! The sun, peeping in at her window, threw his cheering rays upon her face. But besides the sun she saw at this aperture an object that affrighted her—the unlucky face of Quasimodo. She involuntarily closed her eyes, but in vain; she still fancied that she saw through her rosy lids that visage so like an ugly mask. She kept her eyes shut. Presently she heard a hoarse voice saying very kindly: "Don't be afraid. I am your friend. I came to see you sleep. What harm can it do you, if I come to look at you when your eyes are shut? Well, well, I am going. There, now, I am behind the wall. Now you can open your eyes."

There was something still more plaintive than these words in the accent with which they were uttered. The Egyptian, affected by them, opened her eyes. He was actually no longer at the window. She went to it, looked out, and saw the poor hunchback cowering under the wall, in an attitude of grief and resignation. She made an effort to overcome the aversion which he excited. "Come!" said she kindly to him. Observing the motion of her lips, Quasimodo imagined that she was bidding him to go away. He then rose and retired, with slow and halting step and drooping head, without so much as daring to raise his eyes, filled with despair, to the damsel. "Come then!" she cried; but he continued to move off. She then darted out of the cell, ran to him, and took hold of his arm. On feeling her touch, Quasimodo trembled in every limb. He lifted his supplicating eye, and, finding that she drew him toward her, his whole face shone with joy and tenderness. She would have made him go into her cell, but he insisted on staying at her threshold. "No, no," said he, "the owl never enters the nest of the lark."

She then seated herself gracefully on her bed, with her goat at her feet. Both remained for some minutes motionless, contemplating in silence, he so much beauty, she so much ugliness. Every moment she discovered in Quasimodo some new deformity. Her look wandered from his knock-knees to his hunch back, from his hunch back to his only eye. She could not conceive how a creature so awkwardly put together could exist. At the same time an air of such sadness and gentleness pervaded his whole figure that she began to be reconciled with it.

He was the first to break silence. "Did you not call me back?" said he.

"Yes!" replied she, with a nod of affirmation.

He understood the sign. "Alas!" said he, as if hesitating to finish, "you must know, I am deaf."

"Poor fellow!" exclaimed the Bohemian, with an expression of pity.

He smiled sadly. "You think nothing else was wanting, don't you? Yes, I am deaf. That is the way in which I am served. It is terrible, is it not?—while you—you are so beautiful!"

The tone of the poor fellow conveyed such a profound feeling of his wretchedness that she had not the heart to utter a word. Besides, he would not have heard her. He then resumed: "Never till now was I aware how hideous I am. When I compare myself with you I cannot help pitying myself, poor unhappy monster that I am! I must appear to you like a beast.—You, you are a sunbeam, a drop of dew, a bird's song!—I, I am something frightful, neither man nor brute, something harder, more shapeless, and more trampled upon, than a flint."

He then laughed, and scarcely could there be aught in the world more cutting than this laugh. He continued: "Yes, I am deaf: but you will speak to me by gestures, by signs. I have a master who talks to me in that way. And then I shall know your meaning from the motion of your lips, from your look."

"Well, then," replied she smiling, "tell me why you have saved me?"

He looked steadfastly at her while she spoke.

"I understand," rejoined he; "you ask me why I saved you. You have forgotten a wretch who attempted one night to carry you off, a wretch to whom, the very next day, you brought relief on the vile pillory. A draught of water and a look of pity are more than I could repay with my life. You have forgotten that wretch—but he has not forgotten."

She listened to him with deep emotion. A tear started into the eye of the bell-ringer, but it did not fall. He appeared to make a point of repressing it. "Look you," he again began, when he no longer feared lest that tear should escape him—"we have very high towers here; a man falling from one of them would be dead almost before he reached the pavement. When you wish to be rid of me, tell me to throw myself from the top—you have but to say the word; nay, a look will be sufficient."

He then rose. Unhappy as was the Bohemian, this grotesque being awakened compassion even in her. She made him a sign to stay.

"No, no," said he, "I must not stay too long. I am ill at ease. It is out of pity that you do not turn your eyes from me. I will seek some place where I can look at you without your seeing me; that will be better."

He drew from his pocket a small metal whistle. "Take this," said he: "when you want me, when you wish me to come, when you have the courage to see me, whistle with this. I shall hear that sound."

He laid the whistle on the floor and retired.

Gargoyles

Eugene Hirsch

Gargoyles
promenade above
the cathedral,
juggling ugliness
with innocence,
raining joy and fear
upon suppliants below.
From mystic chapels,
from the chancel
down along the nave,
noble monks
soothe fiducial
maladies of faith
while hunchbacks swing
from rafters on ropes
strung from belfries,
chiming life through the air,
nurturing sacrificial loves
found only in great books,
those burned on the altars
of judgement and creed.

The Ear

Lauri Umansky Onek

My child has a birth defect. I hasten to add that it is a mild one, and that it has been corrected in large part by surgery.

But that caveat must not erase the essence of what I have to say.

Her right ear was smaller than the left. It was malformed, turned inward slightly, with two tiny skin tags hanging from it.

The doctors commented on it even as they cleaned her off, as I lay post-cesarean, aching through the middle, hollow with fear.

"The other ear looks fine," they said as they placed the baby in her father's arms.

Then I held her: the sweet damp belly, the eager lips, the reddish ringlets, the ten toes, the clench. And the ear.

"Be grateful," my mother said. "She is beautiful, she is healthy. She is your child. Love her, enjoy her. An ear is a very small part of a life."

As I lay crying for the next two days, specialists came and went from my hospital room, hooking up the baby to machines, reporting with relief and solicitude that her left ear could hear perfectly, that it would compensate for the right, which had no discernible eardrum and was, for all functional purposes, "useless."

The mother of my hospital roommate told me that her son had been born deaf in one ear and that he had never been affected by the shortcoming.

We have seen children so malformed, the nurses told me, that they looked like monsters. Be grateful for what you have.

I am. When I have taken Carenna to the children's hospital for the multiple operations to clear up subsequent complications of the defect, and I have seen the children with heads too large, heads too small, legs twisted, legs absent, hair sparse from chemotherapy, eyes vacant in exaggerated sockets, mobility so limited as to call the definition of living into question, I have known, at the deepest, even cellular level, that all of life is a gift, capricious, precious, momentary.

I understand that my child's birth defect is mild, as such things go. So one ear is a bit smaller than the other. A bit misshapen. After much surgery, my daughter now suffers only a 30% hearing loss in the ear, and that loss has not seemed to have affected her functional hearing in any way. She is a happy, beautiful, dimpled, curly-haired 5-year-old child who belts out the tunes to "The Little Mermaid" with the best of them, who takes on any jungle gym undaunted, who truly believes she is an incarnation of Pippi Longstocking. A normal, spirited child.

I look at Carenna from one angle and say to myself, it is hardly discernible. I look at her from another, and I see the imperfection quite clearly. I fiddle with her hair, never able to cover the ear, because her very curly hair grows out and out, never down. I curse the maternal and paternal genes, silently.

I cry many days about the ear. I wonder what I did wrong during my pregnancy. Was it the photocopy machine? Was it the glass of wine I drank before I knew I was pregnant? On my most difficult days, I wonder if it was the inevitable fate of a child of mine, a reflection of the ineffable wrongness of me.

I feel guilty for indulging this sadness, when indeed the defect is mild. Yet I feel it. Why my child?

It is a cute little ear, really. Not quite formed, it looks fetal, like a curled fern, a glimpse of something sacred. Secretly, I adore the "little ear." I plant kisses around it. It is our miracle ear, once destined never to hear.

It is not that I am ungrateful.

But the ear does not hear fully. And it looks different. And she comes home now from camp with the taunts of the older boys, who bully her into believing that she has no eardrums at all, believing that she is an embodiment of difference and shame. Kids can be ignorant and cruel, we tell her. Everyone has something different about them, some things more obvious than others. Difference can be something positive. We love your ear. It is cute. You have the right to be in the world, however you are, and you have the right to be loved, cherished, and accepted. We love, cherish, and accept you.

"I just want to be normal," she says. "I don't want a magic ear or a cute little ear. I want ears like all the other kids. I don't want them to tease me."

I hold her. She cries and cries. It does not help her to know that there are other children who are worse off, any more than it helps me. Her pain engulfs her. She is only 5. There is so much more to come.

But the next day, she comes to me pertly, having figured it all out. "Those boys don't make any sense. Now, if I had NO eardrums, how could I hear? I have a big ear and a little ear. The big ear hears better. Why do they have such a hard time understanding that?"

"They wonder about themselves," I say.

She nods, sagely.

I hope she will remember that moment of knowing.

I kiss the little ear passionately, and I come incrementally closer to embracing the beleaguered, hungry child that I have always been. The ear *is* little. And it *is* lovable.

Harrison Bergeron

Kurt Vonnegut, Jr.

THE YEAR WAS 2081, and everybody was finally equal. They weren't only equal before God and the law. They were equal every which way. Nobody was smarter than anybody else. Nobody was better looking than anybody else. Nobody was stronger or quicker than anybody else. All this equality was due to the 211th, 212th, and 213th Amendments to the Constitution, and to the unceasing vigilance of agents of the United States Handicapper General.

Some things about living still weren't quite right, though. April, for instance, still drove people crazy by not being springtime. And it was in that clammy month that the H-G men took George and Hazel Bergeron's fourteen-year-old son, Harrison, away.

It was tragic, all right, but George and Hazel couldn't think about it very hard. Hazel had a perfectly average intelligence, which meant she couldn't think about anything except in short bursts. And George, while his intelligence was way above normal, had a little mental handicap radio in his ear. He was required by law to wear it at all times. It was tuned to a government transmitter. Every twenty seconds or so, the transmitter would send out some sharp noise to keep people like George from taking unfair advantage of their brains.

George and Hazel were watching television. There were tears on Hazel's cheeks, but she'd forgotten for the moment what they were about.

On the television screen were ballerinas.

A buzzer sounded in George's head. His thoughts fled in panic, like bandits from a burglar alarm.

"That was a real pretty dance, that dance they just did," said Hazel.

"Huh?" said George.

"That dance—it was nice," said Hazel.

"Yup," said George. He tried to think a little about the ballerinas. They weren't really very good—no better than anybody else would have been, anyway. They were burdened with sashweights and bags of birdshot, and their faces were masked, so that no one, seeing a free and graceful gesture or a pretty face, would feel like something the cat drug in. George was toying with the vague notion that maybe dancers shouldn't be handicapped. But he didn't get very far with it before another noise in his ear radio scattered his thoughts.

George winced. So did two out of the eight ballerinas.

Hazel saw him wince. Having no mental handicap herself, she had to ask George what the latest sound had been.

"Sounded like somebody hitting a milk bottle with a ball peen hammer," said George.

"I'd think it would be real interesting, hearing all the different sounds," said Hazel, a little envious. "All the things they think up."

"Um," said George.

"Only, if I was Handicapper General, you know what I would do?" said Hazel. Hazel, as a matter of fact, bore a strong resemblance to the Handicapper General, a woman named Diana Moon Glampers. "If I was Diana Moon Glampers," said Hazel, "I'd have chimes on Sunday—just chimes. Kind of in honor of religion."

"I could think, if it was just chimes," said George.

"Well—maybe make 'em real loud," said Hazel. "I think I'd make a good Handicapper General."

"Good as anybody else," said George.

"Who knows better'n I do what normal is?" said Hazel.

"Right," said George. He began to think glimmeringly about his abnormal son who was now in jail, about Harrison, but a twenty-one-gun salute in his head stopped that.

"Boy!" said Hazel, "that was a doozy, wasn't it?"

It was such a doozy that George was white and trembling, and tears stood on the rims of his red eyes. Two of the eight ballerinas had collapsed to the studio floor, were holding their temples.

"All of a sudden you look so tired," said Hazel. "Why don't you stretch out on the sofa, so's you can rest your handicap bag on the pillows, honeybunch." She was referring to the forty-seven pounds of birdshot in a canvas bag, which was padlocked around George's neck. "Go on and rest the bag for a little while," she said. "I don't care if you're not equal to me for a while."

George weighed the bag with his hands. "I don't mind it," he said. "I don't notice it any more. It's just a part of me."

"You been so tired lately—kind of wore out," said Hazel. "If there was just some way we could make a little hole in the bottom of the bag, and just take out a few of them lead balls. Just a few."

"Two years in prison and two thousand dollars fine for every ball I took out," said George. "I don't call that a bargain."

"If you could just take a few out when you came home from work," said Hazel. "I mean—you don't compete with anybody around here. You just set around."

"If I tried to get away with it," said George, "then other people'd get away with it—and pretty soon we'd be right back to the dark ages again, with everybody competing against everybody else. You wouldn't like that, would you?"

"I'd hate it," said Hazel.

"There you are," said George. "The minute people start cheating on laws, what do you think happens to society?"

If Hazel hadn't been able to come up with an answer to this question, George couldn't have supplied one. A siren was going off in his head.

"Reckon it'd fall all apart," said Hazel.

"What would?" said George blankly.

"Society," said Hazel uncertainly. "Wasn't that what you just said?"

"Who knows?" said George.

The television program was suddenly interrupted for a news bulletin. It wasn't clear at first as to what the bulletin was about, since the announcer, like all announcers, had a serious speech impediment. For about half a minute, and in a state of high excitement, the announcer tried to say, "Ladies and gentlemen—"

He finally gave up, handed the bulletin to a ballerina to read.

"That's all right—" Hazel said of the announcer, "he tried. That's the big thing. He tried to do the best he could with what God gave him. He should get a nice raise for trying so hard."

"Ladies and gentlemen—" said the ballerina, reading the bulletin. She must have been extraordinarily beautiful, because the mask she wore was hideous. And it was easy to see that she was the strongest and most graceful of all the dancers, for her handicap bags were as big as those worn by two-hundred-pound men.

And she had to apologize at once for her voice, which was a very unfair voice for a woman to use. Her voice was a warm, luminous, timeless melody.

"Excuse me—" she said, and she began again, making her voice absolutely uncompetitive.

"Harrison Bergeron, age fourteen," she said in a grackle squawk, "has just escaped from jail, where he was held on suspicion of plotting to overthrow the government. He is a genius and an athlete, is under-handicapped, and should be regarded as extremely dangerous."

A police photograph of Harrison Bergeron was flashed on the screen— upside down, then sideways, upside down again, then right side up. The picture showed the full length of Harrison against a background calibrated in feet and inches. He was exactly seven feet tall.

The rest of Harrison's appearance was Halloween and hardware. Nobody had ever borne heavier handicaps. He had outgrown hindrances faster than the H-G men could think them up. Instead of a little ear radio for a mental handicap, he wore a tremendous pair of earphones, and spectacles with thick wavy lenses. The spectacles were intended to make him not only half blind, but to give him whanging headaches besides.

Scrap metal was hung all over him. Ordinarily, there was a certain symmetry, a military neatness to the handicaps issued to strong people, but Harrison looked like a walking junkyard. In the race of life, Harrison carried three hundred pounds.

And to offset his good looks, the H-G men required that he wear at all times a red rubber ball for a nose, keep his eyebrows shaved off, and cover his even white teeth with black caps at snaggle-tooth random.

"If you see this boy," said the ballerina, "do not—I repeat, do not—try to reason with him."

There was the shriek of a door being torn from its hinges.

Screams and barking cries of consternation came from the television. The photograph of Harrison Bergeron on the screen jumped again and again, as though dancing to the tune of an earthquake.

George Bergeron correctly identified the earthquake, and well he might have—for many was the time his own home had danced to the same crashing tune. "My God—" said George, "that must be Harrison!"

The realization was blasted from his mind instantly by the sound of an automobile collision in his head.

When George could open his eyes again, the photograph of Harrison was gone.

A living, breathing Harrison filled the screen.

Clanking, clownish, and huge, Harrison stood in the center of the studio. The knob of the uprooted studio door was still in his hand. Ballerinas, technicians, musicians, and announcers cowered on their knees before him, expecting to die.

"I am the Emperor!" cried Harrison. "Do you hear? I am the Emperor! Everybody must do what I say at once!" He stamped his foot and the studio shook.

"Even as I stand here—" he bellowed, "crippled, hobbled, sickened—I am a greater ruler than any man who ever lived! Now watch me become what I *can* become!"

Harrison tore the straps of his handicap harness like wet tissue paper, tore straps guaranteed to support five thousand pounds.

Harrison's scrap-iron handicaps crashed to the floor.

Harrison thrust his thumbs under the bar of the padlock that secured his head harness. The bar snapped like celery. Harrison smashed his headphones and spectacles against the wall.

He flung away his rubber-ball nose, revealed a man that would have awed Thor, the god of thunder.

"I shall now select my Empress!" he said looking down on the cowering people. "Let the first woman who dares rise to her feet claim her mate and her throne!"

A moment passed, and then a ballerina arose, swaying like a willow.

Harrison plucked the mental handicap from her ear, snapped off her physical handicaps with marvelous delicacy. Last of all, he removed her mask.

She was blindingly beautiful.

"Now—" said Harrison, taking her hand, "shall we show the people the meaning of the word dance? Music!" he commanded.

The musicians scrambled back into their chairs, and Harrison stripped them of their handicaps, too. "Play your best," he told them, "and I'll make you barons and dukes and earls."

The music began. It was normal at first—cheap, silly, false. But Harrison snatched two musicians from their chairs, waved them like batons as he sang the music as he wanted it played. He slammed them back into their chairs.

The music began again and was much improved.

Harrison and his Empress merely listened to the music for a while—listened gravely, as though synchronizing their heartbeats with it.

They shifted their weights to their toes.

Harrison placed his big hands on the girl's tiny waist, letting her sense the weightlessness that would soon be hers.

And then, in an explosion of joy and grace, into the air they sprang!

Not only were the laws of the land abandoned, but the law of gravity and the laws of motion as well.

They reeled, whirled, swiveled, flounced, capered, gamboled, and spun.

They leaped like deer on the moon.

The studio ceiling was thirty feet high, but each leap brought the dancers nearer to it.

It became their obvious intention to kiss the ceiling.

They kissed it.

And then, neutralizing gravity with love and pure will, they remained suspended in air inches below the ceiling, and they kissed each other for a long, long time.

It was then that Diana Moon Glampers, the Handicapper General, came into the studio with a double-barreled ten-gauge shotgun. She fired twice, and the Emperor and the Empress were dead before they hit the floor.

Diana Moon Glampers loaded the gun again. She aimed it at the musicians and told them they had ten seconds to get their handicaps back on.

It was then that the Bergerons' television tube burned out.

Hazel turned to comment about the blackout to George. But George had gone out into the kitchen for a can of beer.

George came back in with the beer, paused while a handicap signal shook him up. And then he sat down again. "You been crying?" he said to Hazel.

"Yup," she said.

"What about?" he said.

"I forget," she said. "Something real sad on television."

"What was it?" he said.

"It's all kind of mixed up in my mind," said Hazel.

"Forget sad things," said George.

"I always do," said Hazel.

"That's my girl," said George. He winced. There was the sound of a riveting gun in his head.

"Gee—I could tell that one was a doozy," said Hazel.

"You can say that again," said George.

"Gee—" said Hazel, "I could tell that one was a doozy."

The Diary of an Infidel

RICHARD SELZER

I'VE BEEN GIVEN the run of the monastery. Only the souls of the monks are forbidden me. The complex of buildings is vast and the monks, engaged in their prayers and duties, are largely invisible. A whole day will go by without my meeting one of them. On the occasion that I do, the monumental silhouette floats near, lowers its head, and hurries past with at most a whispered "Buon giorno." More is not permitted.

For one who believes that a good chat is the highest development of civilization, this interdiction of conversation is hardest to bear. I miss that low hum, more audible to the heart than to the ear, by which a lived-in house announces itself. Sometimes while sitting in the park or while writing at my desk, I have the feeling that I am not alone, that others are present. I know they are not. Still I turn around to see. Sometimes I think, "Good Lord. Perhaps the whole of the community who lived here has fled and to the thousand years of spiritual influence now I alone stand heir."

A great drowsiness has come over me, as though the air here were webbed and I trapped within it. I relieve myself of a dozen yawns an hour, as many as a monk does prayers. No sooner is one yawn expelled with jaw-dislocating emphasis than the next bubble gathers in my head. By tomorrow I shall be in a deep coma. In such a convalescent state, for that is what I have diagnosed it to be, I can explore only by small ambitions, hithering and thithering as far as the conclave room for a long solitary sitdown. On to the sacristy, another daydream, then up to the top of the campanile where I feel like I'm a muezzin on a mosque. Once again the abbot has refused to let me work. Oh well, if there's nothing whatever to do here, then I'm just the man to do it.

Every evening I return from a ramble in the cloister to find that my room has been swept clean, the cigarette ashes taken away, and the bed which I had made, remade, according to some fierce precision of which I am ignorant. Who did it? The angels?

Time and again the church coaxes me inside her. I've taken to sitting there at odd hours. Truth to tell, I'm far more attracted to the bells, incense, and statues of a religion than I am to its dogma or Talmud. It is the child in me craving diversion. And this church is brim full of spectacle what with shaggy John the Baptist on the wall, Lazarus half in and half out of his shroud and, of course, St. George in full metallic fig. In the absence of human beings, I am keeping company with the statuary. Today in the church at twilight, a grey angel soared over my head. From its fixed height of fifty feet, I could feel the breeze of its passing. What is this? In the midst of perfection I discovered that one of the host of angels, the third from the left of the main altar, has been imperfectly rendered, one wing being rather too centrally located at the back and more than a little lower in its thoracic attachment than the other wing. The corresponding shoulder droops, giving a type of scoliosis. Such an angel would hover askew, list to the affected side. Here, I think, is a cock-eyed creature, made from a bumpy hunk of marble by hands less skilled than willing. Still, something about its miscreation is endearing, as though her sculptor had not yet learned the dishonesties of art.

I say *her* because of all the race of angels on this island, only this one suggests specificity of gender. Aside from Michael, Gabriel, and the one who wrestles with Jacob, about whose masculinity there has never been any doubt, the other angels are sexually indeterminant. The gender of angels is not readily told. One does not turn them upside to see. Nor is it of the least importance as the whole idea, I gather, is that they be neuter. But this crookback to the left of the altar is, beyond peradventure of doubt, womanly, the female of the species. It is something about the elbows, the knees, whatever. Nor does she have your basic seraph's countenance with plump cheeks and serene brow all framed by ringlets. Instead she is stringy, all wrists and ribs. The face, too, owns a certain gauntness of the feature, the suggestion of fatigue. The mouth is a thin slit. The expression less one of ecstasy than of endurance. This face has witnessed. It has tolerated.

Now and then I have the fleeting thought that I have seen this face before. But where? Whose is it?

It is three midnights later. I awake suddenly and lie there in bed, rummaging about in what I used to call my mind. All at once I'm bolt upright. In a moment I put on my clothes, grab candlestick and matches and am racing along the hallway down a flight of stairs. I push open the side door of the church. It is full still of the sweet smell of incense. And oh, that black that does not hold itself back but comes charging at you like a panther. I light the match, touch it to the taper. But why do my hands tremble so? I watch my shadow become involved with the dormant church as the flame is battered in the draft. The great altar looms, now to the left, one, two, three. And I hold up the candle at arm's length, flashes of gold from chalice and monstrance. The stillness rages in the very pillars. And I know I am certain.

Some months before I left New Haven, a nurse who had worked in the recovery room retired. For thirty-five years each day Frances Bouchet had received into her care dozens of post-operative patients, each of whom shared the single condition of unconsciousness, being either fully anesthetized or in emergence from that state. Upon awakening they would be amnesic for their time spent in this room. While one would flail about in danger of injuring himself, another, driven by some drug-released urge toward violence, would strike out at those who tended him. I remember one of her black eyes. Part of the job, Frances had said afterwards. Still another patient would vomit or choke or suffer cardiac arrest and so must be resuscitated by mouth to mouth breathing and receive a beating upon the chest to coax back the heart. Nor, as I have said, did a single one of her patients remember Frances. Were she later to pass one of them in the street, he would give no sign of recognition. To all of this, Frances presented an unruffled expression. It was more than tolerance or endurance. It was acceptance. It was obedience. Frances Bouchet was a hunchback. Despite the fact of her crooked spine, which was ill-concealed and even accentuated by the thin blue scrub dress she wore at work, there was no awkwardness in her administration. In the recovery room, if nowhere else, she was graceful. When Frances retired, there was a party in the operating room lounge. She was presented with a purse containing $100 collected from the others. The chief of surgery proposed a toast with ginger ale.

"What are you going to do now, Frances?" he asked. "Are you going to travel? Or just loaf?"

"Now?" said Frances with a shy smile. "Now I am going to recover from my own life."

I saw her once after that. There is a small park in the center of New Haven. It is called The Green. In good weather people go there to eat lunch, play chess, or walk their dogs. One day I was crossing The Green on some errand or other when I caught sight of her alone on one of the benches that line the paths. Several people walked by. All at once she rose, walked quickly to catch up with a man who had just passed by. When she had come within arm's length, she reached one hand to touch his sleeve. I saw the man turn, look at her for a moment without expression, then wheel and walk briskly away. After a moment Frances returned to her seat. I stopped to talk.

"Who was that?" I asked her. We were that easy with each other.

"Oh," she said, "someone I thought I knew, but I guess not."

"One of your patients?" I said. Frances smiled and looked at something further and further away from her body.

Later that day, sitting in my office at the hospital, I thought of her again, of how many thousands of people in this city she had steadied and bumped and rubbed, blown into, of all the vomitus, phlegm, and blood with which she had been spattered, all of the prophecies she had sown.

"You're going to be all right. Pretty soon you'll be back in your own bed."

All her crooning, her coaxing back, her padding against mindless battering, all those magic acts of intercession, that endless braiding of tubes and wires about pale, sick faces. And no one could remember having seen her.

Just before I left for Italy, I saw her name in the obituary column. Isn't that just the way? You work all your life and the minute you stop and can begin to enjoy. . .

For a long while, I gazed up at the statue of the angel, the third from the left of the main altar, the hot wax from the taper begloving my hand in tightness and heat which races down the arm and across the chest where the heart beats hard against it. Look! She bends to peer at me, lifts one hand as if to wipe a brow, then slowly relents into marble.

"So, Frances," I say aloud, "I might have known."

Minutes later back in my room, I snuff the taper. There is the sad smell of candlewick and the singing of wings.

Keela, the Outcast Indian Maiden

Eudora Welty

ONE MORNING IN summertime, when all his sons and daughters were off picking plums and Little Lee Roy was all alone, sitting on the porch and only listening to the screech owls away down in the woods, he had a surprise.

First he heard white men talking. He heard two white men coming up the path from the highway. Little Lee Roy ducked his head and held his breath; then he patted all around back of him for his crutches. The chickens all came out from under the house and waited attentively on the steps.

The men came closer. It was the young man who was doing all of the talking. But when they got through the fence, Max, the older man, interrupted him. He tapped him on the arm and pointed his thumb toward Little Lee Roy.

He said, "Bud? Yonder he is."

But the younger man kept straight on talking, in an explanatory voice.

"Bud?" said Max again. "Look, Bud, yonder's the only little clubfooted nigger man was ever around Cane Springs. Is he the party?"

They came nearer and nearer to Little Lee Roy and then stopped and stood there in the middle of the yard. But the young man was so excited he did not seem to realize that they had arrived anywhere. He was only about twenty years old, very sunburned. He talked constantly, making only one gesture—raising his hand stiffly and then moving it a little to one side.

"They dressed it in a red dress, and it ate chickens alive," he said. "I sold tickets and I thought it was worth a dime, honest. They gimme a piece of paper with the thing wrote off I had to say. That was easy. 'Keela, the Outcast Indian Maiden!' I call it out through a pasteboard megaphone. Then ever' time it was fixin' to eat a live chicken, I blowed the sireen out front."

"Just tell me, Bud," said Max, resting back on the heels of his perforated tan-and-white sport shoes. "Is this nigger the one? Is that him sittin' there?"

Little Lee Roy sat huddled and blinking, a smile on his face. . . . But the young man did not look his way.

"Just took the job that time. I didn't mean to——I mean, I meant to go to Port Arthur because my brother was on a boat," he said. "My name is Steve, mister. But I worked with this show selling tickets for three months, and I never would of knowed it was like that if it hadn't been for that man." He arrested his gesture.

"Yeah, what man?" said Max in a hopeless voice.

Little Lee Roy was looking from one white man to the other, excited almost beyond respectful silence. He trembled all over, and a look of amazement and sudden life came into his eyes.

"Two years ago," Steve was saying impatiently. "And we was travelin' through Texas in those ole trucks.—See, the reason nobody ever come clost to it before was they give it a iron bar this long. And tole it if anybody come near, to shake the bar good at 'em, like this. But it couldn't say nothin'. Turned out they'd tole it it couldn't say nothin' to anybody ever, so it just kind of mumbled and growled, like a animal."

"Hee! hee!" This from Little Lee Roy, softly.

"Tell me again," said Max, and just from his look you could tell that everybody knew old Max. "Somehow I can't get it straight in my mind. Is this the boy? Is this little nigger boy the same as this Keela, the Outcast Indian Maiden?"

Up on the porch, above them, Little Lee Roy gave Max a glance full of hilarity, and then bent the other way to catch Steve's next words.

"Why, if anybody was to even come near it or even bresh their shoulder against the rope it'd growl and take on and shake its iron rod. When it would eat the live chickens it'd growl somethin' awful—you ought to heard it."

"Hee! hee!" It was a soft, almost incredulous laugh that began to escape from Little Lee Roy's tight lips, a little mew of delight.

"They'd throw it this chicken, and it would reach out an' grab it. Would sort of rub over the chicken's neck with its thumb an' press on it good, an' then it would bite its head off."

"O.K.," said Max.

"It skint back the feathers and stuff from the neck and sucked the blood. But ever'body said it was still alive." Steve drew closer to Max and fastened his light-colored, troubled eyes on his face.

"O.K."

"Then it would pull the feathers out easy and neat-like, awful fast, an' growl the whole time, kind of moan, an' then it would commence to eat all the white meat. I'd go in an' look at it. I reckon I seen it a thousand times."

"That was you, boy?" Max demanded of Little Lee Roy unexpectedly.

But Little Lee Roy could only say, "Hee! hee!" The little man at the head of the steps where the chickens sat, one on each step, and the two men facing each other below made a pyramid.

Steve stuck his hand out for silence. "They said—I mean, I said it, out front through the megaphone, I said it myself, that it wouldn't eat nothin' but only live meat. It was supposed to be a Indian woman, see, in this red dress an' stockin's. It didn't have on no shoes, so when it drug its foot ever'body could see. . . . When it come to the chicken's heart, it would eat that too, real fast, and the heart would still be jumpin'."

"Wait a second, Bud," said Max briefly, "Say, boy, is this white man here crazy?"

Little Lee Roy burst into hysterical, deprecatory giggles. He said, "Naw suh, don't think so." He tried to catch Steve's eye, seeking appreciation, crying, "Naw suh, don't think he crazy, mista."

Steve gripped Max's arm. "Wait! Wait!" he cried anxiously. "You ain't listenin'. I want to tell you about it. You didn't catch my name—Steve. You never did hear about that little nigger—all that happened to him? Lived in Cane Springs, Miss'ippi?"

"Bud," said Max, disengaging himself, "I don't hear anything. I got a juke box, see, so I don't have to listen."

"Look—I was really the one," said Steve more patiently, but nervously, as if he had been slowly breaking bad news. He walked up and down the bare-swept ground in front of Little Lee Roy's porch, along the row of princess feathers and snow-on-the-mountain. Little Lee Roy's turning head followed him. "I was the one—that's what I'm tellin' you."

"Suppose I was to listen to what every dope comes in Max's Place got to say, I'd be nuts," said Max.

"It's all me, see," said Steve. "I know that. I was the one was the cause for it goin' on an' on an' not bein' found out—such an awful thing. It was me, what I said out front through the megaphone."

He stopped still and stared at Max in despair.

"Look," said Max. He sat on the steps, and the chickens hopped off. "I know I ain't nobody but Max. I got Max's Place. I only run a place, understand, fifty yards down the highway. Liquor buried twenty feet from the premises, and no trouble yet. I ain't ever been up here before. I don't claim to been anywhere. People come to my place. Now. You're the hitchhiker. You're tellin' me, see. You claim a lot of information. If I don't get it I don't get it and I ain't complainin' about it, see. But I think you're nuts, and did from the first. I only come up here with you because I figured you's crazy."

"Maybe you don't believe I remember every word of it even now," Steve was saying gently. "I think about it at night—that an' drums on the midway. You ever hear drums on the midway?" He paused and stared politely at Max and Little Lee Roy.

"Yeh," said Max.

"Don't it make you feel sad. I remember how the drums was goin' and I was yellin', 'Ladies and gents! Do not try to touch Keela, the Outcast Indian Maiden—she will only beat your brains out with her iron rod, and eat them alive!'" Steve waved his arm gently in the air, and Little Lee Roy drew back and squealed. "'Do not go near her, ladies and gents! I'm warnin' you!' So nobody ever did. Nobody ever come near her. Until that man."

"Sure," said Max. "That fella." He shut his eyes.

"Afterwards when he come up so bold, I remembered seein' him walk up an' buy the ticket an' go in the tent. I'll never forget that man as long as I live. To me he's a sort of—well—"

"Hero," said Max.

"I wish I could remember what he looked like. Seem like he was a tallish man with a sort of white face. Seem like he had bad teeth, but I may be wrong. I remember he frowned a lot. Kept frownin'. Whenever he'd buy a ticket, why, he'd frown."

"Ever seen him since?" asked Max cautiously, still with his eyes closed. "Ever hunt him up?"

"No, never did," said Steve. Then he went on. "He'd frown an' buy a ticket ever' day we was in these two little smelly towns in Texas, sometimes three-four times a day, whether it was fixin' to eat a chicken or not."

"O.K., so he gets in the tent," said Max.

"Well, what the man finally done was, he walked right up to the little stand where it was tied up and laid his hand out open on the planks in the platform. He just laid his hand out open there and said, 'Come here,' real low and quick, that-a-way."

Steve laid his open hand on Little Lee Roy's porch and held it there, frowning in concentration.

"I get it," said Max. "He'd caught on it was a fake."

Steve straightened up. "So ever'body yelled to git away, git away," he continued, his voice rising, "because it was growlin' an' carryin' on an' shakin' its iron bar like they tole it. When I heard all that commotion—boy! I was scared."

"You didn't know it was a fake." Steve was silent for a moment, and Little Lee Roy held his breath, for fear everything was all over.

"Look," said Steve finally, his voice trembling. "I guess I was supposed to feel bad like this, and you wasn't. I wasn't supposed to ship out on that boat from Port Arthur and all like that. This other had to happen to me—not you all. Feelin' responsible. You'll be O.K., mister, but I won't. I feel awful about it. That poor little old thing."

"Look, you got him right here," said Max quickly. "See him? Use your eyes. He's O.K., ain't he? Looks O.K. to me. It's just you. You're nuts, is all."

"You know—when that man laid out his open hand on the boards, why, it just let go the iron bar," continued Steve, "let it fall down like that—bang—and act like it didn't know what to do. Then it drug itself over to where the fella was standin' an' leaned down an' grabbed holt onto that white man's hand as tight as it could an' cried like a baby. It didn't want to hit him!"

"Hee! hee! hee!"

"No sir, it didn't want to hit him. You know what it wanted?"

Max shook his head.

"It wanted him to help it. So the man said, 'Do you wanna get out of this place, whoever you are?' An' it never answered—none of us knowed it could talk—but it just wouldn't let that man's hand a-loose. It hung on, cryin' like a baby. So the man says, 'Well, wait here till I come back.'"

"Uh-huh?" said Max.

"Went off an' come back with the sheriff. Took us all to jail. But just the man owned the show and his son got took to the pen. They said I could go free. I kep' tellin' 'em I didn't know it wouldn't hit me with the iron bar an' kep' tellin' 'em I didn't know it could tell what you was sayin' to it."

"Yeh, guess you told 'em," said Max.

"By that time I felt bad. Been feelin' bad ever since. Can't hold on to a job or stay in one place for nothin' in the world. They made it stay in jail to see if it could talk or not, and the first night it wouldn't say nothin'. Some time it cried. And they undressed it an' found out it wasn't no outcast Indian woman a-tall. It was a little clubfooted nigger man."

"Hee! hee!"

"You mean it was this boy here—yeh. It was him."

"Washed its face, and it was paint all over it made it look red. It all come off. And it could talk—as good as me or you. But they'd tole it not to, so it never did. They'd tole it if anybody was to come near it they was comin' to git it—and for it to hit 'em quick with that iron bar an' growl. So nobody ever come near it—until that man. I was yellin' outside, tellin' 'em to keep away, keep away. You could see where they'd whup it. They had to whup it some to make it eat all the chickens. It was awful dirty. They let it go back home free, to where they got it in the first place. They made them pay its ticket from Little Oil, Texas, to Cane Springs, Miss'ippi."

"You got a good memory," said Max.

"The way it *started* was," said Steve, in a wondering voice, "the show was just travelin' along in ole trucks through the country, and just seen this little deformed nigger man, sittin' on a fence, and just took it. It couldn't help it."

Little Lee Roy tossed his head back in a frenzy of amusement.

"I found it all out later. I was up on the Ferris wheel with one of the boys—got to talkin' up yonder in the peace an' quiet—an' said they just kind of happened up on it. Like a cyclone happens: it wasn't nothin' it could do. It was just took up." Steve suddenly paled through his sunburn. "An' they found out that back in Miss'ippi it had it a little bitty pair of crutches an' could just go runnin' on 'em!"

"And there they are," said Max.

Little Lee Roy held up a crutch and turned it about, and then snatched it back like a monkey.

"But if it hadn't been for that man, I wouldn't of knowed it till yet. If it wasn't for him bein' so bold. If he hadn't knowed what he was doin'."

"You remember that man this fella's talkin' about, boy?" asked Max, eying Little Lee Roy.

Little Lee Roy, in reluctance and shyness, shook his head gently.

"Naw suh, I can't say as I remembas that ve'y man, suh," he said softly, looking down where just then a sparrow alighted on his child's shoe. He added happily, as if on inspiration, "Now I remembas *this* man."

Steve did not look up, but when Max shook with silent laughter, alarm seemed to seize him like a spasm in his side. He walked painfully over and stood in the shade for a few minutes, leaning his head on a sycamore tree.

"Seemed like that man just studied it out an' knowed it was somethin' wrong," he said presently, his voice coming more remotely than ever. "But I didn't know. I can't look at nothin' an' be sure what it is. Then afterwards I know. Then I see how it was."

"Yeh, but you're nuts," said Max affably.

"You wouldn't of knowed it either!" cried Steve in sudden boyish, defensive anger. Then he came out from under the tree and stood again almost pleadingly in the sun, facing Max where he was sitting below Little Lee Roy on the steps. "You'd of let it go on an' on when they made it do those things—just like I did."

"Bet I could tell a man from a woman and an Indian from a nigger though," said Max.

Steve scuffed the dust into little puffs with his worn shoe. The chickens scattered, alarmed at last.

Little Lee Roy looked from one man to the other radiantly, his hands pressed over his grinning gums.

Then Steve sighed, and as if he did not know what else he could do, he reached out and without any warning hit Max in the jaw with his fist. Max fell off the steps.

Little Lee Roy suddenly sat as still and dark as a statue, looking on.

"Say! Say!" cried Steve. He pulled shyly at Max where he lay on the ground, with his lips pursed up like a whistler, and then stepped back. He looked horrified. "How you feel?"

"Lousy," said Max thoughtfully. "Let me alone." He raised up on one elbow and lay there looking all around, at the cabin, at Little Lee Roy sitting cross-legged on the porch, and at Steve with his hand out. Finally he got up.

"I can't figure out how I could of ever knocked down an athaletic guy like you. I had to do it," said Steve. "But I guess you don't understand. I had to hit you. First you didn't believe me, and then it didn't bother you."

"That's all O.K., only hush," said Max, and added, "Some dope is always giving me the low-down on something, but this is the first time one of 'em ever got away with a thing like this. I got to watch out."

"I hope it don't stay black long," said Steve.

"I got to be going," said Max. But he waited. "What you want to transact with Keela? You come a long way to see him." He stared at Steve with his eyes wide open now, and interested.

"Well, I was goin' to give him some money or somethin', I guess, if I ever found him, only now I ain't got any," said Steve defiantly.

"O.K.," said Max. "Here's some change for you, boy. Just take it. Go on back in the house. Go on."

Little Lee Roy took the money speechlessly, and then fell upon his yellow crutches and hopped with miraculous rapidity away through the door. Max stared after him for a moment.

"As for you"—he brushed himself off, turned to Steve and then said, "When did you eat last?"

"Well, I'll tell you," said Steve.

"Not here," said Max. "I didn't go to ask you a question. Just follow me. We serve eats at Max's Place, and I want to play the juke box. You eat, and I'll listen to the juke box."

"Well . . ." said Steve. "But when it cools off I got to catch a ride some place."

"Today while all you all was gone, and not a soul in de house," said Little Lee Roy at the supper table that night, "two white mens come heah to de house. Wouldn't come in. But talks to me about de ole times when I use to be wid de circus—"

"Hush up, Pappy," said the children.

About the Authors

Joanna Trautmann Banks, Ph.D., has served for twenty years as Professor of Humanities and Adjunct Professor at Pennsylvania State University College of Medicine in Hershey. She is associate editor of the journal *Literature and Medicine*, and editor of the first and revised editions of *Literature and Medicine: An Annotated Bibliography*.

Donald Barthelme (1931–89), an American writer, is noted for his mocking of American culture and conventions in novels such as *Snow White* (1967) and *The Dead Father* (1975). His short stories have appeared in *The New Yorker* and have been gathered in several collections, including *Sixty Stories* (1981).

Ann Beattie (b. 1947), an American novelist and short story artist, writes of middle class, young suburbanites who are disillusioned and anxious. Her works include *What Was Mine* (1991) and *Picturing Will* (1989).

Harry Beckerman (b. 1913), active in inventing rehabilitation devices for the handicapped, has been sponsored by NASA and the plastics industry.

Elisabeth A. Bednar is executive director of AboutFace, a Canadian-based organization that assists individuals with facial deformities worldwide.

Ray Bradbury (b. 1920) is an American writer of science fiction and fantasy. The author of *The Martian Chronicles* (1950), *The Illustrated Man* (1951), and *Fahrenheit 451* (1953), he has also published several collections of short stories. His work has appeared in over eight hundred anthologies.

Jonathan Sinclair Carey, a theologian and ethicist, is Director of the Institute of Ethics of Surgery in London, England, and ethics consultant to the Center for Craniofacial Disorders of Montefiore Medical Center.

Raymond Carver (1938–88) was a poet and short story writer noted for his realism and sparse style. His collections of poems and stories include *Will You Please be Quiet, Please?* (1976), *What We Talk About When We Talk About Love* (1981), and *Cathedral* (1983). A selection of Carver's stories, *Short Cuts*, was made into the 1993 Robert Altman film by the same name.

John Ciardi (1916–86) was poetry editor and essayist for *The Saturday Review*, director of the Bread Loaf Writers' Conference, popular translator of Dante, and author of several volumes of poetry and essays.

Jack Coulehan (b. 1943), physician/poet, is Professor of Medicine at SUNY-Stony Brook, where he is developing the program in clinical ethics. His poetry has been published widely in such journals as *Poetry Journal, Prairie Schooner,* and *Hiram Poetry Review,* and has been collected in *The Knitted Glove* (1991).

Marilyn Davis has taught English at Dyke College.

Dallas Denny (b. 1949) is well known for her work on transgender issues, gender dysphoria, and nontraditional gender roles. She has a masters degree in psychology and is working on her doctorate in special education at Vanderbilt University. She is the author of *Gender Dysphoria: A Guide to Research* (1994) and *Identity Management in Transsexualism* (1994).

Andre Dubus (b. 1936), a Louisiana-born writer now in New England, was the winner of the prestigious MacArthur Fellowship in 1988, the same year his *Selected Stories* was published.

Leslie Fiedler (b. 1917), literary critic known for his attacks on established canon, is currently the SUNY Distinguished Professor at the State University of New York in Buffalo. Some of his critical works include *An End to Innocence: Essays on Culture and Politics* (1955), *What Was Literature?* (1982), *Love and Death in the American Novel* (1966), and *Freaks: Myths and Images of the Secret Self* (1978).

Lucia Cordell Getsi has published four collections of poetry, and her poems, fiction, and essays have appeared in literary magazines. *Intensive Care,* a collection of poems about her daughter's battle with Guillain-Barre Syndrome, won the 1990 Capricorn Poetry Prize. Her other works include translations of Georg Trakl's poetry (1973), *No One Taught This Filly To Dance* (1989), and *Bottleships: For Daughters* (1986).

Ellen Gilchrist (b. 1935), a short-story writer focusing on adolescents and women, won the 1984 American Book Award for Fiction with *Victory Over Japan.* Other collections of her stories include *In the Land of Dreamy Dreams* (1981), *The Annunciation* (1983), and *The Anna Papers* (1988).

Patricia Goedicke (b. 1931) teaches creative writing at the University of Montana at Missoula. An award-winning poet, she has published more than eleven books of poems, including *The Tongues We Speak* (1989) and *Paul Bunyan's Bearskin* (1991).

Robert M. Goldwyn, M.D., is Clinical Professor of Surgery at the Harvard Medical School and head of the Division of Plastic Surgery at Beth Israel Hospital, Boston.

Pamela White Hadas (b. 1946) is a writer and lecturer, staff member of the Bread Loaf Writers' Conferences, winner of several awards and fellowships, and author of several books, including *Designing Women* (1979) and *Beside Herself: Pocahantas to Patty Hearst* (1983).

J. L. Haddaway, who has published poetry in a number of journals, is working on her Ph.D. at Bowling Green State University, Bowling Green, Ohio.

Nathaniel Hawthorne (1804–64), a leader in the development of the short story, began writing historical sketches and allegorical tales of moral significance in his native New England. The author of *The Scarlet Letter* (1850) and *The House of Seven Gables* (1851), he also wrote a number of short stories, collected in *Twice-Told Tales* (1837) and *Mosses from an Old Manse* (1846).

Eugene Hirsch (b. 1932) is Clinical Associate Professor of Medicine at the University of Tennessee Graduate School of Medicine at Knoxville. Active in interdisciplinary literature and medicine programs, he is also a widely published poet.

William Hoskin (b. 1921), a physician and poet, has devoted his retirement from medical practice to writing and helping those with learning disabilities.

Victor Hugo (1802–85) led the Romantic movement in French literature. A poet, novelist, dramatist, essayist, and critic, his works include *Notre-Dame de Paris* (1831) and *Les Misérables* (1862).

Franz Kafka (1883–1924), an Austrian novelist, wrote psychological and metaphorical fiction that dealt with the alienation of twentieth-century Western society. His novels include *Metamorphosis* (1915) and *The Trial* (1925), and his short stories have been collected in *The Complete Stories* (1976).

John L'Heureux (b. 1934) is an American novelist, a short story writer, contributing editor to *The Atlantic Monthly,* and Professor of English at Stanford. His many published works include a novel, *An Honorable Profession* (1991), as well as *Desires* (1981) and *Comedians* (1990), two collections of short stories.

Pär Lagerkvist (1891–1974) was a Swedish novelist, playwright, and poet, whose work, in addition to prose fantasy, tells of life deprived of meaning and hope. He won the Nobel Prize for literature in 1951.

Arlette Lefebvre, M.D., Fellow Royal College of Physicians, Canada, is a staff psychiatrist at the Hospital for Sick Children in Toronto, Ontario, Canada.

Barbara McFarland is founder of the Eating Disorders Recovery Center in Cincinnati, Ohio, and co-author of *Feeding the Empty Heart* (1988).

Frances Cooke Macgregor, M.A., is Clinical Associate Professor of Surgery (Sociology) at the Institute of Reconstructive Plastic Surgery, New York University Medical Center, and Consultant in Social Psychology in the Plastic Surgery Division at the Manhattan Eye, Ear, and Throat Hospital, New York.

Mary Briody Mahowald is a philosopher and professor at the University of Chicago in the Department of Obstetrics and Gynecology. She is also Associate Director for Clinical Medical Ethics. Her many publications include *Women and Children in Health Care: An Unequal Majority* (1993).

Toni Morrison (b. 1931), Nobel laureate and winner of the 1987 Pulitzer Prize for her novel *Beloved*, has written several novels that portray the African American struggle for identity and meaning.

Flannery O'Connor (1925–64) was a Southern writer of grotesque figures who often have distorted ideas of religion. Her novels include *Wise Blood* (1952) and *The Violent Bear It Away* (1960), and her short story collections include *A Good Man Is Hard To Find* (1955) and *Everything That Rises Must Converge* (1965).

Sharon Olds (b. 1942), a prolific poet, writes with candor about family and extremes of emotion. A winner of two awards for her 1984 collection, *The Dead and the Living*, she published *The Father*, a powerful collection of poetry about the death of her father, in 1992.

Lauri Umansky Onek teaches history and women's studies at Suffolk University in Boston.

Edgar Allan Poe (1809–49), American poet and short-story writer, is known for creating the American Gothic tale as well as detective fiction genre. His publications include *Tales of the Grotesque and Arabesque* (1840), *The Raven and Other Poems* (1845), and numerous short stories.

Bernard Pomerance (b. 1940), American playwright, screenwriter, and novelist now living in London, is best known for *The Elephant Man* (1979).

Rainer Maria Rilke (1875–1926), Austrian poet and novelist, is considered one of the greatest lyrical poets of German literature. He published his first volume of lyrical verse, *Leben und Lieder*, in 1894. His poetry in English includes *Translations from the Poetry of Rainer Maria Rilke* (1938), *Sonnets to Orpheus*, and *Duino Elegies* (both 1922).

Richard Selzer (b. 1928), former surgeon and Professor of Surgery at Yale, has written several books of essays and stories, including *Rituals of Surgery* (1974), *Taking the World in for Repairs* (1986), and the autobiographical *Down From Troy* (1992).

Karl Shapiro (b. 1913) is a poet, literary critic, essayist, and novelist, whose work has been published over more than fifty years, from *Poems* (1935) to *Reports of My Death* (1990).

Rennie Sparks (b. 1965) earned her MFA from the University of Michigan.

Ronald P. Strauss, DMD, Ph.D., is professor of both Dental Ecology and Social Medicine at the University of North Carolina, Chapel Hill.

Carol Tavris earned her Ph.D. in the interdisciplinary social psychology program at the University of Michigan. Her publications include *Anger: The Misunderstood Emotion* (1989) and *The Longest War: Sex Differences in Perspective* (1984) as well as the award-winning *Mismeasure of Woman* (1992).

Rawdon Tomlinson is a Denver poet whose most recent book is *Deep Red* (1995). He is an editor of an anthology of works by poets recovering from alcohol and drug addiction.

John Updike (b. 1932) is an award-winning novelist (the Rabbit series), short-story writer, and chronicler of middle- and upper-middle class lives, broken marriages, and frustrated searches. A frequent contributor to *The New Yorker*, he is well known for his perceptive reviews and criticism.

Kurt Vonnegut, Jr. (b. 1922), science fiction writer with penetrating insights into the human condition, is the author of many novels, the most famous of which is *Slaughterhouse Five* (1969). His short stories are collected in *Canary in the Cat House* (1961) and *Welcome to the Monkey House* (1968).

Alice Walker (b. 1944) won the Pulitzer Prize and the American Book Award for her novel, *The Color Purple* (1982). In addition to other novels, she has written several collections of short stories, such as *In Love and Trouble: Stories of Black Women* (1973) and *You Can't Keep a Good Woman Down* (1981).

Eudora Welty (b. 1909) is a wry Mississippi writer of wonderful characters rooted in their place—usually small Mississippi towns. Her stories appeared in *The New Yorker* and *The Atlantic* before being collected and published as *The Collected Stories of Eudora Welty* in 1980.

Miller Williams (b. 1930), a scientist and poet who directs the University of Arkansas Press, is the winner of the 1990 Poets' Prize and the Prix de Rome of the American Academy of Arts and Letters. His poetry collections include *Living on the Surface: New and Selected Poems* (1989).

Monica Wood (b. 1953) has had her short stories published in *North American Review, Redbook,* and *Yankee* as well as the anthology *Sudden Fiction.*

Harry Yeide, Jr., Ph.D., is Professor and Chairman of the Department of Religion, George Washington University, Washington, D.C.

Permissions Acknowledgments

❧

Donald Barthelme: "The President" from *Sixty Stories* (1981). Copyright © 1968 by Donald Barthelme. Reprinted with the permission of Wylie, Aitken & Stone, Inc.

Ann Beattie: "Dwarf House" from *Distortions,* by Ann Beattie. Reprinted by permission of International Creative Management, Inc. Copyright © 1974 by Ann Beattie.

Harry Beckerman: "To: The Access Committee" by Harry Beckerman. Previously published in *Kaleidoscope: International Magazine of Literature, Fine Arts, and Disability* 20 (Winter–Spring 1990): 16. Reprinted by permission of author.

Ray Bradbury: "The Dwarf" from *October Country* by Ray Bradbury. Reprinted by permission of Don Congdon Associates, Inc. Copyright © 1954, renewed 1981 by Ray Bradbury.

Jonathan Sinclair Carey: "The Quasimodo Complex: Deformity Reconsidered" by Jonathan Sinclair Carey, including all responding essays, from *The Journal of Clinical Ethics* 1, no. 3 (Fall 1990): 212–36. Reprinted with permission of *The Journal of Clinical Ethics, Inc.*

Raymond Carver: "Fat" from *Will You Please Be Quiet, Please?* by Raymond Carver. Reprinted by permission of Tess Gallagher. Copyright © 1971 by Tess Gallagher.

John Ciardi: "Washing Your Feet" from *Selected Poems* by John Ciardi. Copyright © 1984 by John Ciardi. Reprinted by permission of the University of Arkansas Press, Fayetteville, AR.

Jack Coulehan: "The Six Hundred Pound Man" by Jack Coulehan. Originally published in *Poets & Writers* magazine. Copyright © 1993. Reprinted with permission of Jack Coulehan.

Marilyn Davis: "Song for My Son" from *Towards Solomon's Mountain,* by Marilyn Davis. Reprinted with permission of Temple University Press.

John L'Heureux: "The Anatomy of Desire" from *Desires* by John L'Heureux. Reprinted by permission of John L'Heureux. Copyright © 1981 by John L'Heureux.

Mary Briody Mahowald: "To Be or Not Be a Woman: Anorexia Nervosa, Normative Gender Roles, and Feminism," *The Journal of Medicine and Philosophy* 17 (1992): 233–51. Reprinted by permission of author.

Barbara McFarland and Tyeis Baker-Baumann: excerpts from *Shame and Body Image: Culture and the Compulsive Eater* by Barbara McFarland and Tyeis Baker-Baumann. Reprinted by permission of Health Communications, Inc.

Toni Morrison: excerpt from *Sula*, by Toni Morrison. Reprinted by permission of International Creative Management, Inc. Copyright © 1973 by Toni Morrison.

Flannery O'Connor: "Good Country People" from *A Good Man Is Hard To Find And Other Stories*, Copyright © 1955 by Flannery O'Connor and renewed 1983 by Regina O'Connor. Reprinted by permission of Harcourt Brace & Company.

Sharon Olds: "The Meal" from *The Gold Cell* by Sharon Olds. Copyright © 1987 by Sharon Olds. Reprinted by permission of Alfred A. Knopf, Inc.

Sharon Olds: "The Pull" from *The Father* by Sharon Olds. Copyright © 1992 by Sharon Olds. Reprinted by permission of Alfred A. Knopf, Inc.

Laurie Umansky Onek: "The Ear" from *JAMA* 269 (1993): 918, by Laurie Umansky Onek. Reprinted by permission of the American Medical Association.

Edgar Allan Poe: "Hop Frog," reprinted by permission of the publishers from *The Collected Works of Edgar Allan Poe*, edited by Thomas Olive Mabbott, Cambridge, Mass.: Harvard University Press. Copyright © 1969, 1978 by the President and Fellows of Harvard College.

Bernard Pomerance: Scenes 3 and 18 from *The Elephant Man* by Bernard Pomerance. Copyright © 1979 by Bernard Pomerance. Used by permission of Grove-Atlantic, Inc.

Rainer Maria Rilke: "The Song the Dwarf Sings" from *Selected Poems of Rainer Maria Rilke*, edited and translated by Robert Bly. Copyright © 1981 by Robert Bly. Reprinted by permission of HarperCollins Publishers, Inc.

Richard Selzer: Excerpt from *Diary of an Infidel* by Richard Selzer. Permission granted by author.

Karl Shapiro: "The Leg" from *Collected Poems* by Karl Shapiro. Copyright © 1944, 1987 by Karl Shapiro by arrangement with Wieser & Wieser, Inc., New York.

Index

❧